Longitudinal research in human development requires more careful planning than do cross-sectional studies, and is demanding theoretically and organizationally. This volume focuses on methods of data treatment, emphasizing the importance of careful matching of methodology to the substantive problem under consideration. It deals particularly with concepts of stability and change which are central to personality and developmental research.

The ultimate goal for developmental research is to understand and explain the developmental process underlying an individual's way of thinking, feeling, acting and reacting at any stage of the life process. Contributors to this volume explore the methodology and scope of life-span longitudinal studies in a variety of contexts, including intellectual and cognitive development, transitions such as that from childhood to early adult life, social mobility, behavioral genetics, and psychological disorders, particularly depression.

Stressing the advantages of the prospective approach, and providing detailed analysis of the methodologies available, this volume is based on a workshop sponsored by the European Science Foundation. It will be of particular interest to social and behavioral scientists, and to research workers in disciplines such as psychology, psychiatry and epidemiology where longitudinal studies have an important place in the study of human development.

Problems and methods in longitudinal research: Stability and change

European Network on Longitudinal Studies on Individual Development (ENLS).

The European Science Foundation (ESF) is an association of 50 research councils and scientific academies in 20 European countries. The member organizations represent all scientific disciplines – in natural sciences, in medical and biosciences, in social sciences and in humanities. One of its main modes of operation is establishing scientific networks.

In this frame the European Network on Longitudinal Studies on Individual Development (ENLS) was established. By organizing a series of workshops on substantive and methodological topics the network has brought together several hundred scientists from very different fields – criminology, developmental biology, epidemiology, pediatrics, psychiatry, psychology, sociology, statistics and others – all actively involved in longitudinal research. By distributing fellowships to young researchers and twinning grants to researchers for planning common projects and by the development and administration of an inventory covering all major longitudinal projects in Europe, longitudinal research has been further supported and stimulated.

Chairman: David Magnusson
Coordination Committee Members: Paul Baltes, Paul Casaer, Alex Kalverboer, Jostein Mykletun, Anik de Ribaupierre, Michael Rutter, Fini Schulsinger, Martti Takala, and Bertil Törestad.

Already published:

1. *Michael Rutter*, ed., Studies of psychosocial risk: The power of longitudinal data
2. *Anik de Ribaupierre*, ed., Transition mechanisms in child development: the longitudinal perspective
3. *David Magnusson and Lars R. Bergman*, eds., Data quality in longitudinal research
4. *Paul B. Baltes and Margret M. Baltes*, eds., Successful aging: Perspectives from the behavioral sciences
5. *David Magnusson, Lars R. Bergman, Georg Rudinger and Bertil Törestad*, eds., Problems and methods in longitudinal research: Stability and change
6. *Michael Rutter and Paul Casaer*, eds., Biological risk factors for psychosocial disorders

Problems and methods in longitudinal research: Stability and change

Edited by

DAVID MAGNUSSON,
LARS R. BERGMAN,
Department of Psychology, University of Stockholm

GEORG RUDINGER
Psychologisches Institut, University of Bonn

and

BERTIL TÖRESTAD
Department of Psychology, University of Stockholm

EUROPEAN SCIENCE FOUNDATION
E·S F

CAMBRIDGE
UNIVERSITY PRESS

Published by the Press Syndicate of the University of Cambridge
The Pitt Building, Trumpington Street, Cambridge CB2 1RP
40 West 20th Street, New York, NY 10011–4211, USA
10 Stamford Road, Oakleigh, Melbourne 3166, Australia

First published 1991
First paperback edition 1994

British Library cataloguing in publication data

Problems and methods in longitudinal research: stability
and change. – (European Network on Longitudinal Studies on
Individual development).
1. Man. Development
I. Magnusson, David II. Series
155

Library of Congress cataloguing in publication data

Problems and methods in longitudinal research: stability and change /
edited by David Magnusson . . . [et al.].
p. cm. – (European Network on Longitudinal Studies on
Individual Development ; 5)
Texts emanate from workshops organized by the European Network on
Longitudinal Studies on Individual Development.
Includes indexes.
ISBN 0-521-40195-X
1. Longitudinal method. 2. Psychology – Research – Methodology.
3. Psychology – Longitudinal studies. 4. Developmental psychology –
Longitudinal studies. I. Magnusson, David. II. European Network
Longitudinal Studies on Individual Development. III. Series:
European Network on Longitudinal Studies on Individual Development
(Series) ; 5.
BF76.6.L65P76 1991
150'.72 – dc20 90-25490CIP

ISBN 0 521 40195 X hardback
ISBN 0 521 46732 2 paperback

Transferred to digital printing 2003

UY

Contents

Contributors to this volume ix
Foreword xiii
Preface xv

1. Studying individual development: problems and methods 1
Lars R. Bergman, Gunnar Eklund and David Magnusson

2. Modeling individual and average human growth data from childhood to adulthood 28
Roland C. Hauspie, Gunilla W.-Lindgren, James M. Tanner and Hanna Chrzastek-Spruch

3. Intraindividual variability in older adults' depression scores: some implications for developmental theory and longitudinal research 47
John R. Nesselroade and David L. Featherman

4. Now you see it, now you don't – some considerations on multiple regression 67
George W. Brown, Tirril O. Harris and Louise Lemyre

5. Differential development of health in a life-span perspective 95
Leiv S. Bakketeig, Per Magnus and Jon Martin Sundet

6. Assessing change in a cohort-longitudinal study with hierarchical data 107
Dan Olweus and Françoise D. Alsaker

7. Statistical and conceptual models of 'turning points' in developmental processes — 133
Andrew Pickles and Michael Rutter

8. Qualitative analyses of individual differences in intra-individual change: examples from cognitive development — 166
Eberhard Schröder, Wolfgang Edelstein and Siegfried Hoppe-Graff

9. Application of correspondence analysis to a longitudinal study of cognitive development — 190
Jacques Lautrey and Philippe Cibois

10. Event-history models in social mobility research — 212
Hans-Peter Blossfeld, Alfred Hamerle and Karl Ulrich Mayer

11. Behavioral genetic concepts in longitudinal analyses — 236
Nancy L. Pedersen

12. Genetic and environmental factors in a developmental perspective — 250
Peter C. M. Molenaar, Dorret I. Boomsma and Conor V. Dolan

13. Structural equation models for studying intellectual development — 274
Georg Rudinger, Johannes Andres and Christian Rietz

14. Longitudinal studies for discrete data based on latent structure models — 308
Erling B. Andersen

15. Stability and change in patterns of extrinsic adjustment problems — 323
Lars R. Bergman and David Magnusson

Index — 347

Contributors to this volume

Dr Françoise D. Alsaker
Department of Personality Psychology, University of Bergen, Øysteingate 3, N-5007 Bergen, Norway

Professor Erling B. Andersen
Department of Statistics, University of Copenhagen, Studiestraede 6, DK-1455 Copenhagen, Denmark

Dr Johannes Andres
Department of Psychology, University of Kiel, Kiel, Germany

Professor Leif S. Bakketeig
Department of Epidemiology, National Institute of Public Health, Geitmyrsveien 75, N-0462 Oslo 4, Norway

Professor Lars R. Bergman
Department of Psychology, University of Stockholm, S-106 91 Stockholm, Sweden

Professor Hans-Peter Blossfeld
Department of Political and Social Studies, European University Institute, Badia Fiesolana, Via dei Roccettini 5, I-50016 San Domenico die Fiesole, Florence, Italy

Dr Dorret I Boomsma
Department of Experimental Psychology, Free University, De Boelelaan 1115, NL-1081 HV Amsterdam, The Netherlands

Professor George W. Brown
Department of Social Policy and Social Science, Royal Holloway and Bedford New College, University of London, 11 Bedford Square, London WC1B 3RA, England

Dr Hanna Chrzastek-Spruch
Institute of Pediatrics of the Medical Academy, Lublin, Poland

Dr Philippe Cibois
Laboratoire d'Information pour les Sciences Humaines, CNRS, 54 BVD Raspail, F-75 006 Paris, France

Dr Conor V. Dolan
Department of Psychology, University of Amsterdam, Weesperplein 8, NL-1018 XA Amsterdam, The Netherlands

Professor Wolfgang Edelstein
MPI for Human Development and Education, Lentzeallee 94, D-1000 Berlin 33, Germany

Professor David L. Featherman
Social Science Research Council, 605 Third Avenue, New York, NY 10158, USA

Professor Alfred Hamerle
Fakultät für Wirtschaftswissenschaften und Statistik, Universtat Konstanz, Postfach 5560, D-7750 Konstanz, Germany

Dr Tirril O. Harris
Department of Social Policy and Social Science, Royal Holloway and Bedford New College, University of London, 11 Bedford Square, London WC1B 3RA, England

Dr Roland C. Hauspie
National Fund for Scientific Research (Belgium), Laboratory of Anthropogenetics, Free University of Brussels, Pleinlaan, B-1050 Brussels, Belgium

Dr Siegfried Hopp-Graff
University of Heidelberg, Heidelberg, Germany

Professor Jacques Lautrey
Laboratoire de Psychologie Différentielle, Universite de Paris V, 41 Rue Gay-Lussac, F-75 005 Paris, France

Dr Louise Lemyre
Department of Social Policy and Social Science, Royal Holloway and Bedford New College, University of London, 11 Bedford Square, London WC1B 3RA, England

Dr Gunilla W.-Lindgren
Department of Educational Research, Stockholm Institute of Education, PO Box 34103, S-100 26 Stockholm, Sweden

Dr Per Magnus
Department of Epidemiology, National Institute of Public Health, Geitmyrsveien 75, N-0462 Oslo 4, Norway

Professor David Magnusson
Department of Psychology, University of Stockholm, S-106 91 Stockholm, Sweden

Professor Karl Ulrich Mayer
MPI for Human Development and Education, Lentzeallee 94, D-1000 Berlin 33, Germany

Professor Peter C. M. Molenaar
Department of Psychology, University of Amsterdam, Weesperplein 8, NL-1018 XA Amsterdam, The Netherlands

Professor John R. Nesselroade
The Center for the Study of Child and Adolescent Development, The Pennsylvania State University, S-106 Human Development Building, University Park, PA 16802, USA

Professor Dan Olweus
Department of Personality Psychology, University of Bergen, Øysteingate 3, N-5007 Bergen, Norway

Dr Nancy Pedersen
Department of Environmental Hygiene, The Karolinska Institute, PO Box 60400, S-104 01 Stockholm, Sweden

Dr Andrew Pickles
MRC Child Psychiatry Unit, Institute of Psychiatry, DeCrespigny Park, Denmark Hill, London SE5 8AF, England

Dr Christian Rietz
Department of Psychology, Technical University Berlin, Berlin, Germany

Professor Georg Rudinger
Department of Psychology, University of Bonn, Romerstrasse 164, D-5300 Bonn, Germany

Professor Michael Rutter
MRC Child Psychiatry Unit, Institute of Psychiatry, DeCrespigny Park, Denmark Hill, London SE5 8AF, England

Dr Eberhard Schröder
MPI for Human Development and Education, Lentzeallee 94, D-1000 Berlin 33, Germany

Dr Jon Martin Sundet
Department of Psychology, University of Oslo, Oslo, Norway

Professor James M. Tanner
Insititute of Child Health, University of London, London, England

Foreword

This book is the fifth in a series of volumes, emanating from the workshops organized by the European Network on Longitudinal Studies on Individual Development (ENLS) within the framework of the European Science Foundation.

The normal process in which an individual develops from birth through the life course is of interest in itself as a subject for research. Understanding and explaining that process is also fundamental for understanding what contributes to physical and mental health and for revealing the causes of mental, social and physical problems during the life course. As has been convincingly demonstrated in the earlier content-oriented volumes in this series, the development of individuals cannot be adequately and effectively investigated without using a longitudinal research strategy (see, e.g., Baltes & Baltes, 1990; Magnusson & Bergman, 1990; de Ribaupierre, 1990; Rutter, 1988; Rutter & Casaer, 1991, as listed on p. iv; see also Magnusson (1988) on p. 27 of this volume).

Individual development can be described as a multidetermined, stochastic process in a lifetime perspective, a process in which psychological and biological factors in the individual and factors in the environment are actively involved. In that perspective, important aspects of the process of individual development cannot be investigated, understood and explained efficaciously without following the same individuals across time; i.e., without conducting longitudinal research. Longitudinal research puts special claim on the researcher in terms of careful planning of all steps in the process from the formulation of a problem to the presentation of the results.

Of special concern in longitudinal research is the choice and application of adequate methods for treatment of data that can yield effective answers to the problems under investigation. Few areas of research on individual functioning, be it research in education, demography, pediatrics, psychology or sociology, are as full of methodological traps in this respect as longitudinal research.

A whole arsenal of methods, some of them technically advanced, are at the disposal of those conducting longitudinal research. However, the level of technical sophistication can be a fallible guide for the choice of methods of data treatment in longitudinal study, as in any other research area. What is, of course, relevant when we choose methods for data treatment is only how appropriate they are with respect to the question formulated and to the level of individual functioning at which it is located. Thus there is an indispensable link between the correct method for data treatment and the explicit formulation of the problem. The aim of the present volume is to emphasize the importance of this link. A combination of careful analysis of the relevant phenomena and an explicit formulation of the problem becomes a first step in longitudinal research. Such a combination is required in order for a longitudinal research strategy to contribute to understanding and explaining individual development.

We hope that this volume will draw attention to and extend the claim of longitudinal study as a prerequisite for future scientific progress in understanding individual development.

David Magnusson
Chairman of the ENLS Coordination Committee

Preface

Longitudinal research is the main road to fundamental and valid knowledge of living organisms' development. Because the longitudinal approach implies collecting data about the same subjects across time, the demands on the researchers to be accurate and scrupulous are high for several reasons. First, a mistake made at one assessment occasion can seldom be satisfactorily remedied at a later stage. Second, the complexity of information makes it necessary to treat and analyze data with special care.

The importance of issues of methodology and research strategy in longitudinal research is evident from the fact that two of the eight workshops organized by the European Science Foundation's Network on Longitudinal Studies on Individual Development have exclusively dealt with methodology. The first of these was concerned with data quality and resulted in one of the volumes that have come out of the workshop series (see page iv).

This volume emanates from the second methodology workshop, which was held at Soria Moria conference center in Oslo, Norway, April 2–5, 1989. It concentrates on issues that have to do with the intricate task of applying methodological tools which are appropriate to the problem at hand. Two overriding and related concepts are central to longitudinal research: stability and change. In this book these concepts subsume multiple aspects of the human condition: for example, depression, health development, cognitive development, behavior genetics, and adjustment problems. An array of statistical methods is introduced and discussed in relation to the content areas and the problems studied.

The original contributions to the workshop have been thoroughly revised by the authors. Many additions, reformulations, and new ideas were sparked by vivid and stimulating discussions in and out of sessions. Some of the contributions by invited discussants at the workshop have been re-written and appear in this volume.

There are fifteen chapters in the book. The first one, an introductory chapter, has been written by the two first editors in collaboration with

Professor Gunnar Eklund. An organizing principle for the chapter sequence was not self-evident. What we have tried to do is to order the chapters according to degree of complexity of the models presented and to place chapters dealing with similar areas close to each other.

We are most grateful to many people who have contributed to organizing the workshop and to editing this volume. First, thanks are due to the other members of the Longitudinal Network's Co-ordination Committee. We also want to thank Dr Jostein Mykletun for his efforts to make the workshop arrangements go well. He was efficiently assisted by Mrs Luki Hagen-Norberg who took on most of the secretarial duties.

D.M.
L.R.B.
G.R.
B.T.

1 Studying individual development: problems and methods

LARS R. BERGMAN, GUNNAR EKLUND AND DAVID MAGNUSSON

INTRODUCTION

The ultimate goal for developmental research is to understand and explain the developmental process underlying an individual's way of thinking, feeling, acting and reacting at a certain stage of the life process.

In order for empirical research to contribute effectively to this goal there are three crucial aspects of the research strategy which are important:

1. the problem under consideration,
2. the data used to reflect the structures and processes involved, and
3. the methods applied for data treatment.

An important prerequisite for the formulation of relevant problems is a careful analysis of the phenomena, in this case the functioning of the individual at the appropriate level of the structures and processes relevant for the problem. Too often problems are formulated with reference to theories which have not been anchored in careful observation and analysis of the phenomena, a circumstance which has contributed to much artificial theorizing and meaningless empirical research.

The crucial importance of using data relevant to the character of the problem, with respect to reliability, validity, level of generalization, etc., was comprehensively dealt with in an earlier volume in this series (Magnusson & Bergman, 1990).

The focus of this volume is on methods for data treatment. The emphasis is on the importance of careful linking of methods for data treatment to the character of the substantive problem under consideration in the specific case. The choice of method for data treatment should always be made with reference to an analysis of the structures and processes relevant to the problem under consideration. Too often the choice of method is made on the basis of its technical sophistication.

During the last decades a series of technically sophisticated methods for data treatment have been developed (LISREL, path analysis, log linear analysis, etc.). It has become a fashion to use such methods, sometimes without investigating if the assumptions made by the methods are really met. The value system sometimes seems to reward technical sophistication in data treatment independent of its effectiveness in answering substantive questions. It is self-evident that no sophisticated method for data analysis can save bad data or contribute to better knowledge of the developmental process if it does not match relevant problems anchored in the world of real phenomena.

Each correct use of a method for data treatment is dependent on a set of specific conditions or assumptions, which must be met. Such assumptions pertain to the phenomena under study, to the theoretical concepts used and to the properties of the data. To the extent that these assumptions are not met, the empirical results will give false answers to the questions. The important fact that the method for data treatment applied in the specific case can determine the outcome, is cogently illustrated by Brown, Harris and Lemyre in Chapter 4.

THE CHARACTER OF THE DEVELOPMENT PROCESS

An individual functions currently and develops as a totality in which each specific aspect gets its functional meaning from its role in the totality. Developmental research is concerned with which psychological and biological factors in the individual and which factors in the distal and proximal environment are involved and operating in the developmental process. An essential feature of the process is that these factors are in constant, reciprocal interaction.

All aspects of the total functioning of an individual cannot be successfully investigated in one or a few studies. In each specific case it is necessary to break down the totality into substructures and subprocesses which form the frame of reference for the formulation and elucidation of the problem under consideration. In this breakdown of the total process it is essential for the interpretation of empirical results that the subspace under consideration is defined with consideration to the functioning of related subspaces and to the functioning of the totality.

Over time the process in which an individual is involved and develops has the characteristic features of a multidetermined, stochastic process, i.e., there are many factors operating and we deal with probabilities (Magnusson, 1988). In this process many factors contribute to the existence of individual differences in functioning at a certain chronological age. Two circumstances are of particular interest.

1. The multidetermined, stochastic character of the process itself contributes to individual differences. For example, significant events (Magnusson & Törestad, in press) and independent factors in the environment may have as a consequence 'turning points' as discussed by Pickles and Rutter in Chapter 7.

For our understanding of their role in individual functioning and in interindividual differences, it is important to observe that such events occur at different ages for different individuals. This fact may lead to different impacts in different individuals, owing to differences in preparedness and the role it plays in the total functioning of the individual.

For the central topic of this volume, namely the importance of choosing methods for data treatment with reference to the character of the phenomena, the multidetermined, stochastic feature of the developmental process has a crucial implication: when certain aspects of individual functioning are regarded and treated as nomothetic variables in statistical analysis, the relations among variables across individuals most often are nonlinear (cf. Hinde & Dennis, 1986; see Chapter 15 of this volume, by Bergman and Magnusson).

2. The second important factor contributing to individual differences in individual functioning in a certain situation at a certain chronological age is the existence of sometimes large individual differences in growth rate (Magnusson, 1985). Such differences occur not only for biological but also for cognitive–emotional aspects, such as language development, intelligence, etc. Certain deviances from the normal rate of development indicate a lower final stage of functioning while others are only indications of a delayed development with a later catch up.

What has briefly been summarized above has essential consequences in developmental research for the choice of methods for data treatment in each specific case, and for research strategy. It affects the choice between categorical and continuous data and between variable-oriented methods and profile-oriented methods in treatment of data. These consequences will be discussed later in this chapter.

Here one important implication for developmental research should be emphasized, namely the necessity of conducting longitudinal research, i.e., following the same individuals across time. The inappropriateness of a cross-sectional approach for the study of development as a stochastic, multidetermined process, with the implications briefly summarized above, should be obvious. Longitudinal research is demanding: it not only needs consistent funding over long periods of time; it also requires more careful planning than cross-sectional studies, theoretically, organizationally, and administratively. Following the same individuals over time, wherever they have moved, is demanding, and the personal involvement and engagement over time, along with long periods of waiting for the results and possible rewards, make longitudinal research less attractive. Cross-sectional studies most often yield data which contain enough linear variance to show statistical significance. However, if we really want to understand and explain individual development as a process, there is no alternative to longitudinal research.

STABILITY AND CHANGE IN THE DEVELOPMENTAL PROCESS

During the last decades a central issue for debate, both in personality and in developmental research, has been the issue of *personality consistency*. In developmental research consistency has often been discussed in terms of stability and change. One cause of confusion in the debate about personality consistency has been the lack of clear conceptualization. It is possible to distinguish four basic meanings of the concept.

1. *Absolute stability*. According to this definition, an individual is assumed to function with respect to a certain aspect in the same way in an absolute sense across different situations and across time. No one argues seriously that this would be the case for specific manifest behaviors. However, it seems to be implied at the trait level to some extent in some extreme trait theorizing.

2. *Relative stability*. This is a statistical definition of cross-situational and temporal personality consistency. According to it, an individual is stable with respect to a certain aspect of individual functioning if he/she retains – across situations and across time – his/her position in the rank order of individuals in the sample to which he/she belongs. This meaning of developmental stability for a certain aspect of individual functioning is usually expressed in a coefficient for the stability of rank orders obtained at two different points in time.

Formulations of the interpretation of high stability coefficients sometimes imply that they mean high temporal consistency in the absolute sense, as discussed under point 1. However, it must be kept in mind that correlation coefficients expressing relative stability for a certain aspect of individual functioning do not say anything about stability in terms of the absolute level of functioning.

A survey of the literature on temporal stability shows that the overwhelming number of empirical studies on which the discussion of stability and change in development is based report figures for relative stability, i.e., for personality consistency in statistical, relative terms.

Of course, correlation coefficients expressing the stability of rank orders for a sample of individuals for a certain aspect of individual functioning reflect the extent to which the individuals retain their rank orders from time to time. However, it should be kept in mind that when time refers to chronological age, stability coefficients may be unduly deflated by two factors:

(a) data for the variable under study may not express 'the same' latent variable at time 1 and time 2, even if they superficially have the same character as indicated by being based on data from the same instrument, and

(b) individual growth curves, though having exactly the same shape, may have different onsets and peaks for different individuals (cf. Magnusson, 1985).

Both absolute and relative stability are definitions of personality consistency in statistical terms.

For discussing personality consistency in a cross-situational and in a temporal perspective, respectively, the terms *coherence* and *lawful continuity* have been introduced (cf. Magnusson & Törestad, in press).

3. *Coherence.* Across situations each individual's way of functioning in all respects is characterized by coherence, i.e., it is coherent and explainable, without necessarily being stable in either absolute or relative terms for each aspect. The basis for the assumption of coherent patterning of manifest behaviors across situations is the coherent way in which an individual interprets the information that the environment offers in each specific occasion/situation, and how he/she uses this information as a basis for inner and outer activity.

4. *Lawful continuity.* According to the definition of personality consistency in terms of lawful continuity, individual development is lawful and consistent in the sense that the total functioning of an individual at a certain stage of development and any change in this respect takes place against the background of, and is lawfully connected with, the individual's earlier history of maturation and experience. Any change in the individual's way of functioning is a lawful consequence of the state of the organism, psychologically and biologically, and its way of dealing with external events and their consequences. This view on stability and change in individual development has implications for the choice of data for the elucidation of a certain problem and for the choice of methods for data treatment in longitudinal research (see Bergman and Magnusson, Chapter 15 of this volume).

PROSPECTIVE AND RETROSPECTIVE APPROACHES TO LONGITUDINAL RESEARCH

An important distinction with respect to longitudinal research strategy is the one between a prospective and a retrospective type of analysis. An example may be helpful to clarify the distinction. Let us assume that the problem under consideration is a hypothesis concerning the developmental background to adult criminality. A *prospective* analysis of this problem takes its starting point in data referring to an early age, say ten years of age, for factors that are assumed to be of relevance, e.g., aggressiveness, hyperactivity, intelligence, and social background. The answer to the question if and to what extent these factors are operating in the developmental process leading to adult criminality will then be sought in data for adult criminality. A *retrospective* analysis of the same problem takes its starting point in data for adult criminality and investigates the hypothesis about the relevance of the given set of variables in the development process by comparing those who have committed crimes at adult age and those who have not, using data from the early age for the hypothesized variables.

A prospective approach means looking forward to the outcome of the process, a retrospective approach means looking backwards to the antecedents. When the two approaches have been discussed and evaluated, the general conclusion has been that a prospective approach is more effective than a retrospective. This conclusion is often based on the deficiences in retrospective *data* which have been elucidated in empirical research (cf. Janson, 1990). However, this means a confounding of two issues, namely the research strategy and the type of data.

Four aspects of data used in longitudinal analyses should be distinguished (Janson, 1981, 1990; Magnusson, 1988).

1. *The reference point in time.* The particular occasion or age level in a person's life that a datum refers to.
2. *The coding point in time.* The point in time when the observation is coded into a datum. For example, the observations that a teacher makes about a pupil can be expressed in a datum in direct connection with the observation or ten years later.
3. *The collection point in time.* The point in time when the researcher collects the datum. For example, a register datum for a certain individual may refer to a specific age level and has been coded at the same time that it refers to but is collected by the researcher much later.
4. *The usage point in time.* The point in time when the researcher uses the data for calculation.

A common mistake is that it is the collection point in time that determines whether data are prospective or retrospective: if data are collected at the end of the process, they are regarded as retrospective data, if they are collected during the process they are regarded as prospective. However, the collection point in time is of no relevance for the distinction between prospective and retrospective data. What is decisive is the relation between the *reference point* in time and the *coding point* in time. If the reference point in time and the coding point in time coincide a datum is not retrospective, independent of the points in time for the collection and usage. If they do not coincide, the datum is retrospective. In principle, both a retrospective and a prospective analysis can use both prospective and retrospective data.

Thus, the problems concerning a prospective and a retrospective approach to longitudinal studies and concerning prospective and retrospective data in these analyses are two different problems. That retrospective data often have lower quality than prospective data does not invalidate the retrospective research strategy per se. Prospective and retrospective analyses of developmental problems elucidate the same kind of problems by studying such problems in different ways. In principle both of them can use both prospective and retrospective data as in the example given above. What is decisive for the choice between a prospective and a retrospective analysis in any specific case is the problem under consideration, the character of the sample for which data are available, and the properties of the data. Indeed, in situations with an outcome variable that is rare, for example, when the object of interest is an illness with a low frequency of occurrence, the only feasible approach may be a *case-control study* in which a sample with the rare condition and a control group are studied retrospectively.

PROBLEMS IN STUDYING STABILITY AND CHANGE

Do both quantity and quality change with time?

As briefly mentioned earlier, studying change or growth in a single variable when the variable measured is not really 'the same' at the different ages poses difficulties. Even if the same operationalized measure is used at different points in time, the measures may not be indicators of the same theoretical concept. For instance, a test consisting of simple mathematical problems may primarily measure inductive–deductive ability at the age of ten but numerical ability at age 15. (The problem of changing meaning of measures with age is discussed by, for instance, Wohlwill, 1973.) This situation may create all kinds of interpretation and analytic problems as discussed in Bergman (1972) and Harris (1963).

The above-stated implications for the study of individual development are, of course, different depending on the character of the variables under investigation. When studying how one aspect of behavior evolves into another aspect of behavior at a later age (heterotypic continuity), the problems to handle are different from studying an aspect of behavior which maintains its character over time (homotypic continuity). It is of foremost importance that the researcher is explicit about what theoretical concepts the studied variables measure and to what extent the operationalized measures change their meaning with age.

It often appears to be sound advice that one should avoid measures of change when studying individual development and instead consider 'the same variable', measured at different points in time as different but related variables. This advice has implications both for the choice of measurement procedures and the choice of statistical methods (Cronbach & Furby, 1970).

The situation is different if the aim is not to study 'the same thing' at different ages. In certain approaches the attempt is not to measure the same variables at the different ages but rather to measure indicators of relevant (and partly different) concepts at the different ages (cf. Magnusson, 1988, and Bergman & Magnusson, Chapter 15 of this volume).

Matching concepts and measurement models

The above argument also highlights the importance of using appropriate measures that really reflect the concepts one wants to study. Again and again it has been pointed out that an explicit measurement model is needed in which the theoretical concepts are linked to the observed variables (Magnusson, 1988; Rudinger & Wood, 1990; Rutter & Pickles, 1990).

The type of scale appropriate for the measurement model is, of course, entirely dependent on the problem area. For instance, it is a misunderstanding that a continuous scale, whenever it is obtainable, is always preferable to a discrete or categorical scale. Some phenomena are naturally discrete or categorical and are distorted if they are described by a continuous variable. This is exemplified by Brown *et al.* in Chapter 4.

Making causal inferences

Ethical and practical problems usually prohibit the use of powerful random control experiments when studying individual development of human beings, forcing the researcher to use non-experimental data. The difficulties involved in making causual inferences using such data are well known (see, e.g., Cook & Campbell, 1979). It is also well known that the situation in this regard can be more favorable in a longitudinal context than in a cross-sectional context since the time-ordering of the variables in the former context gives information that can be used when building causal models. This use of time-ordering is exemplified in several chapters in this volume, for example by Pickles and Rutter in Chapter 7, concerning the effects on adult adjustment of childhood factors, by Rudinger, Andres and Rietz in Chapter 13, concerning the growth of intelligence, and by Molenaar, Boomsma and Dolan in Chapter 12, concerning the operation of genetic factors at different ages.

Confirmation versus exploration

It has often been stated that a confirmatory approach is preferable to an exploratory one. In a confirmatory approach a specific theory is tested by examining whether or not the observed data are consistent with those that are predicted from a statistical model generated by the theory. In an extreme form this means that the theory and statistical model are formulated beforehand and the data set is only used for the binary decision of retaining or rejecting the theory. This approach has been contrasted to another extreme; an exploratory approach in which the researcher performs various analyses on data and explores within a more vague theoretical framework, using the findings for hypothesis generation which can be tested empirically on another set of data. The dangers in this second approach are obvious.

However, within the context of studying individual development, the limitations of a confirmatory approach should be recognized.

First, it should be noted that a high-quality longitudinal data base is very difficult to obtain. It requires a great deal of time, money, and effort, especially if the study covers a long time period. Such a data base is simply too valuable to be used for a theoretical one-shot (cf. Bergman, 1988).

Second, in many areas of individual development the issues are very complex and no thoroughly sound body of theory exists. This means that theories that can be made before looking at the data are bound to be over-simplified and the rejection of such a theory does not provide much information.

Third, using a confirmatory approach may increase the danger of confirmation bias (Greenwald *et al.*, 1986) by which is meant that the procedures, testing and reporting are too much geared towards fitting into the existing theoretical framework.

Of course we do not advocate an atheoretical explorative approach of merely stocking facts; exploration should be aided by a theoretical framework and should result in new theoretical formulations (Bergman, 1988; Magnusson, 1990). In this connection the need for replication and cross-validation should be stressed, as has been done by others (Rutter & Pickles, 1990).

Somewhere along the line, the common-sense aspect of knowing the facts before theorizing has been lost in many cases. The consequences of this loss are more expensive in the longitudinal field than in most other fields, and research about individual development would, in our opinion, do well by emphasizing careful observation, description and micro-theorizing and dwell less on more formal confirmatory approaches.

SOME VARIABLE-ORIENTED METHODS: ASSUMPTIONS AND APPLICATIONS

The variable-oriented approach

In this section the assumptions and applications of some variable-oriented methods will be discussed. By 'variable-oriented methods' we mean those methods in which the main conceptual and analytical unit is the variable. For instance, the focus of interest is on mean differences for a certain variable or on the relationships among variables (latent or manifest). Several such approaches are illustrated in this volume addressing various problems in studying individual development. The uses of modern, powerful analytical tools are illustrated within different areas such as the study of the development of intelligence by Rudinger, Andres and Rietz, in Chapter 13 (structural equation modeling using LISREL), gene-environment contributions to phenotypic variance in a developmental perspective by Molenaar, Boomsma and Dolan in Chapter 12 and Pedersen in Chapter 11 (time-series analysis using LISREL). Blossfeld, Hamerle and Mayer in Chapter 10 illustrate the use of event history analysis for studying social mobility. In other chapters, means or variances of key variables are compared between groups of subjects over time (this is done by Olweus and Alsaker in Chapter 6 using a cohort-longitudinal approach with hierarchical data and by Nesselroade and Featherman in Chapter 3 focusing on intraindividual variability in depression scores).

In these chapters, some attention is given to the assumptions and conditions necessary for the adequate use of the methods. This is a complex issue, dependent on both the nature of the phenomena to be studied and on the specific methods to be used. In the following, the issue is discussed in some detail for some rather simple situations. In this way the reader is given examples of some ways of thinking about assumptions and conditions for applying a statistical method that, it is our hope, provide a base for understanding these issues in more complex situations.

Assumptions and applications in some simple cases

In an ordinary longitudinal study, subject matter knowledge and theory give a basis for a model. With access to appropriate data a statistical analysis is carried out in order to answer relevant questions. However, as a rule it is necessary to impose some assumptions, for example, that some of the correlations are assumed to be zero, that the relationship between included variables is linear, that no bias due to suspected confounder is present, etc.

Example: Suppose that we are investigating the relation between the number of years of education, y, and the corresponding ones of the parents, x_1, and x_2. It seems justified to look upon y as a random variable and to regard x_1 and x_2 as predetermined non-random variables (predictors). The relationship can be specificed in many ways. In the simple type of linear multiple regression it is often written

$$y = B_0 + B_1x_1 + B_2x_2 + E \qquad (1)$$

where B_i are parameters and E is random error mainly due to unknown disregarded factors. It is evident that even for subjects with identical x_1 and x_2 the value of y may differ as a consequence of different E-values.

In this connection the imposed assumptions can be as follows.

1. x_1 and x_2 are observed non-random variables.
2. x_1 and x_2 have variances greater than zero and the correlation between them is less than 1.
3. x_1 and E are independent or at least uncorrelated and the same is valid for x_2 and E.
4. The variance of E is expected to be the same for all x_1 and x_2 and for all combinations between them.
5. The E-values are 'pure' random errors and thus uncorrelated.
6. E follows the Gaussian distribution with a mean of zero and a fixed variance in situations where y is continuous. If y is binary, a binomial or Poisson distribution is usually assumed.

If the linear model is regarded as too simple it is allowable to add new variables x_3 and x_4 assumed to follow the same assumptions as x_1 and x_2, e.g., $x_3 = x_1^2$, and $x_4 = x_1 \cdot x_2$ with the model

$$y = B_0 + B_1x_1 + B_2x_2 + B_3x_3 + B_4x_4 + E. \qquad (2)$$

In this way polynomial relationships and interactions can be taken into account. The relationship is still additive in equation (2) and the coefficients B_0, B_1, B_2, B_3, and B_4 can be estimated with the help of data on y, x_1, and x_2.

If the specification of the model is adequate and if the assumptions 1–3 are valid the (point) estimates obtained by ordinary regression analysis are unbiased. If also the assumptions 4–6 are valid, adequate confidence intervals of B_i can be estimated as well as prediction intervals. Thus, if only the assumptions 1–3 are true it is still possible to produce point estimates of B_i – which often implies that the main purpose of the study is fulfilled.

How is it possible to test if the assumptions must be rejected? This is very simply done with respect to assumption 2. If the observed variances of x_1 and x_2 are greater than zero and if the numerical value of the correlation is less than 1 it is confirmed that this assumption is valid.

By analyzing the residuals in equation (1), i.e., by studying the residual expression for each subject, where

$$\text{residual} = y - B_0 - B_1 x_1 - B_2 x_2, \tag{3}$$

the assumptions 4–6 can be tested.

- Are the residuals Gaussian distributed (test of assumption 6) according to a test of goodness of fit?
- Is the variance of the residuals greater for large x_1-values or for large x_2 than for small ones (test of assumption 4)?
- Are the residuals, ordered according to the magnitude of x_1 and x_2, autocorrelated (test of assumption 5)?

It is often more problematic to test assumption 1 and 3, because they can hardly be tested without additional data. However, the independency in assumption 3 can be rejected if at least one of the correlations between the residuals (3) and the independent variables differs significantly from zero. For binary y-values the presence of an interaction between x_1 and x_2 can indicate that x_1 or/and x_2 is stochastic.

What happens if we must admit that assumption 3 is not valid? As E is then correlated to y as well as to x (x_1 or x_2 or both), E takes the same position as a confounder, and as a consequence the point estimates of the B_i-values become biased.

What happens if assumption 1 in (1) is not true for one of the variables, x_1, and x_1 is a random variable? If x_1 can be written $x_1 = x_{1\,\text{true}} + e$, where e is a random variable and if $y = B_0 + B_1 x_{1\,\text{true}} + B_2 x_2 + E$, equation (1) must be substituted by $y = b_0 + b_1 x_1 + b_2 x_2$ because the true x_1 value is hidden. The numerical value of the estimate, b_1, then underestimates the numerical value of B_1. However, if there are two parallel determinations of the true x_1-value

$$x_1' = x_{1\,\text{true}} + e' \quad \text{and} \quad x_1'' = x_{1\,\text{true}} + e'',$$

where e' and e'' are uncorrelated, then the bias can be corrected.

Besides the six assumptions it remains to scrutinize what happens if the specified function in (1) and (2) is adequate or not. Instead of writing y as an additive function, y can more generally be expressed as

$$Y = F(x_1, x_2) + E \tag{4}$$

i.e., y is written as a sum of a systematic part, F, and a random part, E. F

can be written in many ways, such as in equations (5)–(7):

$$y = e^{A+B_1x_1+B_2x_2} \quad (5)$$

$$y = \frac{e^{A+Bx_1}}{1+e^{A+Bx_1}} \quad (6)$$

$$y = (A + B_1x_1 + B_2x_2)^{0.5}. \quad (7)$$

The separation into one F-part and another E-part in (4) is justified from a pure statistical point of view (Nelder & Wedderburn, 1972). The preference for linear relations as in equation (1) or for polynomial as in equation (2) is often mathematically motivated by reference to Taylor's theorem. A common reason to doubt the specification of the F-part is that the residual variance is great or the multiple correlation coefficient, R, is low. In this situation it is recommended to test other specifications of the function F and compare their R-values or other related indicators (Harvey, 1983). Another way to detect specification errors in equation (2) is possible if the magnitude of a coefficient is specified in advance, for example, the sign of B_1 is positive or $B_2 = 0$ or $B_1 > B_3$. Then, something must be wrong if the estimates of B_i are not in agreement with the prespecified conditions.

If the y-variable is binary it is possible that the residual variance is so small that it is in agreement with the variance expected if a Poisson or binomial distribution were valid, and thus the model specification and assumptions ought so far to be accepted.

If the model is more complicated than in the example above, the first step is still to try to identify the sources of error: the deviations from the assumptions. A next step could be to modify the equation model, to use other methods of analysis and/or to include additional data from the present or some other data set. An overview of some suggested ways of approaching various fallacies is presented in Table 1.1, which is partly illuminated by the *path model* shown in Figure 1.1. From the figure it is evident that a simplified situation is being discussed. Thus, Table 1.1 is relevant in relatively simple applications.

Illustrating example. The implications of the survey in Table 1.1 are exemplified by a follow-up study based on a large health screening in the Swedish county of Värmland in 1971. The screening included about 90 000 subjects and was carried out in 1962–5. It has been followed-up with respect to death, cause of death, and cancer incidence, almost without drop-outs. One of many aspects is exemplified here, namely the effect of blood pressure and excess weight on death rate 15–25 years after the screening. The data gathered refer to one single occasion (during the period 1962–5) and include laboratory values, and data concerning blood pressure, weight, height, cholesterol

Table 1.1. *Assumption oriented sources of error; How to identify? How to clear? Consequences?*

Source of error	How to notice by statistical analysis	Consequence of inactivity	How to clear?		
			Additional data	Modified model	Analysis method
1. Function, systematic part wrongly specified	a. R^2 'too low' b. Estimates of B senseless	Dubious estimates Inoptimal model?	Add predictors	Other functions Add interactions	Try other functions (cf. eqs 4–7)
2. Confounders	a. Residual to y (eq. 3) and to x correlated b. xZ interaction[a] c. Extreme residual	Bias in B_x	Try to identify confounder Include confounder Include instrumental variable (v)	Use correlations between confounders and predictors from external studies	
3. Random error in x	Interaction between[a] correlated x_0 and Z	B_x too small	Two determinations of x, x_0' and x_0''	Use correlations between x variables from other studies	
4. Isolated predictor	R^2 low or residual var. large	Standard errors somewhat too large. No bias	Include isolated predictor u		
5. Dependency between the predictor x and E_y	a. x^2 and y-residual correlated b. Zx and y-residual correlated	B_x difficult to interpret	Include confounder if possible to identify	Add z-terms Add Zx-term	
6. Dependency between E_x and E_y	Residuals $y - A_1 - B_x x$ and $x - a - bZ$ correlated	Bias in B_x	Try including instrumental variable (v)	Try more complicated relation, e.g., $y = b_0 + B_1 x + Cx^2 + E_u$	
7. E pure random series	Observed auto-correlation	Standard error of B too low	Aggregate adjacent observations	Use ARMA-procedure	
8. Homoscedasticity	Residual variance correlated to a predictor	Prediction interval and possibly confidence interval biased		Transform y in order to reduce hetero-scedasticity	Introduce e.g., Var. $(E) = A + Bx$

9. Normal distribution	Goodness of fit test	Prediction interval and in small materials, confidence interval biased		Transform y	Try other distribution assumptions
10. Predictor's causality	Estimates of B senseless	Bias in all estimates	Instrumental variable	Eliminate false predictors such as Q_1 and Q_2 in Figure 1.1	

[a] Relevant if y is binary. By B and by estimate is here meant an estimate corresponding to an arrow in the path model in Figure 1.1 (cf. B-values in eqs 1 and 2).

Notes to Table 1.1: (The numbering refers to source of error.)

2. The assumption: no correlation between some factors (variables) and especially confounders. Such an assumption concerning correlations is often necessary in order to obtain demanded estimates.

It can be argued that such assumptions are chosen for statistical reasons rather than on the basis of subject matter knowledge. It is very difficult to base the assumptions on empirical or theoretical knowledge, especially as it is a common experience that at least weak correlations often exist even between variables that are not supposed to be correlated. With respect to hidden confounders – nominated or anonymous – almost nothing can be done if they are not recorded. It is well known that the identification and recording of previously overlooked confounders is a common type of progress in the non-experimental study of the relationship between one factor and its suggested effect.

However, it is possible that bias due to assumed null-correlations is a minor problem, as the supposed correlations are often weak compared with the requested target correlation. If so, a sensitivity analysis ought to be performed in order to verify that small deviations from zero for assumed null-correlations do not give rise to a sizeable bias in the demanded estimates.

The use of instrumental (exogenous) variables (such as variable v in Figure 1.1) is still one of the few approaches to eliminate bias due to unknown confounders recommended in spite of the fact that it is difficult to identify such variables.

3. That a variable has measurement errors is a common situation. If some double determinations for at least a subsample are available, the correlation between them can be used for attenuation. In the more advanced form x_0 is a 'proxy' for the unknown x (see Figure 1.1) with a relation such as $x_0 = a_0 + b_0x + E_0$ where $b_0 = 1$. Even here an additional proxy, x, is meaningful in order to estimate the (partial) correlation between x and y, if $x_1 = a_1 + b_1x + E_1$, where E_0 and E_1 are assumed to be uncorrelated.

5, 6. The residual $x - a - bz$ is obtained by regression analysis with x as dependent variable. According to the path model, E_x and E_y are independent as well as z and E_y. The last assumptions are important in the ordinary multiple regression analysis. The data-based suspicion that these assumptions are not valid leads to a recommendation, which aims at eliminating the notified confounders.

7. Autocorrelation is a common problem in the analysis of time series, especially if distributed legs are included in the model. For example, late occurrences of various kinds of cancer and heart, disease, y, can be related to exposure to an etiological factor, x, 5–25 years before the diagnosis. Thus, y at time t, $y(t)$ can be expressed as

$$y(t) = A + B_5x_{t-5} + B_6x_{t-6} + \cdots + B_{25}x_{t-25} + E_t$$

In such a distributed lag relationship the autocorrelation, i.e., the correlation between the error terms, E_t and E_{t-1}, complicates the estimation of the standard error of the B-variables.
The procedure ARMA (auto regression moving average) is a way to take autoregression into consideration (Sögaard, 1983).

in serum, sialin acid in serum, etc. (Värmland, 1971). No data concerning smoking habits were collected.

The path model for the Värmland study is illustrated in Figure 1.1, with the symbols having the following meaning.

- y Dependent variable with the observed values 0 or 1, alive or dead.
- x_0 Observed systolic blood pressure at a single occasion expressed in quintile group 1 to 5, lowest to highest, respectively.
- x Mean blood pressure (quintile group) over the relevant induction period. This variable is in the focus of interest, but is not recorded. The length of the induction period is unknown; it is supposed to be 5–30 years before death.
- Z Body mass index = weight/height^2 at a single occasion. Assumed to be a relatively stable variable. Defined from 1–5 according to quintile group.
- U Sialin acid at a single occasion, quintiles.
- W Smoking habits during the relevant induction period.

y, x_0, Z, and U are recorded for about 90 000 subjects. Standardization with respect to age is applied. Males and females are analyzed separately.

The causal relationships in Figure 1.1 are in agreement with theory and earlier results. Figure 1.1 needs some comments:

Because y is a binary variable it is appropriate to specify a log-linear model as a first approach:

$$y = e^{A+B_0x_0+B_ZZ} + E,$$

where E follows a Poisson-related distribution, i.e., the non-random part can be written

$$\log y = A + B_0x_0 + B_ZZ. \tag{8}$$

By combining the quintiles of x_0 and Z, 25 groups are obtained. A, B_0 and B_Z are estimated and after that the expected death risk, y, for each combination can be compared with the observed death rate. After calculating goodness of fit by chi-square it may be evident that the model in equation (8) is not perfect as the residual variance is larger than the variance expected if E were Poisson-distributed. The model has to be modified, e.g., by including an interaction term:

$$\log y = A + B_0x_0 + B_ZZ + Bx_0Z. \tag{9}$$

The values of the estimated coefficients are reasonable and statistically significant but the goodness of fit may still not be acceptable – the presence of an extra Poisson variance cannot be denied. In the next step we substitute the interaction term and transfer the predictors x_0 and Z into 4 + 4 dummy variables, one for each quintile except for the fifth quintile which is used as reference. The new nine coefficients may be

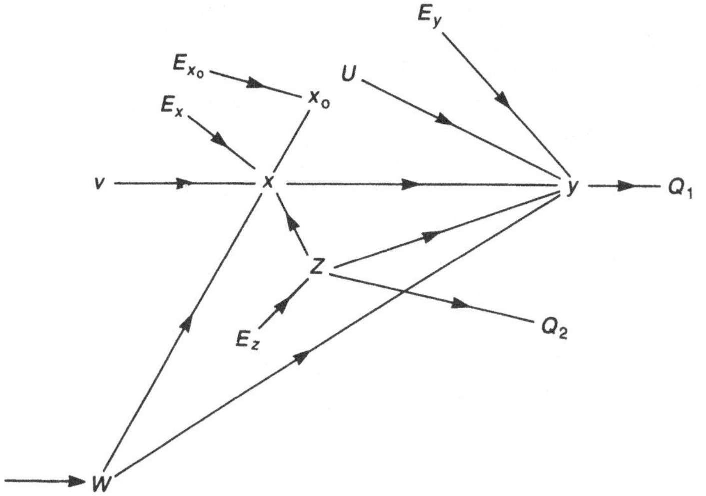

Observed variables	Random components not observed directly	Not observed variables, characterized as	Source error in Table 1.1
y, x, Z, U	E_y, E_x, E_Z	W = confounder	2
y, x, Z, U, v = instrumental	E_y, E_x, E_Z	W = confounder	2
y, x, Z, U, W	E_y, E_x, E_Z, E_{x_0}	x = genuine factor	3
y, x, Z, W	E_y, E_x, E_Z	U = isolated variable	4, 1
y, x, Z, W	E_y, E_x, E_Z		6
y, x, Z, W, Q_1 or Q_2	E_y, E_x, E_Z		10

Figure 1.1. Path model.

reasonable but, still, the goodness of fit is not good enough. We can go further by including interactions between x_0- and Z-quintiles and in this way reach perfect goodness of fit (but no degrees of freedom).

However, it seems better to search for other sources of error. Could it, for example, be useful to include isolated variables such as U in Figure 1.1 (sialin acid in the example). The answer is 'no', because y is a binary variable; if it had been continuous, the answer would have been 'yes'.

What about confounders? Smoking habit is in the example an already-identified confounder. Data could be added from a contemporary study including about 1% of the population which is sufficient for estimates of correlations between smoking habits and other predictors. It should be noticed that the correlation between x and Z and, as a consequence, between x_0 and Z, in combination with the significant interaction between x_0 and Z (equation 9), may indicate that a confounder is present or – as we already know – that x has been substituted.

The source of error due to substitution of x by x_0 (the relevant factor x is substituted by a single occasion determination, x_0) could have been corrected if repeated annual determinations year after year had been available. As such a recording has not been carried out and a contemporary double determination is lacking, another study has been used. In this study, determinations of x_0 had taken place at an interval of two years, and the correlation was calculated between the two determinations. The crucial question is whether or not such an interval corresponds to the relevant induction period. Further, even if a two year period is accepted as an appropriate interval, it is not clear how the goodness of fit in equations (8) and (9) should be adjusted since access to an attenuation correction formula is lacking.

If one had access to an instrumental variable, an unbiased estimate could be obtained. The instrumental variable corresponds in Figure 1.1 to v and is characterized by a strong effect on x (relevant blood pressure level) but without *direct* relationship to other variables in the path model. Blood pressure medication could be such a variable v. However, the main indication for such a medicine is just increased blood pressure, i.e., blood pressure can be regarded as both cause and effect. Further, no such effective medicine was on the market as early as 1965; the variance of v equals zero.

There are other known confounders such as 'fat-indicators', e.g., cholesterol level which was recorded and, thus, can and ought to be included (the same position in Figure 1.1 as W).

Another source of error relevant in this example concerns the dependency between errors of measurement for the measured variables. Such errors may be correlated because the recording is carried out on one occasion (one day) and thus not representative for a long period. It is evident from this example that there are many ways to illuminate and reduce or eliminate errors.

Design aspects of specification and testing of assumptions

The statistical testing of the assumptions above cannot, of course, be carried out until data are collected. However, it is important to predict already in the design phase what type of objections and biases are to be expected in the analysis phase and which type of measures ought to be prepared. This is especially important in long-term longitudinal studies because supplementary data collection ex post is beyond reach.

SOME PROFILE-ORIENTED METHODS: ASSUMPTIONS AND USES

There is a fundamental difference between studying individual development using a variable-oriented approach and using a person-oriented approach (Block, 1971; Magnusson, 1985). The latter approach can take many forms but often emphasizes the importance of focusing on an information profile or gestalt as the basic piece of information. Pairwise relationships among the measured variables, which often are the basic data that are analyzed using a variable-oriented method such as, for instance, structural equation modeling, are not considered to contain sufficient information about the individuals. The profile of the individuals' values must be studied as a unit.

In certain cases a classification is produced and analyzed using a profile-oriented method but in other cases all profiles are retained throughout the analysis and in the results. A basic distinction is made between descriptive methods and methods that provide a model for the data.

In the sequel, some profile-oriented methods are described to give the reader an idea of the variety and usefulness of such methods.

Descriptive methods

By descriptive methods are here meant methods where profile development in terms of patterns is described with a minimum of model-imposing on the data. This is, of course, both a strength and a weakness. It is a strength in that there is less chance that an inadequate model blocks the view of aspects of reality not covered by the model. It is a weakness in that the guiding power of a sound model is lost as is the possibility of testing that model. However, what we here call a descriptive method can, of course, be used for theory testing.

In the next two sections, two different descriptive approaches are discussed as illustrations of the use of a descriptive methodology.

Longitudinal applications of cluster analysis

The term 'cluster analysis' is often used as a name for a number of different methods for grouping subjects on the basis of the profile similarity (Everitt, 1974). Cluster analysis can be used for studying individual development in different ways. Two common approaches are as follows.

1. Performing cluster analysis at different ages for a longitudinal sample and linking the age-specific cluster solutions using cross-tabulation techniques: this is discussed and exemplified by Bergman and Magnusson in Chapter 15 of this volume.
2. Performing a longitudinal cluster analysis on the complete data set from all points in time.

It should be noted that two basic assumptions in cluster analysis are (a) that it is sufficient to consider the similarities between all pairs of subjects and (b) that an adequate measure of the degree of similarity is used. Concerning (a) it is probably fair to say that the limitation as to pairs is not a severe limitation. It is usually less severe than the limitation to relationships between pairs of measured variables in many variable-oriented analyses since the number of pairs of subjects usually is much larger than the number of pairs of variables thus providing a richer information.

Concerning (b) it is undeniable that the interpretation of the results of a cluster analysis stands or falls on the assumption that the degree of (dis)similarity between the subjects is adequately represented by the chosen measure. The adequacy of the similarity measure has at least two aspects. The first is that the scale level of the involved variables must match the measure used, and the second aspect is that the similarity measure must correspond to the aspects of similarity or dissimilarity that are of interest. For instance, if only profile form is of interest, then certain kinds of measures are adequate (e.g. the correlation coefficient), whereas if both profile form and profile level are of interest, then other measures are adequate (e.g. squared Euclidean distance). The practical importance of the choice of similarity measure is illustrated in Figure 1.2. There it can be observed that the similarity between the objects *A* and

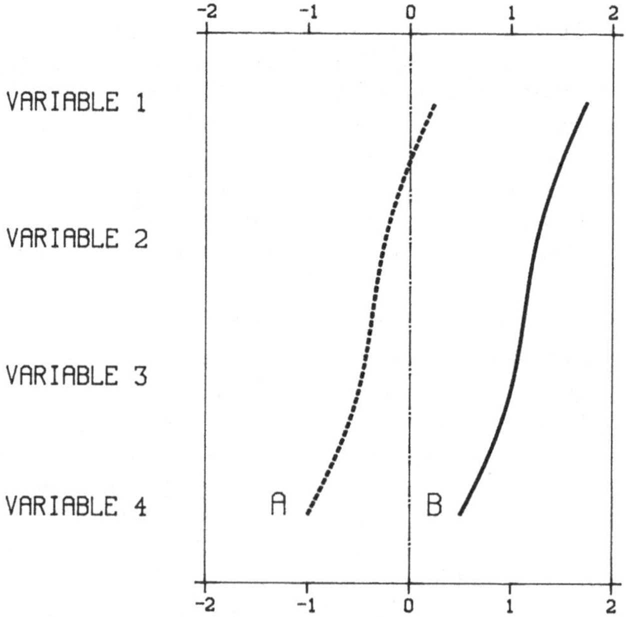

Figure 1.2. The value profiles of two objects *A* and *B*.

B is total according to form ($r = 1.00$), but much less than total if level is taken into account (average squared euclidean distance = 2.25). The choice of similarity measure has been discussed repeatedly in the literature and the reader is referred to Cronbach & Glesser (1953).

It has been claimed that the fact that different cluster analytic methods sometimes give different descriptions shows that such methods are of limited value and should be avoided. This argument is discussed by Bergman and Magnusson in Chapter 15 of this volume and they conclude that the argument does not generally hold; used appropriately, cluster analysis can be a very useful technique for studying individual development. They also conclude that forming a residue of unclassified deviant objects which are analyzed separately can be very useful.

So far only the cross-sectional use of cluster analysis has been discussed. Cross-sectional cluster analysis naturally forms the basis also for longitudinal approaches, but these also have their special features and problems. With regard to approach 1 above, one can graphically, or in cross-tabulations, follow the longitudinal streams and see how individuals develop from belonging to one cluster at age 1 to another cluster at age 2, and so on (Bergman & Magnusson, 1987). This is illustrated in Figure 15.1 in Chapter 15 by Bergman and Magnusson. A problem with this approach is, of course, the simplification of individual pattern development that must be made in order to present comprehensive developmental streams. If many ages are analyzed, even this approach gives a complicated picture, though this drawback is probably unavoidable considering the complexity of the phenomena that are analyzed.

From the viewpoint of comprehensiveness, it is an attractive feature of approach 2, above, that the complete longitudinal data set is analyzed in the same analysis. This approach was followed by Block (1971) when searching for a longitudinal typology of personality development (although he used Q-factor analysis as the classification method). However, in addition to the ordinary problems of cluster analysis, there are special problems involved: for example, the problem of discriminating between individuals' having similar patterns during a large part of their development but a different outcome; and individuals' starting out very differently but then having a similar pattern of development. Most measures of similarity would tend to find both types of individuals similar to each other, and they may come out in the same longitudinal cluster. However, from a substantive viewpoint one often wants such individuals to belong to different clusters.

Sometimes a modified form of approach 2 is used in which in a first step an ordination procedure is applied to reduce the number of dimensions (e.g. by performing a principal component analysis and computing the factor scores). The factor scores are then used as a basis for grouping individuals through cluster analysis (see, e.g., Mumford & Owens, 1984).

Longitudinal applications of studying all possible patterns

If the variables involved only take on a few values it is a natural descriptive approach to study all possible developmental patterns. Some cases involving continuous variables can also be studied in this way if it makes sense to, for instance, dichotomize the variables. However, it should be kept in mind that the number of possible patterns grows very rapidly with the number of variables measured at each occasion, the number of values each variable can take, and the number of measurement occasions. For instance, with two dichotomous variables measured at two points in time there are 16 possible value patterns and with four variables taking four values measured at four points in time there are 4.3 billion possible value patterns. Thus, the scope of a study of all possible patterns has to be limited. Nevertheless, this kind of study has many attractive features, the main one being its closeness to the basic data profile in the analysis and presentation.

Two main variants of analyzing all possible patterns are:

1. The study of higher-order cross-tabulations of categorical variables. This method has mainly been developed within sociology but is used in many disciplines. Certain aspects of the findings can be tested using ordinary chi-square analysis. Log-linear modeling can also be applied (see the next section about model-oriented methods). An illustrative example of the potency of this approach is given by Brown, Harris, and Lemyre in Chapter 4 of this volume. The main problem of the approach is the small number of variables and measurement occasions that can be handled.

2. Somewhat less restrictive in the number of variables that can be treated is the pattern analysis of Zubin (1937), which has been further developed by Lienert (1969) and Krauth & Lienert (1982), and has been given the name configural frequency analysis (CFA). Here all possible pattern combinations are listed and the frequency of each observed pattern is compared with the corresponding expected frequency (usually computed assuming a model of total randomness). If the observed frequency is significantly in excess of what could be expected, the value pattern is called a significant type. This model for hypothesis testing has been shown to have limitations since trivial or competing dependencies can create significant types. However, this deficiency can be amended by the choice of more appropriate procedures, and CFA holds great potential as a heuristic tool for understand-

ing what there is in one's data set. Various kinds of extensions have been made expanding the general idea into longitudinal applications (Lienert & zur Oeveste, 1985; Kohnen & Lienert, 1987; Lienert & Bergman 1985).

Model-based methods

A basic set of model-based methods that can be used for analyzing longitudinal profile data are log-linear models. The logarithm of a cell frequency (corresponding to a specific pattern) can then be modeled as depending on a sum of effects of the single variables and on interaction terms between them (see, e.g., Bishop, Feinberg & Holland, 1975). This technique can be very useful if the profile consists of a few variables taking on a few values (often categorical variables). Different model specifications can be tested and the study of the residuals between the frequencies produced by a model and the observed frequencies is often very informative. In this sense, log-linear modeling also contains a basic description. The use of this kind of modeling is exemplified by several authors in this volume. A related set of methods, logit analysis, can be used for modeling the log-odds ratio of a dichotomous outcome variable after a value profile in independent variables pertaining to an earlier age.

In the 1950s, Paul Lazarsfeld introduced latent structure analysis (LSA; Lazarsfeld, 1950; Lazarsfeld & Henry, 1968). Starting from a population being measured by a number of dichotomous variables it is assumed in LSA that there exists a small number of latent classes or subpopulations that explain all the observed relationships between the variables. Within a latent class the variables are independent. This ingenious idea has been expanded to other types of variables and can also be applied in a longitudinal setting (see, e.g., Goodman, 1979; Mårdberg, 1967). In this kind of methodology, the identification of the latent classes is complicated and involves subjective decisions. Also the evaluation of the quality of a model specification is not always straightforward. Nevertheless, the elegance of the basic idea makes LSA-oriented methods very attractive in situations when one can have clear expectations about latent classes (cf. Gangestad & Snyder, 1985).

SUMMARIZING DISCUSSION

The common theme in this volume is the matching of problems and methods in longitudinal research. Two main aspects of this match are those between method and theory and between method and data.

It was earlier emphasized that a complex issue when studying change or development is to what degree the same quality has been measured at the different ages. It has to do with the essential issue about the relation between data and phenomena and the need for data to reflect the phenomena under study at the right level (this topic was discussed in volume 3 in this series).

Another issue is the scale properties of the involved variables in relation to the statistical methods that are used. How well do the properties of the numbers correspond to the mathematical operations that are performed on them? Research practice is rather permissive of some mismatch between scale level and the statistical methods used. From a statistical viewpoint it may be permissible to use a certain statistical method on a data set as long as the assumptions about distributional form, random sampling, etc. are fulfilled, even if there is a mismatch between the scale level and the mathematical operations performed when using the method (cf. Lord's (1953) argument, in which he coined the catchy phrase 'the numbers don't remember where they came from', p. 751). However, from a substantive perspective the results in such a case are difficult to interpret and, in our opinion, a reasonably good match should be demanded (Townsend & Ashby, 1984).

In previous sections, aspects of the matching of theoretical problem formulation and the choice of statistical method were discussed. In this volume, many examples are given of ways to achieve a good match within different problem areas. Earlier it was contended that sometimes sophisticated methods are not congruent with the problem formulation that is the focus of the study. The easy availability of powerful statistical methods for data treatment creating testable models of the data have lead to an over-emphasis on a confirmatory, theory-testing approach. It was argued that this, in many respects commendable, approach has drawbacks when studying individual development in fields where our knowledge is very incomplete. Thus, an important and often overlooked first step is the careful description and observation of individual development and the longitudinal data set as a precursor to the formulation of realistic theories. A symptom of this state of affairs is the emergence of quasi-confirmatory studies in which the published report is a confirmatory study but where a fair amount of unreported exploration was first performed.

There is now a widespread consensus that the rejection of a statistical model for data on the basis of a significant misfit can be less interesting than the comparison between the fit of different models and also the power of the model in explaining the observed variation (Dillon & Goldstein, 1978). As was pointed out earlier, even if a model fits the data perfectly, it may be of very limited value if a large part of the variation in the dependent variable(s) is 'explained' by error terms in the model. Physicists' demand that a model should both fit the data and have small error terms makes good sense. The relaxed attitude towards this issue in the life sciences may have contributed to the over-use and over-interpretation of developmental models tested on cross-sectional data. A good model fit may be obtained in this situation, but the model may include very large error variance components. Important explanatory factors from other ages in the subjects' lives are excluded, and the variance these factors create is entered in the cross-sectional model largely as error variance.

The use of appropriate statistical methods on longitudinal data of individual development has been facilitated by new statistical methods and by modern computer technology. These advances carry great potential for understanding and explaining the developmental process beyond current knowledge. But the concepts, variables, and measures used must also be expanded to deal directly with change and development and be rooted in a process-oriented analysis of the phenomena.

REFERENCES

Bergman, L. R. (1972). Change as the dependent variable. Reports from the Psychological Department, University of Stockholm, supplement 14.

Bergman, L. R. (1988). You can't classify all of the people all of the time. *Multivariate Behavioral Research, 23,* 425–441.

Bergman, L. R. & Magnusson, D. (1987). A person approach to the study of the development of adjustment problems: An empirical example and some research strategy considerations. In D. Magnusson and A. Öhman (eds.), *Psychopathology: An interactional perspective.* Orlando, Florida: Academic Press.

Bergman, L. R. & Magnusson, D. (1990). General issues about data quality in longitudinal research. In D. Magnusson & L. R. Bergman (eds.), *Data quality in longitudinal research.* New York: Cambridge University Press.

Bishop, Y. M. M., Feinberg, S. E. & Holland, P. W. (1975). *Discrete multivariate analysis: Theory and practice.* Cambridge, Mass: MIT Press.

Block, J. (1971). *Lives through time.* Berkley: Bancroft Books.

Cook, T. D. & Campbell, D. T. (1979). *Quasi-experimentation: Design and analysis issues for field settings.* Skokie, IL: Rand McNally.

Cronbach, L. J. (1975). Beyond the two disciplines of scientific psychology. *American Psychologist, 30,* 116–127.

Cronbach, L. J. & Furby, L. (1970). How we should measure 'change' – or should we? *Psychological Bulletin, 74,* 68–80.

Cronbach, L. J. & Glesser, G. C. (1953). Assessing similarity between profiles. *Psychological Bulletin, 50,* 456–473.

Dillon, W. R. & Goldstein, M. (1978). On the performance of some multinominal classification rules. *Journal of the American Statistical Association, 73,* 305–313.

Everitt, B. (1974). *Cluster analysis.* London: Heinemann.

Gangestad, S. & Snyder, M. (1985). 'To carve nature at its joints': On the existence of discrete classes in personality. *Psychological Review, 92*(3), 317–349.

Goodman, L. A. (1979). On the estimation of parameters in latent structure analysis. *Psychometrika, 44*(1), 123–128.

Greenwald, A. G., Pratkanis, A. R., Lieppe, M. R. & Baumgardner, M. H. (1986). Under what conditions does theory obstruct research progress? *Psychological Review, 93*(2), 216–229.

Harris, C. W. (1963). *Problems in measuring change.* Madison, Wisconsin: University of Wisconsin Press.

Harvey, A. C. (1983). *The econometric analysis of time series.* Oxford: Philip Allan.

Hinde, R. A. & Bateson, P. (1984). Discontinuities versus continuities in behavioral development and the neglect of process. *International Journal of Behavioral Development, 7*, 129–143.

Hinde, R. A. & Dennis, A. (1986). Categorizing individuals: An alternative to linear analysis. *International Journal of Behavioral Development, 9*, 105–119.

Janson, C.-G. (1981). The longitudinal approach. In F. Schulsinger, S. A. Mednick & J. Knop (eds.), *Longitudinal research: Methods and uses in behavioral science.* Boston: Nijhoff.

Janson, C.-G. (1990). Retrospective data, undesirable behavior, and the longitudinal perspective. In D. Magnusson and L. R. Bergman (eds.), *Data quality in longitudinal research.* New York: Cambridge University Press.

Kohnen, R. & Lienert, G. A. (1987). Interactional research in human development approached by interactive configural frequency analysis. In D. Magnusson & A. Öhman (eds.), *Psychopathology: An interactional perspective.* New York: Academic Press.

Krauth, J. & Lienert, G. A. (1982). Fundamentals and modifications of configural frequency analysis (CFA). *Interdisciplinaria, 3*, issue 1.

Lazarsfeld, P. F. (1950). The logical and mathematical foundation of latent structure analysis. In S. A. Stouffer *et al.* (eds.), *Measurement and prediction.* Princeton University Press.

Lazarsfeld, P. F. & Henry, N. W. (1968). *Latent structure analysis.* New York: Houghton Mifflin.

Lienert, G. A. (1969). Die 'Konfigurationsfrequenzanalyse' als Klassifikationsmittel in der klinischen Psycholgie. In M. Irle (ed.), *Bericht über den 26. Kongress der Deutschen Gesellschaft für Psychologie.* Tübingen, Göttingen: Hogrete, pp. 244–253.

Lienert, G. A. & Bergman, L. R. (1985). Longisectional interaction structure analysis (LISA) in psychopharmacology and developmental psychopathology. *Neuropsychobiology, 14*, 27–34.

Lienert, G. A. & zur Oeveste, H. (1985). Configural frequency analysis as a statistical tool for developmental research. *Educational and Psychological Measurement, 45*, 301–307.

Lord, F. M. (1953). On the statistical treatment of football numbers. *American Psychologist, 8*, 750–751.

Magnusson, D. (1985). Implications of an interactional paradigm for research on human development. *International Journal of Behavioral Development, 8*(2), 115–137.

Magnusson, D. (1988). Individual development from an interactional perspective. A longitudinal study. Vol. 1 in D. Magnusson (ed.), *Paths through life.* Hillsdale, N. J.: Lawrence Erlbaum.

Magnusson, D. (1990). Personality development from an interactional perspective. In L. A. Pervin (ed.), *Handbook of personality: Theory and research.* New York: Guilford Publications.

Magnusson, D. & Bergman, L. R. (eds.) (1990). *Data quality in longitudinal research.* New York: Cambridge University Press.

Magnusson, D. & Törestad, B. (in press). The individual as an interactive agent. In W. B. Walsh, K. Craik & R. Price (eds.), *Person-environment psychology: Models and perspectives.* Hillsdale, N. J.: Erlbaum

Mumford, M. D. & Owens, W. A. (1984). Individuality in a developmental context: Some experimental and theoretical considerations. *Human Development, 27*, 84–108.

Mårdberg, B. (1967). Arbetspsykologisk klassificering (classification in industrial psychology) Report No. 42. Stockholm: P. A.-rådet.

Nelder, J. A. & Wedderburn, R. W. M. (1972). Generalized linear models. *Journal Royal Statistic Society A, 135*(3), 370.

Rudinger, G. & Wood, P. K. (1990). *N*'s, times and numbers of variables in longitudinal research. In D. Magnusson & L. R. Bergman (eds.), *Data quality in longitudinal research.* New York: Cambridge University Press.

Rutter, M. & Pickles, A. (1990). Improving the quality of psychiatric data: Classification, cause and course. In D. Magnusson & L. R. Bergman (eds.), *Data quality in longitudinal research.* New York: Cambridge University Press.

Søgaard, J. (1983). Socio-economic change and mortality: A multivariate coherency analysis of Danish time series., In J. John *et al.* (eds.), Influence of economic instability on health. Proceedings, Berlin, Mimeograph, pp. 85–112.

Townsend, J. T. & Ashby, F. G. (1984). Measurement scales and statistics: The misconception misconceived. *Psychological Bulletin, 96*(2), 394–401.

The Värmland Study (1971). Allmänna Förlaget, Stockholm.

Wohlwill, J. F. (1973). *The study of behavioral development.* London: Academic Press.

Zubin, J. (1937). The determination of response patterns in personality adjustment inventories. *Journal of Educational Psychology, 28*, 401–413.

2 Modeling individual and average human growth data from childhood to adulthood

ROLAND C. HAUSPIE, GUNILLA W.-LINDGREN, JAMES M. TANNER AND HANNA CHRZASTEK-SPRUCH

INTRODUCTION

The first longitudinal growth study dates back to 1759 when Count de Montbeillard measured the body length of his son from birth to 18 years (Scammon, 1927; Tanner, 1962). Actually, when studying growth, there are two basically different approaches: longitudinal and cross-sectional studies. In longitudinal growth studies, we measure the same children over several years at regular intervals (as was done by de Montbeillard) in order to be able to establish individual growth patterns. In cross-sectional growth studies, we measure children of different ages only once. A plot of the average height obtained at each age (or age group) depicts the average growth pattern in the sample. One should realize that the shape of the curve seen in an average growth pattern is different from the shape of individual growth curves (Hauspie, 1989). The information provided by the longitudinal and cross-sectional approaches is quite different. Both methods have their advantages and limitations. Whether the data concerns individual or average growth patterns, we are dealing with a series of measures of size (height or average height, for example) at particular ages, either precise chronological ages (in case of longitudinal studies) or mid-points of age classes (in case of cross-sectional studies). However, the researcher is quite often interested in determining the underlying continuous process of growth, from which he wants to derive certain characteristics, such as the age at maximum velocity at adolescence, for example.

This chapter deals with some aspects of growth modeling, a technique which allows us to estimate a smooth curve passing through the observed growth data. Several models have been proposed to achieve this goal. Some of them describe the whole growth process, others deal with only a part of the growth process (Hauspie, 1989). We will discuss some of the features, advantages and limitations of a few models, capable of representing human growth data for height from birth or childhood to adulthood on the basis of applications on a single individual and on average growth data for the Swedish population.

INDIVIDUAL GROWTH PATTERN

Figure 2.1 (upper part) shows a graph of the measurements of height attained at successive ages, from birth to 18 years, of a single child (girl nr. 7 from the Lublin Longitudinal Growth Study: Chrzastek-Spruch, Susanne, Hauspie and Kozlowska, 1989). The child was measured at regular intervals, monthly from birth to 1 year, 3-monthly between 1 and 7 years (with some missing measurement occasions), and yearly thereafter. Altogether, there are 42 measurements of height. The lower

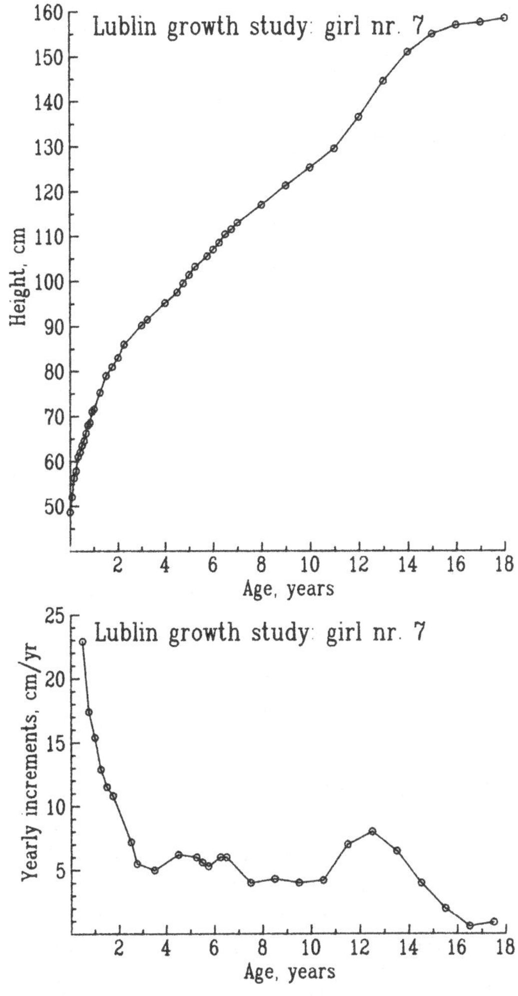

Figure 2.1. Attained height (upper graph) and yearly increments (lower graph) of girl nr. 7 from the Lublin Longitudinal Growth Study (Chrzastek-Spruch *et al.*, 1989).

Table 2.1. *Height (cm) for age (years) and whole-year increments of height (cm/year) for age (mid-point of the one-year interval, in years) for girl nr. 7 of the Lublin Longitudinal Growth Study*

Age	Height	Age	Height	Age	Increments
0.000	48.6	6.000	107.0	0.500	22.9
0.083	52.0	6.250	108.5	0.750	17.4
0.167	56.3	6.500	110.4	1.000	15.4
0.250	57.8	6.750	111.5	1.250	12.9
0.333	61.0	7.000	113.0	1.500	11.5
0.417	62.0	8.000	117.0	1.750	10.8
0.500	63.5	9.000	121.3	2.500	7.2
0.583	64.5	10.000	125.3	2.750	5.5
0.667	66.2	11.000	129.5	3.500	5.0
0.750	68.0	12.000	136.5	4.500	6.2
0.833	68.5	13.000	144.5	5.250	6.0
0.917	71.0	14.000	151.0	5.500	5.6
1.000	71.5	15.000	155.0	5.750	5.3
1.250	75.2	16.000	157.0	6.250	6.0
1.500	78.9	17.000	157.6	6.500	6.0
1.750	80.9	18.000	158.5	7.500	4.0
2.000	83.0			8.500	4.3
2.250	86.0			9.500	4.0
3.000	90.2			10.500	4.2
3.250	91.5			11.500	7.0
4.000	95.2			12.500	8.0
4.500	97.5			13.500	6.5
4.750	99.5			14.500	4.0
5.000	101.4			15.500	2.0
5.250	103.2			16.500	0.6
5.750	105.5			17.500	0.9

part of Figure 2.1 shows the growth velocity or yearly increments in height, i.e. the amount of growth achieved over one-year intervals. For example, the first point on this graph is the difference between height at one year and at birth, i.e. $71.5 - 48.6 = 22.9$ cm, plotted at the mid-point of the interval, i.e. 0.5 years of age. The second whole-year increment could be calculated over the interval of 0.25–1.25 years (mid-point at 0.75 years), i.e. 17.4 cm. In order to avoid the effect of seasonal variation in growth velocity and to reduce the effect of measurement error, it is recommended to calculate increments over yearly, or nearly yearly, increments. The latter is usually the case when children are not measured at exact birthdays or precise intermediate target ages. Tanner & Davies (1985) state that in such situations increments can be taken over 0.85 to 1.15 years and then converted to whole-year increments. Table 2.1 shows the raw data of height for age (distance data) and the yearly increments for the case shown in Figure 2.1.

The graphical plot of the growth data as shown in Figure 2.1 illustrate the main features of the human growth pattern. The velocity curve is more informative than the distance (attained height) curve. The first two years after birth (early childhood) are characterized by a relatively high, but steadily decreasing, growth velocity. This period is followed by a period of more or less constant growth rate (childhood), which is eventually interrupted by a small mid-childhood spurt (Tanner & Cameron, 1980; Meredith, 1981). Recently, Butler, McKie & Ratcliffe (1989) even suggested the existence of a series of small spurts during childhood. The present example clearly shows the presence of at least one, perhaps two, mid-childhood spurts. Finally, the childhood period is followed by the adolescent growth spurt, a phenomenon present in all healthy children.

In the analysis of longitudinal growth data we shall often be interested in determining 'biological parameters' of the growth process, such as the age (T), size (H) and velocity (V) at particular milestones along the growth process, like the onset (or take-off) and peak of a spurt. For this chapter we have defined the following biological parameters:

$T1'$	age at take-off of mid-childhood spurt
$H1'$	size at take-off of mid-childhood spurt
$V1'$	velocity at take-off of mid-childhood spurt
$T2'$	age at maximal velocity of mid-childhood spurt
$H2'$	size at maximal velocity of mid-childhood spurt
$V2'$	velocity at maximal velocity of mid-childhood spurt
$T1$	age at take-off of adolescent growth spurt
$H1$	size at take-off of adolescent growth spurt
$V1$	velocity at take-off of adolescent growth spurt
$T2$	age at maximal velocity of adolescent growth spurt
$H2$	size at maximal velocity of adolescent growth spurt
$V2$	velocity at maximal velocity of adolescent growth spurt

Graphical analysis of the data, as shown in Figure 2.1, will sometimes require a certain amount of subjectivity to locate the peak or the onset of a spurt. This is particularly the case when the data are somewhat irregular, owing to measurement error for example. The growth data may also suggest that certain events are located between two measurement occasions, which may force us to estimate biological parameters by means of some interpolation technique. This problem is even more likely to occur when the serial growth data contains gaps (missed measurement occasions). To some extent, these problems can be overcome by fitting a mathematical model to the growth data. The growth pattern is then represented by a continuous curve, which smooths out the noise in the empirical data and short-term variations in growth rate. The mathematical first derivative of the fitted curve provides a good picture of the instantaneous growth velocity. Biological parameters are then, analytically or numerically, derived from the fitted curve rather than from the raw data.

CURVE FITTING

Before discussing the characteristics of some models describing human growth, let us remind ourselves about some basic principles of curve fitting. The most simple growth model is a first-degree polynomial or straight line ($y = bx + a$), whereby y (size) increases or decreases linearly as a function of x (age). Indeed, for some non-skeletal body dimensions we can expect negative growth in some age periods (skinfold thickness, for example). This simple model has two parameters: b, the slope of the line, and a, the intercept (value of y when x equals 0). Our goal is to find the 'best fitting' line, i.e. the line which describes most closely our observations. Generally, this consists in finding the values of a and b for which the sum of squared deviations (sum of the differences between the observed values and the fitted curve) are minimal (least squares method). There is one set of values of a and b which meet that criterion. Remember that fitting a straight line is a problem of linear regression, which can be easily handled by practically any statistical software.

The sum of squared deviations (or residuals) divided by the number of degrees of freedom is called the residual variance, which is a measure of the goodness of fit. The number of degrees of freedom is the number of observations minus the number of parameters estimated (two in the case of a first-degree polynomial). Since the chosen model is supposed to represent a true picture of the trend (growth pattern, for example), the deviations are often considered as noise in the data, or error terms. It is a policy to compare the square root of the residual variance (standard error of estimate) with the measurement error of the dependent variable (y), which is a way of verifying this hypothesis.

By fitting a mathematical model (in this case a straight line), we actually summarize the original raw data (the set of x–y values) into a limited number of constants, the estimated function parameters (a and b). With these values to hand, we can easily draw the best fitting line, estimate values of y for new values of x, or compare several curves in terms of their slope or intercept. Indeed, the estimated function parameters have the same meaning for all fitted curves.

In human growth data, the use of a straight line as a model is only valid when dealing with fairly narrow age ranges. Sometimes second- or third-degree polynomials are more appropriate. These polynomials require the estimation of respectively three and four function parameters, but they still do not allow us to describe accurately human growth data over broad age ranges.

Whenever interest lies in characterizing the growth pattern over age ranges of several years (the childhood period, adolescence or the whole growth cycle, for example), we have to rely on more complex models, which are usually nonlinear in their constants. These models require nonlinear least squares methods, which can be handled by statistical packages such as SPSS (Nie *et al.*, 1975) or subroutines such as the VA05A from the Harwell Subroutine Library (Powell, 1969).

(a) (b)

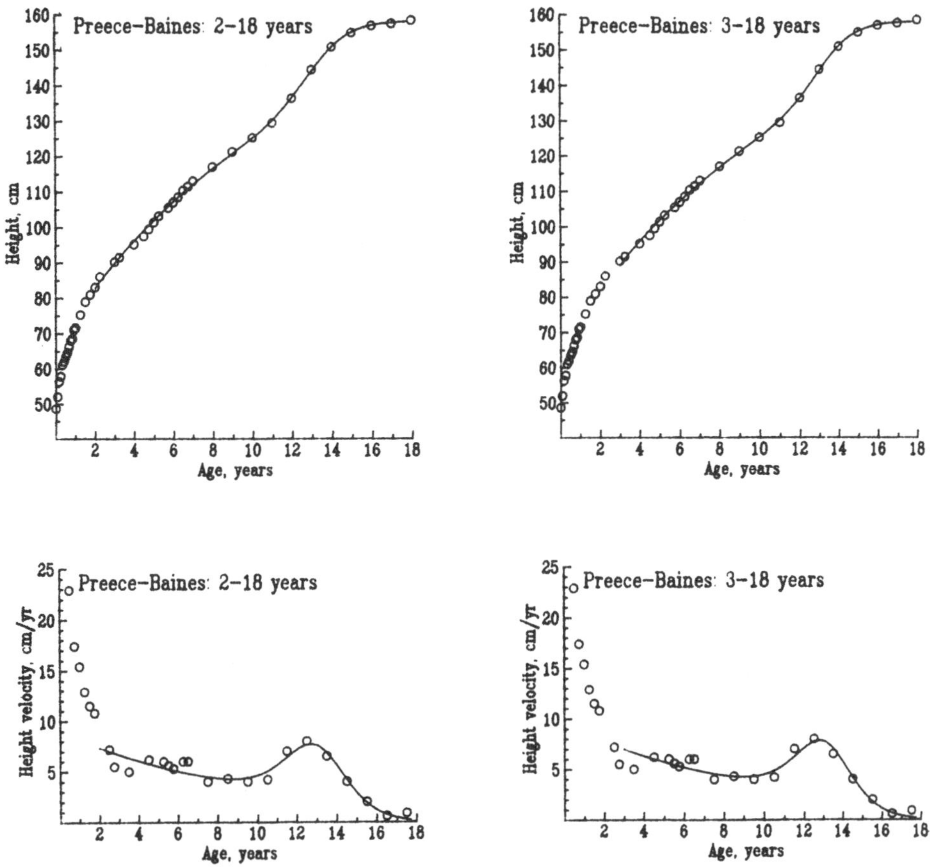

Figure 2.2. The Preece–Baines model fitted to the attained height for age for girl nr. 7 from the Lublin Longitudinal Growth Study (upper graph in each part a–d). First derivative of the Preece–Baines model and yearly increments for height (lower graph in each part a–d) (Chrzastek-Spruch *et al.*, 1989).

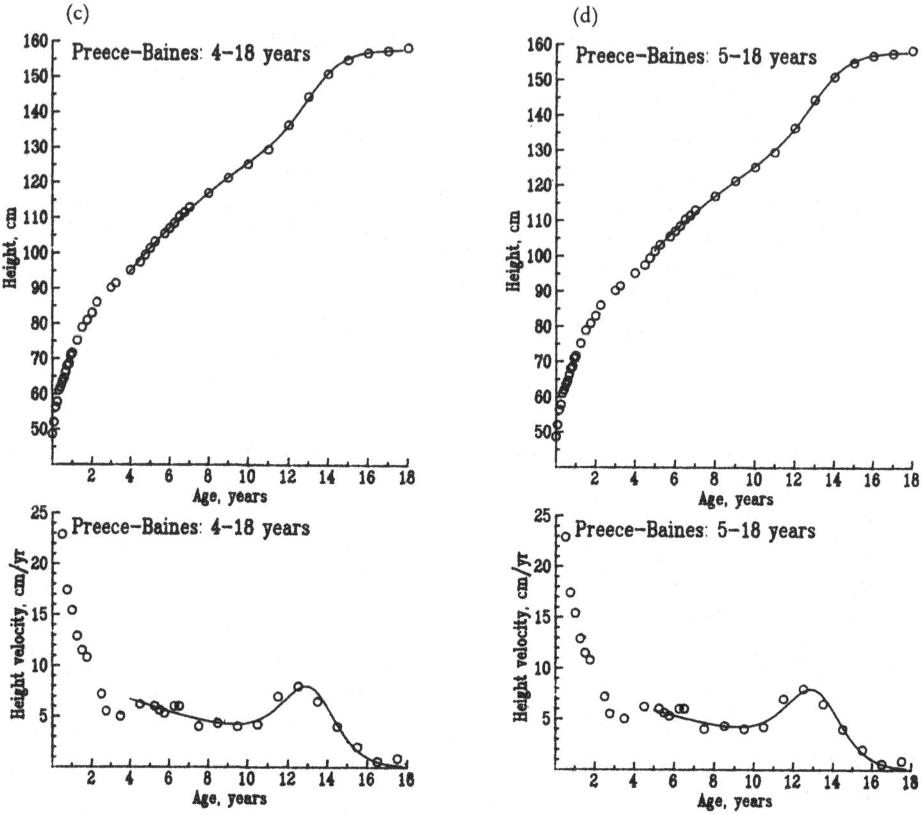

Figure 2.2. *(cont.)*.

PREECE–BAINES MODEL

Preece & Baines (1978) proposed the following multiplicative exponential-logistic model:

$$y = h_1 - \frac{2(h_1 - h_\theta)}{e^{s_0(t-\theta)} + e^{s_1(t-\theta)}}$$

where y = size, t = age, and h_1, h_θ, s_0, s_1 and θ are the parameters. This model has five parameters, one of which is adult size (h_1). Parameter θ is a time parameter, locating the peak of the adolescent spurt along the time axis, while h_θ is size at age θ. The parameters s_0 and s_1 are growth rate constants, defining respectively childhood and adolescent growth velocity. The model is characterized by a gradually decreasing growth velocity during childhood followed by the adolescent growth spurt. However, the model does not allow for a mid-childhood spurt. So, even if such a spurt is shown by the empirical data, it will be smoothed out

Table 2.2. *Function parameters of the Preece–Baines model fitted to different sections of the serial growth data for height of girl nr. 7 of the Lublin Longitudinal Growth Study. Residual variance and degrees of freedom (d.f.)*

	Age ranges			
Parameters	2–18	3–18	4–18	5–18
h_1	158.3223	158.1461	157.9445	158.0060
h_θ	145.6129	145.8993	146.3108	146.1146
s_0	0.0973	0.1011	0.1071	0.1043
s_1	1.0662	1.1323	1.2254	1.1908
θ	13.1937	13.2335	13.2945	1.3266
Residual var.	0.51	0.39	0.22	0.19
d.f.	21	19	17	14

by the fit of the Preece–Baines model. Otherwise, the model describes fairly well the overall growth pattern of height and several other skeletal body dimensions from about 1–2 years of age to adulthood (Hauspie, Das, Preece and Tanner, 1980; Brown & Townsend, 1982).

Figure 2.2 shows the results of the fit of the Preece–Baines model to various sections of the serial data of the same subject as in Figure 2.1: (a) 2–18 years, (b) 3–18 years, (c) 4–18 years and (d) 5–18 years. The upper graph in each part shows the complete series of raw data for height attained at each age together with the Preece–Baines curve plotted over the interval which was used to do the curve fitting. The lower graph in each part shows the empirical yearly increments together with the mathematical first derivative of the fitted curve (instantaneous velocity). Table 2.2 shows the function parameters and the residual variances obtained for these four fits. Table 2.5 shows the biological variables concerning the adolescent growth spurt for the same four fits of the Preece–Baines model, compared with the biological variables derived from a graphical analysis of the empirical distance and velocity curve. This analyis on a single child shows that the estimation of the adolescent growth spurt is not greatly affected by the amount of preadolescent data included in the curve fitting procedure. Actually, this example illustrates the findings of Hauspie *et al.* (1980*b*), who showed that the Preece–Baines model is fairly robust to fit longitudinal growth data for height where the first measurement is located somewhere between 1–2 years of age and some age before the onset of the adolescent growth spurt. In general, the first measurement should be at least one year before take-off of the adolescent growth spurt in order to obtain a reliable fit. As for all other models discussed in this paper, the empirical data should also show that mature size is almost reached. If not, the value of the b_1 parameter (adult size) may be quite misleading. Since the Preece–Baines model does not comprise parameters to represent a mid-childhood spurt, we may expect the largest residuals in that age period. This is particularly visible in Figure 2.5a. The model can not cope with the sharp drop in growth velocity during the first two years of life, and hence extrapolations into this age range on the basis of a fitted curve do not make sense.

JPPS MODEL

More recently, Jolicoeur, Pontier, Pernin & Sempé (1988) have developed a new 7-parameter asymptotic growth model, which passes through the origin and fits human growth data from birth to adulthood (see also : Pontier, Jolicoeur, Abidi and Sempé, 1988; Pontier, Jolicoeur,

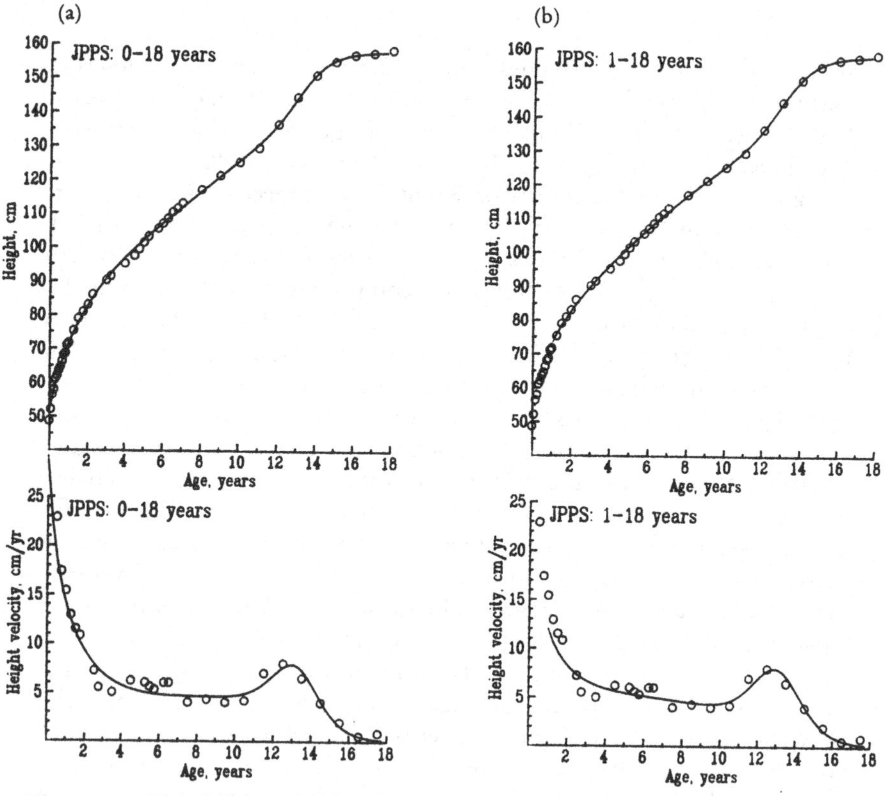

Figure 2.3. The JPPS model fitted to the attained height for age for girl nr. 7 from the Lublin Longitudinal Growth Study (upper graphs). First derivative of the JPPS model and yearly increments for height (lower graphs). (Chrzastek-Spruch *et al.*, 1989).

Pernin, Abidi and Sempé, 1988):

$$y = A\left\{1 - \frac{1}{1 + (t/D_1)^{C_1} + (t/D_2)^{C_2} + (t/D_3)^{C_3}}\right\}$$

where y = size, t = age, and A, D_1, D_2, D_3, C_1, C_2, and C_3 are the function parameters. Parameter A is adult size. Parameters D_1, D_2 and D_3 are three positive time-scale factors; C_1, C_2 and C_3 are three positive dimensionless exponents, reflecting respectively the shape of the initial, central and final section of the growth curve. The model is not able to depict the mid-childhood spurt either. While most other models use *postnatal age* (measured from the day of birth), the JPPS model uses *total age* (measured from the day of conception), which is practically obtained by correcting postnatal age with the average duration of pregnancy (0.75 years).

Figure 2.3 shows, in the same style as for Figure 2.2, the graphical representation of the JPPS model fitted to the data: (a) 0–18 years and (b) 1–18 years. Attempts to fit the model to data sets in which the lower age bound was greater than or equal to two years were not successful. The corresponding function parameters are given in Table 2.3, the biological parameters in Table 2.5. The JPPS model estimates age at peak velocity (T2) about 0.5 years later than the empirically obtained value. One of the advantages of the JPPS model is that it can cope with the dramatic change in growth velocity in early childhood and so give a fairly good picture of the growth process from birth to maturity. From

Table 2.3. *Function parameters of the JPPS Model fitted to different sections of the serial growth data for height of girl nr. 7 of the Lublin Longitudinal Growth Study. Residual variance and degrees of freedom (d.f.)*

	Age ranges	
Parameters	0–18	1–18
A	157.991010	158.146800
C_1	0.629566	0.511546
C_2	4.199605	3.012662
C_3	19.107433	17.577177
D_1	2.392040	2.432397
D_2	10.152432	9.078520
D_3	12.839947	12.652202
Residual var.	0.96	0.55
d.f.	35	23

the experience on this single child, it seems that the fitting of the JPPS model might be quite sensitive towards variations in the lower age bound of the data range. The model has not yet been fully tested, but according to Pontier *et al.* (1988*a*,*b*) it performs well in both normal and pathological growth.

TRIPLE LOGISTIC MODEL

Finally, Bock and Thissen (1980) proposed the triple logistic model. The model is based on the idea that mature size is a summation of three processes, each of which can be represented by a logistic function (see also Bock, 1986):

$$y = a_1\left\{\frac{1-p}{1+e^{-b_1(t-c_1)}} + \frac{p}{1+e^{-b_2(t-c_2)}}\right\} + \frac{a_2}{1+e^{-b_3(t-c_3)}}$$

where y = size, t = age, and a_1, b_1, c_1, a_2, b_2, c_2, b_3, c_3 and p are the function parameters. Parameter a_1 reflects the contribution of pre-adolescent growth to mature size. Parameters b_1 and c_1 govern the shape of the curve in the early childhood period, while b_2 and c_2 do so for the mid-childhood period, and b_3 and c_3 for the adolescent period. Parameter a_2 is the contribution of the adolescent component to mature size. El Lozy (1978) gives a critical analysis of the triple logistic model.

The triple logistic model requires quite extensive data since there are nine parameters to be estimated. However, it describes the human growth pattern for height from birth to maturity, allowing for a mid-childhood spurt as well. Figure 2.4 shows the graphical representation of the triple logistic model fitted to the data: (a) 0–18 years and (b) 1–18 years. As for the JPPS model, the fit of the triple logistic model to data sets excluding height measurements below two years of age failed. The function parameters for the triple logistic fit are given in Table 2.4, the biological parameters in Table 2.5. The low values of the residual variance indicate, indeed, that the triple logistic model fitted the data very well, even when data from birth onwards are included in the fitting procedure. The plotted distance and velocity curve fit the empirical data remarkably well and the biological parameters are very close to those obtained from the graphical analysis. So, it seems that, if the investigator has enough serial data at hand, starting from below two years of age, the triple logistic model is a very appropriate model to describe the growth process.

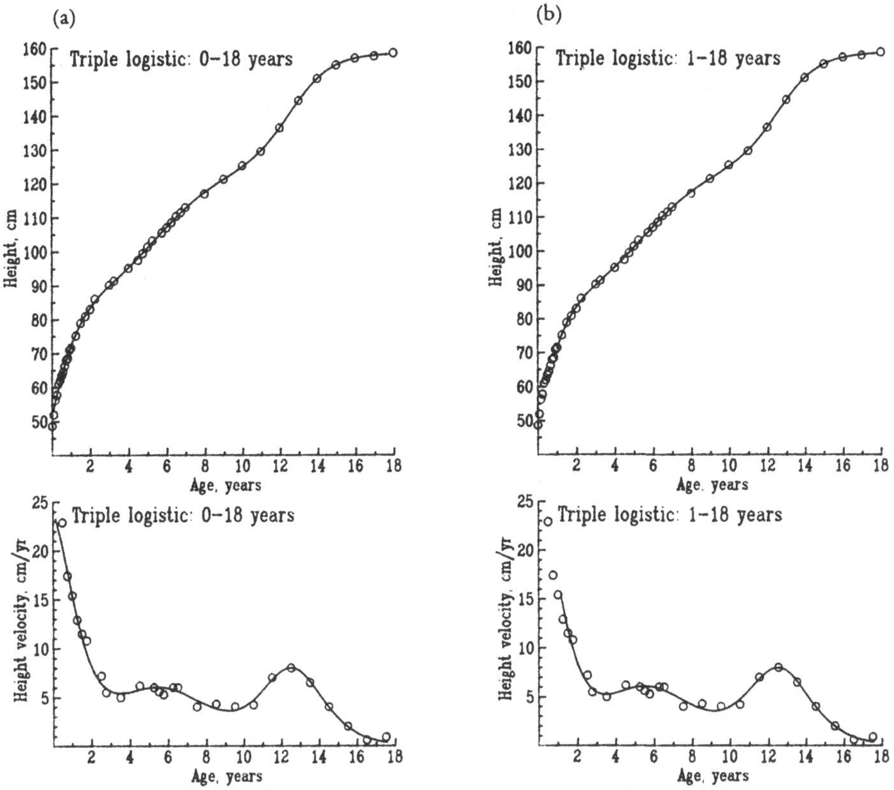

Figure 2.4. The triple logistic model fitted to the attained height for age for girl nr. 7 from the Lublin Longitudinal Growth Study (upper graphs). First derivative of the triple logistic model and yearly increments for height (lower graphs). (Chrzastek-Spruch *et al.*, 1989).

CURVE FITTING OF AVERAGE GROWTH: AN EXAMPLE

Although human growth models are usually applied to individual longitudinal growth data, they can also be used as a smoothing technique to represent average growth patterns. In this section we will deal with such an application on data of Swedish school children born in 1955 and 1967 (Lindgren & Hauspie, 1989). The Preece–Baines model was chosen to describe the average growth pattern for height obtained in these two surveys. Tanner, Hayashi, Preece & Cameron (1982) previously used this technique to describe trends of cross-sectional means, for the purpose of comparing populations. Vercauteren (1984), Hauspie & Wachholder (1986), and Wachholder & Hauspie (1986) applied the same model to fit centile values in order to produce smooth centile lines.

Table 2.4. *Function parameters of the triple logistic model fitted to different sections of the serial growth data for height of girl nr. 7 of the Lublin Longitudinal Growth Study. Residual variance and degrees of freedom (d.f.)*

Parameters	Age ranges 0–18	1–18
a_1	125.050950	124.265540
b_1	1.155183	1.216845
c_1	−0.347534	−0.210679
a_2	33.461461	34.276313
b_2	0.570143	0.604909
c_2	5.527326	5.565885
b_3	0.911166	0.895470
c_3	12.574188	12.542760
p	0.330622	0.317425
Residual var.	0.31	0.13
d.f.	32	20

Table 2.5. *Biological parameters obtained by graphical analysis and by various mathematical models fitted to the serial growth data for height of girl nr. 7 of the Lublin Longitudinal Growth Study (for explanations of abbreviations, see text)*

Parameters	Graphical	PB 2–18	PB 3–18	PB 4–18	PB 5–18	JPPS 0–18	JPPS 1–18	Tr. log. 0–18	Tr. log. 1–18
$T1'$	3.5	—	—	—	—	—	—	3.5	3.5
$H1'$	92.7	—	—	—	—	—	—	92.5	92.5
$V1'$	5.0	—	—	—	—	—	—	5.4	5.2
$T2'$	5.5	—	—	—	—	—	—	5.4	5.5
$H2'$	104.2	—	—	—	—	—	—	103.8	104.3
$V2'$	6.0	—	—	—	—	—	—	6.1	6.1
$T1$	9.5	8.7	9.0	9.3	9.2	8.9	9.4	9.2	9.2
$H1$	123.2	119.6	120.9	122.8	122.0	120.6	123.1	121.9	121.8
$V1$	4.0	4.3	4.2	4.2	4.2	4.6	4.4	3.6	3.5
$T2$	12.5	12.7	12.8	12.9	12.9	13.0	12.9	12.5	12.5
$H2$	140.5	142.0	142.5	143.2	142.9	143.6	143.0	140.5	140.5
$V2$	8.0	7.7	7.9	8.1	8.0	7.9	8.0	8.0	8.0

In the Swedish study, the fit of the Preece–Baines model to the averages for height at each age were successful in all instances, yielding fairly low residual variances. The square root of the residual variances (standard error of estimate) was of the order of magnitude of, or below, the standard error of the respective sample means. Increments in mean height were calculated over one-year intervals, the values being plotted at the mid-point of each interval. Figure 2.5 shows the results for attained height (left) and yearly increments (right) for boys (top) and girls (bottom).

It seems that average growth in height for boys has slightly increased in the 1967 sample, compared with the 1955 sample. For girls, the change in mean height over the same age range is almost nil. The age ranges of the data were unfortunately not sufficient to make accurate inferences about adult height in either sample. Age at maximal increment in height during puberty was estimated according to Tanner

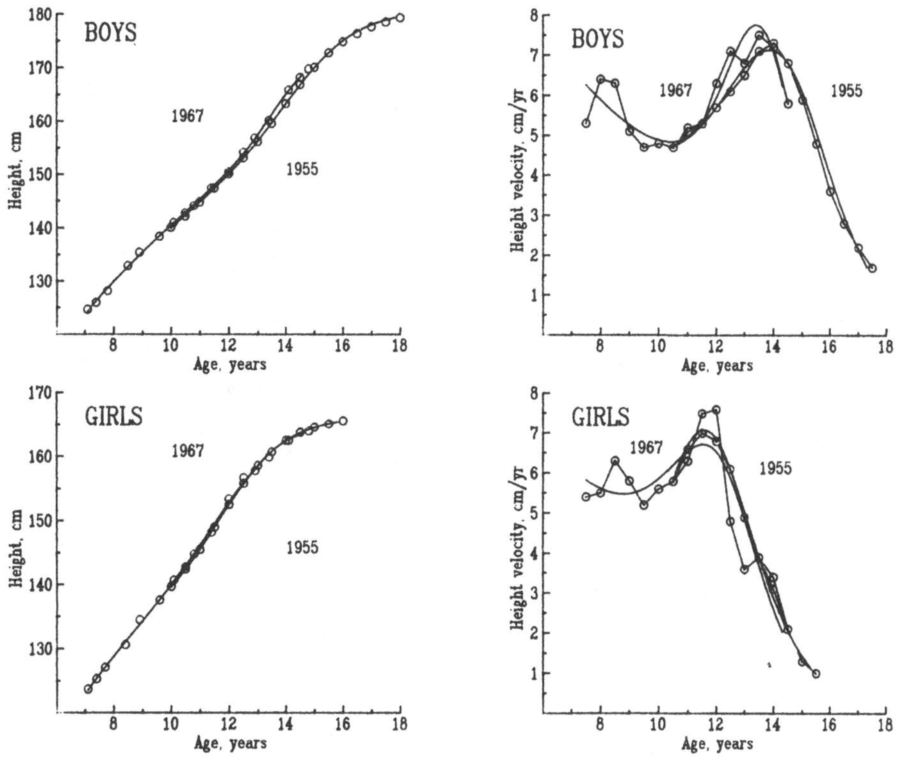

Figure 2.5. Attained height (left) and yearly increments (right) for boys (top) and girls (bottom): Sweden (Lindgren & Hauspie, 1989). The Preece–Baines model fitted to attained height is plotted on the distance data, the mathematical first derivative on the yearly increments.

Table 2.6. *Fitting of the Preece–Baines model to the yearly mean values of height for Swedish boys and girls born in 1955 and 1967*

	Boys		Girls	
	1955	1967	1955	1967
h_1	180.8235	174.3479	166.3629	165.2661
h_θ	167.0512	164.0021	149.7116	155.1186
s_0	0.0924	0.1310	0.0057	0.1382
s_1	0.8876	1.2929	0.8452	1.0680
θ	14.5405	13.8534	11.6008	12.3588
Residual variance	0.19	0.10	0.00	0.21
Degrees of freedom	12	12	8	12
Age at maximum increment: Preece–Baines (years)	13.8	13.4	11.6	11.5

et al. (1982) as the age at maximal velocity of the fitted curve (cf. Table 2.6). It appears that, for boys, maximal increment in height occurs about 0.4 years earlier in the 1967 sample while, for girls, it is only 0.1 years earlier. As can be seen for the girls (Figure 2.5), the raw height increments show a maximum of 7.6 cm/year at age 12 years, but the value of 11.5 years is very close (7.5 cm/year), so that the 'best estimate' of age at maximal increment is likely to lie between 11.5 years and 12 years, which reduces slightly the difference between the 1955 and the 1967 samples. In conclusion, the results indicate that, for girls, there is a slight positive secular trend in the mean height in the age range 10–15 years between the 1955 and 1967 samples. This trend is more marked for the boys. About the maturational rate, expressed as age of maximal increment in height during adolescence, it seems that the trend in height for boys is partly, if not wholly, attributable to an earlier maturation of the boys in the 1967 sample. For the girls, this seems to be of a lesser degree.

Mean peak height velocity (PHV) ages have, for the 1955 sample, been estimated earlier by Lindgren (1976) using a rather simple 'mid-year velocity' method on individuals. Those estimates were for the boys' PHV-age 14.1 years, and for the girls' PHV-age 11.9 years. Thus comparing these results estimated from individual growth data with the estimates obtained by the Preece–Baines model on the same data, treated cross-sectionally, it is interesting to notice that the Preece–Baines' estimates for PHV-age are 0.3 years earlier for both boys and girls. The reason for this could either be the error of ±0.25 years when estimating peak height velocity by the 'mid-year method', or an effect of peak height velocity's regression on age – that is, the earlier the PHV-age, the higher the peak height velocity. In the latter case, we might have to add 0.3 years to the PHV-ages obtained by the Preece–Baines model fitted to yearly mean values in height? The real 'true' values for PHV-ages for Swedish youth of today can, however, only be estimated by individual velocity curves – that is, a current longitudinal study of a representative sample.

DISCUSSION AND CONCLUSION

Describing the human growth pattern in terms of a limited number of constants (the parameters of a mathematical model) is the main goal of curve fitting. The success of this technique depends on the choice of an appropriate model for the kind of data to be fitted (type of variable, age interval, number of observations in the series, etc.).

Most models are capable of describing only a part of the growth curve, like the Jenss model (Jenss & Bayley, 1937), the Count model (1942; 1943) and the Reed model (Berkey & Reed, 1987) for the period of infancy and childhood, or the logistic model (Marubini & Milani, 1986) and the Gompertz model (Deming, 1957) for the adolescent period. The number of parameters to be estimated in these models varies between three and four.

The models described in this chapter have a larger number of parameters (5–7) and are more complex in their mathematical expression, but they can cope with a broader age interval. Increasing the number of parameters also increases the flexibility of the curve to describe more detailed features of the growth process. However, there is a price to pay to that: fitting a nine-parameter model like the triple logistic function, for example, requires a large number of observations in order to obtain a reliable fit. Even with a large number of parameters, there may always be certain events or short-term variations in growth rate which will not be shown by the fitted curve, simply because the mathematical function does not allow for it. So, the Preece–Baines and the JPPS models will smooth out the mid-childhood spurt, and the triple logistic model will show only one mid-childhood spurt, even if the empirical mid-childhood velocity curve shows two small peaks.

The models for human growth discussed in this paper are called structural models since they imply a certain shape on the growth data. They all expect the presence of a clear adolescent growth spurt in the data such as is seen in all skeletal body dimensions. Consequently, they may be quite inappropriate to fit head dimensions, for example, which show little or no adolescent growth spurt. They also all assume a monotonous increase of size as a function of age and have an upper asymptote (mature size). Therefore, these growth models are not necessarily appropriate to fit variables, which may show negative as well as positive growth. Indeed, the fit of such a model to an individual's serial data of weight, for example, can not account for a sudden gain or loss in weight as a result of a change in diet or a disease. If the effect of such factors results in an empirical growth curve which differs considerably from the shape expected by the applied model, then the resulting fit may be biased or erroneous. In such situations, a plot of the fitted model on the empirical growth data will usually be helpful to decide whether the smooth curve gives an acceptable picture of the growth process.

In pathological situations, the growth of skeletal dimensions, such as body length or leg length, for example, may be characterized by periods of delayed growth and catch-up growth, also resulting in a pattern which can not be fully described by the chosen model. However, it might be interesting to investigate to what extent, in such situations, examination of the residuals can be a tool to demonstrate the short-term effect of a disease and subsequent treatment on the growth of a child. Otherwise, pathological situations affecting the overall shape of the growth pattern may be interpreted in terms of the function parameters.

In conclusion, the usefulness of growth models mainly lies in the fact that they summarize growth data in a rather limited number of growth curve parameters (or constants), which can be directly or indirectly related to particular growth events, such as adult size, peak velocity, pre-adolescent growth, etc. In fact, the biological justification of these models is typically no more than a crude physical justification of how growth rate is related to growth achieved, which is itself a knowledge empirically derived from the known pattern of serial growth data (Goldstein, 1984).

REFERENCES

Berkey, C. S. & Reed, B. (1987). A model for describing normal and abnormal growth in early childhood. *Human Biology*, *59*, 973–987.

Bock, R. D. (1986). Unusual growth patterns in the Fels Data. In A. Demirjian (ed.), *Human growth, a multidisciplinary review* (pp. 69–84). London: Taylor & Francis.

Bock, R. D. & Thissen, D. M. (1980). Statistical problems of fitting individual growth curves. In F. E. Johnston, A. F. Roche & C. Susanne (eds.), *Human physical growth and maturation* (pp. 265–290). New York: Plenum Press.

Brown, T. & Townsend, G. C. (1982). Adolescent growth in height of Australian Aboriginals analysed by the Preece–Baines function. *Annals of Human Biology*, *9*, 495–505.

Butler, G. E., McKie, M. & Ratcliffe, S. G. (1989). An analysis of the phases of mid-childhood growth by synchronization of growth spurts. In J. M. Tanner (ed.), *Auxology 88: Perspectives in the science of growth and development (selected papers from the Fifth International Auxology Congress, UK, July 1988)* (pp. 77–84). Smith-Gordon/Niigata-Shi: Nishimura.

Chrzastek-Spruch, H., Susanne, C., Hauspie, R. C. & Kozlowska, M. A. (1989). Individual growth patterns and standards for height and height velocity based on the Lublin Longitudinal Growth Study. In J. M. Tanner (ed.), *Auxology 88: Perspectives in the science of growth and development (selected papers from the Fifth International Auxology Congress, UK, July 1988)* (pp. 161–166). Smith-Gordon/Niigata-Shi: Nishimura.

Count, E. W. (1942). A quantitative analysis of growth in certain human skull dimensions. *Human Biology, 14,* 143–165.

Count, E. W. (1943). Growth patterns of the human physique: an approach to kinetic anthropometry. *Human Biology, 15,* 1–32.

Deming, J. (1957). Application of the Gompertz curve to the observed pattern of growth in length of 48 individual boys and girls during the adolescent cycle of growth. *Human Biology, 29,* 83–122.

El Lozy, M. (1978). A critical analysis of the double and triple logistic growth curves. *Annals of Human Biology, 5,* 389–394.

Goldstein M. J. (1984). Current developments in the design and analysis of growth studies. In J. Borms, R. Hauspie, A. Sand, C. Susanne & M. Hebbelinck (eds.), *Human growth and development* (pp. 733–752). New York: Plenum Press.

Hauspie, R. C. (1989). Mathematical models for the study of individual growth patterns. *Revue d'Epidémiologie et de Santé Publique, 37,* 461–476.

Hauspie, R. C. & Wachholder, A. (1986). Clinical standards for growth velocity in height of Belgian boys and girls, aged 2 to 18 years. *International Journal of Anthropology, 1,* 339–348.

Hauspie, R. C., Das, S. R., Preece, M. A. & Tanner, J. M. (1980*a*). A longitudinal study of the growth in height of boys and girls of West Bengal (India), aged six months to 20 years. *Annals of Human Biology, 7,* 429–441.

Hauspie, R. C., Wachholder, A., Baron, G., Cantraine, F., Susanne, C. & Graffar, M. (1980*b*). A comparative study of the fit of four different functions to longitudinal data of growth in height of Belgian girls. *Annals of Human Biology, 7,* 347–358.

Jenss, R. M. & Bayley, N. (1937). A mathematical method for studying the growth of a child. *Human Biology, 9,* 556–563.

Jolicoeur, P., Pontier, J., Pernin, M.-O. & Sempé, M. (1988). A lifetime asymptotic growth curve for human height. *Biometrics, 44,* 995–1003.

Lindgren, G. (1976). Height, weight and menarche in Swedish urban school children in relation to socio-economic and regional factors. *Annals of Human Biology, 3,* 501–528.

Lindgren, G. W. & Hauspie, R. C. (1989). Heights and weights of Swedish school children born in 1955 and 1967. *Annals of Human Biology, 16,* 397–406.

Marubini, E. & Milani, S. (1986). Approaches to the analysis of longitudinal data. In F. Falkner & J. M. Tanner (eds.), *Human growth vol. 3:*

Methodology, ecological, genetic, and nutritional effects on growth (pp. 79–94). New York: Plenum Press.

Meredith, H. V. (1981). An addendum on presence and absence of a mid-childhood spurt in somatic dimensions. *Annals of Human Biology, 8,* 473–476.

Nie, N. H., Hull, C. H., Jenkins, J. G., Steinbrenner, K. & Bent, D. H. (1975). SPSS: *Statistical package for the social sciences.* New York: McGraw-Hill.

Pontier, J., Jolicoeur, P., Abidi, H. & Sempé, M. (1988*a*). Croissance staturale chez l'enfant: le modèle JPPS. *Biométrie et Praximétrie, 28,* 27–44.

Pontier, J., Jolicoeur, P., Pernin, M.-O., Abidi, H. & Sempé, M. (1988*b*). Modélisation de la courbe de croissance staturale chez l'enfant: le modèle JPPS. *Cahiers d'Anthropologie et Biométrie Humaine (Paris), 6,* 71–85.

Powell, M. J. D. (1969). Harwell Subroutine Library. Routine VA05A, AERA.

Preece, M. A. & Baines, M. K. (1978). A new family of mathematical models describing the human growth curve. *Annals of Human Biology, 5,* 1–24.

Scammon, R. E. (1927). The first seriatim study of human growth. *American Journal of Physical Anthropology, 10,* 329–336.

Tanner, J. M. (1962). *Growth at adolescence* (pp. 1–3). Oxford: Blackwell Scientific.

Tanner, J. M. & Cameron, N. (1980). Investigation of the mid-growth spurt in height, weight and limb circumferences in single-year velocity data from the London 1966–67 growth survey. *Annals of Human Biology, 7,* 565–577.

Tanner, J. M. & Davies, P. W. (1985). Clinical longitudinal standards for height and height velocity for North American children. *The Journal of Pediatrics, 107,* 317–329.

Tanner, J. M., Hayashi, T., Preece, M. A. & Cameron, N. (1982). Increase in length of leg relative to trunk in Japanese children and adults from 1957 to 1977: a comparison with British and Japanese Americans. *Annals of Human Biology, 9,* 411–423.

Vercauteren, M. (1984). Evolution séculaire et normes de croissance chez des enfants belges. *Bulletin de la Sociéte royale belge d'Anthropologie et de Préhistoire, 95,* 109–123.

Wachholder, A. & Hauspie, R. C. (1986). Clinical standards for growth in height of Belgian boys and girls, aged 2 to 18 years. *International Journal of Anthropology, 1,* 327–338.

3 Intraindividual variability in older adults' depression scores: some implications for developmental theory and longitudinal research

JOHN R. NESSELROADE AND DAVID L. FEATHERMAN

INTRODUCTION

Research focus

A salient aspect of research on adult development and aging is the use of general dimensions of interindividual differences to classify elderly persons into diagnostic groups, to predict longevity, morbidity, mortality, and other conditions, and to theorize about the nature of development and change. Among the more prominent variables that social and behavioral scientists are using currently for these purposes are measures of morale, life satisfaction, autonomy and control, adjustment, and depression. Of these, depression has become a major focus of concern because of both its probable association with the variety of losses that older adults are apt to experience (spouse, job, status, health, etc.) and its mediating role between the onset of traumatic events and the person's subsequent adaptation. An aspect of research conducted with depression and other relatively broad interindividual differences dimensions that has yet to be integrated into either theoretical or methodological concerns generally are the various phenomena of *intraindividual variability* or short-term changes.

Although greater and greater levels of sophistication in measurement, research design, and data analyses are being reached in longitudinal approaches (see, e.g., Goldstein, 1979; Nesselroade & Baltes, 1979; Schaie, Campbell, Meredith & Rawlings, 1988), many promising ideas and innovations do not readily filter into substantive research efforts. An encouraging conception and accompanying set of findings that researchers in adult development and aging have not yet sufficiently taken into account concern the nature, scope, and correlates of intraindividual variability and the implications that arise therefrom both for explanatory purposes and for the classification and prediction objectives mentioned above (Nesselroade, 1990). Here, we will first examine the concept of intraindividual variability in the more general context of individual differences research. We will then briefly report a short-term longitudinal study of elderly adults' self-reported depression scores that was designed to throw light on both the character of depression and the potential importance of recognizing day-to-day intraindividual variability in trying to understand more fully adult development and aging.

Many different kinds of intraindividual variability have received at least some consideration by social and behavioral researchers (see, e.g., Cattell & Scheier, 1961; Featherman, 1979; Featherman & Petersen, 1986; Fiske & Rice, 1955; Luborsky & Mintz, 1972; Nesselroade, 1988; Zevon & Tellegen, 1982). These include emotions, moods, states, circadian rhythms, seasonal rhythms, socially mediated rhythms, and, of course, stochastic indeterminancy. No doubt these different kinds of intraindividual variability and their various manifestations overlay each other in a web of relationships that contributes to the complexity of behavior patterns observable in human beings. It is against such a dynamic, active background that stabilities, other kinds of changes, and interindividual differences that interest researchers occur and, we argue, need to be examined if the validity of inference is to improve. Through this lush jungle of intraindividual variability and interindividual differences we have sought to hack a trail by designing a study that would provide two kinds of information: (1) estimates of the magnitude and nature of intraindividual variability manifested in a week-to-week measurement protocol; and (2) the nature of similarities and differences in patterns of intraindividual variability among persons.

Admittedly, choosing an interval for repeating measurements is something like selecting a sieve or a strainer for use; you may lose some pieces you would like to keep because the holes (intervals between measurements) are too large or retain some that you don't want because the holes are too small. Nevertheless, in order to implement a study such choices must be made, and the weekly interval we chose offered the promise of capturing short-term intraindividual variability of considerable magnitude without disrupting the lives of our elderly participants to such an extent that their response patterns would have had no temporal generality.

There is no doubt that the measurements we made will reflect some of most of the kinds of intraindividual variability mentioned above. It is also likely that variability due to learning, habituation, boredom, and perhaps fatigue will have some involvement. It is our belief, however, that a major portion of the intraindividual variability reflected in the data represents variability that can be reliably measured, is of essentially constant magnitude from time to time for a particular group of individuals, and has important correlates in other behavioral manifestations. The concept of state variability (Cattell & Scheier, 1961; Nesselroade, 1988) comes close to capturing the interpretation that we wish to convey in describing the variability on which we are focusing, and will be relied on for that purpose.

Stability and change concepts

Both stability and change concepts are central features of contemporary research and theory in the study of individual differences. The two are not always integrated, however. Rather, one conception often is pitted against the other as an alternative way to characterize phenomena of interest. The discussion by Costa & McCrae (1980), for example, focused on whether stability or change dominates adult personality development. Moreover, empirical findings suggest the value of discriminating between two kinds of changes: short-term, more or less reversible changes (intraindividual variability) and smoother, longer-term intraindividual changes (Nesselroade, 1988; Nesselroade & Ford, 1985). These two kinds of intraindividual changes are represented pictorially in Figure 3.1 using the weaving of cloth as a metaphor for their integration. There, intraindividual variability is depicted analogously to the woof (or weft) and intraindividual change is represented as the warp in the fabric of individual development. In this chapter we will focus principally on intraindividual variability phenomena.

Central to the present discussion is the juxtaposition of *intraindividual variability* and relatively stable *interindividual differences.* The key notion is that the variation that is found among individuals' scores on some attribute at any given occasion of measurement is composed of both intraindividual change and interindividual differences variance. Individuals differ from each other at any given time of measurement in part because they always differ from each other (interindividual differences) but also in part because each one of them is himself different from one time to another (intraindividual variability). Because there is no particular reason to assume that intraindividual variability is in any way synchronous over individuals, such intraindividual variability contributes to the differences manifested among individuals at a given point in time, thus confounding estimates of the magnitude of interindividual differences variance (Steyer, 1987; Wittmann, 1988).

The trait–state distinction

One way that psychologists have tried to formalize differences between intraindividual variability and stable interindividual differences is with the *trait–state* distinction (Cattell & Scheier, 1961; Nesselroade, 1988;

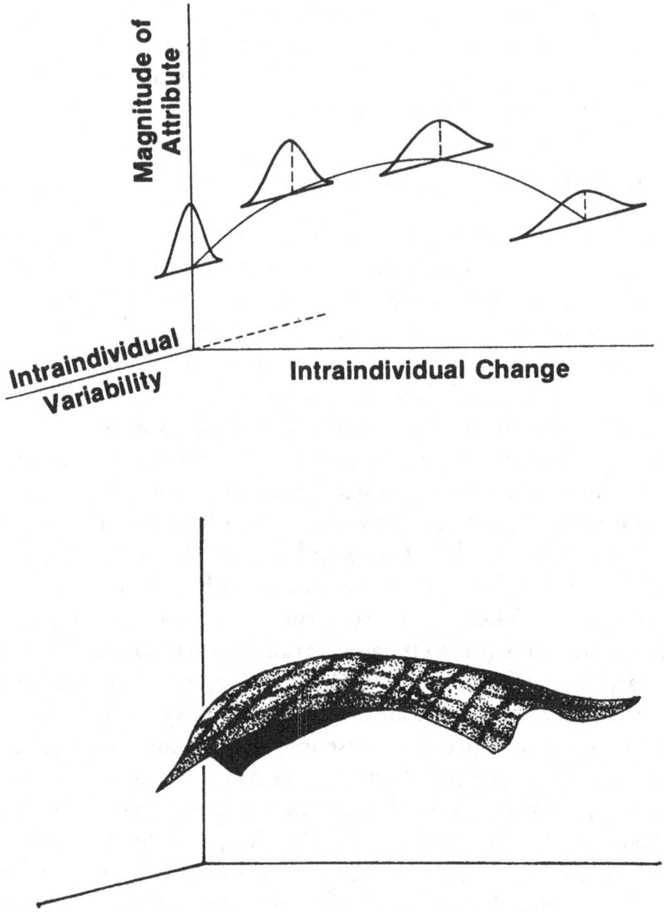

Figure 3.1. Intraindividual variability and intraindividual changes as the woof and warp of the fabric of development (from Nesselroade, 1990).

Singer & Singer, 1972; Spielberger, Gorsuch & Lushene, 1969). The differentiation of state and trait is, in fact, quite old. Eysenck (1983), for example, pointed out that in 45 BC the Roman Cicero, in characterizing behavior patterns, distinguished between *traits,* relatively permanent and enduring behavioral dispositions such as irascibility, and *states,* relatively changeable attributes such as anger. In recent times, this categorization has been highly valued by some (e.g., Cattell, 1973; Cattell & Scheier, 1961; Spielberger, Gorsuch & Lushene, 1969; Zuckerman, 1983) who have sought to operationalize it with measurement devices, and quite skeptically regarded by others (e.g., Allen & Potkay, 1981; Magnusson, 1980).

Traits and stability. Trait concepts exemplify the relatively stable interindividual differences dimensions pertinent to our discussion. They have a somewhat stormy history. The advent of concern with the rigorous definition and measurement of human abilities (see, e.g., Spearman, 1904) brought a new emphasis to the study of trait-like attributes; a concern that soon embraced other kinds of individual differences concepts such as temperament attributes. Refinement of these concepts by writers such as Allport (1937) and Cattell (1946) and subsequent challenges to their validity (e.g., Mischel, 1968) have been met in turn with renewed efforts to establish their scientific worth and generality (see, e.g., Block, 1977). Resolution of the salient issues is yet to occur but, at the very least, these arguments have led to more careful thinking and conceptualization of the nature of interindividual differences dimensions and the roles they play in determining behavior (see, e.g., Magnusson & Endler, 1977).

States and intraindividual variability. States exemplify the intraindividual variability aspects of concern in this chapter. In the study of personality, however, states have not enjoyed the attention that traits have, no doubt for several reasons. One of the central ones seems to be that the interindividual differences on such dimensions, even though they can be substantial at a given point in time, do not lend themselves to the traditional prediction paradigm of the behavioral sciences. For example, if behavior Y at time $t + 1$ is to be predicted from trait X measured at time t, it is important to know that the value of X obtained at time t still holds at time $t + 1$ if the prediction of Y from X is to be accurate. No matter how highly correlated X and Y are at time t, individual differences on X measured at time t that do not accurately reflect the status of individuals on X at time $t + 1$, can not be depended on to be valid predictors of Y at time $t + 1$.

It is the case that measures of intraindividual variability dimensions with quite reasonable psychometric properties have been developed (see, e.g., Curran & Cattell, 1976; Spielberger, Gorsuch & Lushene, 1969; Watson & Tellegen, 1985) and are used to assess a variety of changes. However, largely as a consequence of the prediction emphasis and the appeal of classical test theory, psychological measurement has tended to downplay, ignore, or relegate to 'error' the intraindividual variability that is often detectable in repeated measurement situations. This attitude is prevalent in much of this century's writing concerning the nature of psychological attributes. For example, Gulliksen (1950) in discussing the estimation of reliability said, '. . . the major difficulty with reliability obtained by the successive administration of parallel forms is that it is too high. This is because there is no possibility for the variation due to *normal daily variability* [italics added] to lower the correlation between parallel forms' (p. 357). Others have made similar remarks concerning the interrelationship of intraindividual variability and interindividual differences. Indeed, there is considerable recognition of the existence (often seen as troublesome) of intraindividual variability (Nesselroade, 1988).

Discussion of methods and conceptualizations that might enable students of behavior to capture, to account for, and to capitalize on intraindividual variability include research and theory on state and state variation, largely in the temperament domain. Research in other domains, however, also bears on the study of intraindividual variability. Horn (1966), for example, in describing the outcome of analyses of intraindividual variability in human ability performance remarked, 'The results illustrated how fluid intelligence (as well as other attributes of intellectual test behavior) varies functionally *within persons* [italics added] and also represents a stable pattern of performances that distinguishes one person from another' (p. 47). Thus, what Horn (1966) found in the very same data reflecting ability performances were both stable interindividual differences and intraindividual variability.

Some research implications of intraindividual variability concepts

Despite the reservations that some writers have expressed, from both substantive and methodological points of view, the distinction between trait and state dimensions has had a number of positive effects on the study of behavior. From a substantive perspective, researchers have been led to scrutinize the concepts of stability and traits more closely. One needs to distinguish, for example, between personality attributes in terms of their ranges and degrees of temporal stability. That stability, in turn, reflects on an attribute's suitability for describing the status of individuals and their value for predicting later events from earlier ones. In those cases where measured differences among individuals are used to classify individuals, diagnose conditions, and predict (and understand) behavior, we need to understand better not only the stable interindividual differences but also the changes that individuals manifest over time and situations. To the extent that the latter is confounded with the former, classification and prediction will be limited in their validity.

From a methodological perspective, the distinction between trait and state has led to some important innovations in the conceptualization, development, and evaluation of measurement instruments, the design and implementation of research, and the analysis of data. Among the methodological issues that have been identified at least in part because of work stemming from the study of intraindividual variability are the recognition of the need for more sensitive measure devices, clearer distinctions between reliability and stability, an emphasis on repeated measurement designs and the construction of scores for individuals that reflect occasion-to-occasion variability as well as occasion-to-occasion central tendency, and analysis techniques for studying the nature of intraindividual variability and between-persons differences and similarities therein. However, we contend that additional concern for the implications of the presence of intraindividual variability in data are needed, including in the design and conduct of longitudinal research. One line of methodological development that holds much promise in this regard is P-technique factor analysis and its derivatives.

P-technique and intraindividual variability

P-technique methodology is one of several covariation techniques defined within the context of the data box (Cattell, 1952, 1966*a*). Cattell, who participated in the first published account of P-technique use over a half century ago (Cattell, Cattell & Rhymer, 1947), systematically described the nature, purpose, and further application of P-technique in a series of papers (Cattell, 1952, 1963, 1966*b*). Bereiter (1963) dubbed P-technique 'the logical way to study change'.

What is P-technique? It is a covariation technique that focuses on the individual rather than the group by confining measurement or observation and the determination of covariation patterns to one participant at a time. Thus, for instance, a participant might be measured on a battery of 40 tests or measures once each day for 100 days to produce 100×40 score matrix. The P-technique data can then be analyzed by, for example, intercorrelating the 40 scores over the 100 occasions and factoring them to identify covariation patterns over time for that individual. This is in contrast to the more familiar R-technique where 40 variables would be intercorrelated over 100 persons, each person measured with the battery of 40 measures only one time. With R-technique one focuses on among-persons variation but, as was noted above, some of the among-persons variation is doubtless within-person variability as manifested at that particular measurement occasion. Obviously, with P-technique the only variation available is within-person variation because only one person is involved.

The rationale underlying P-technique is that the occasion-to-occasion scores of the individual vary systematically as a function of events, both internal and external. To the extent that common influences are involved in 'producing' the individual's scores then the scores will covary over the occasions of measurement. Studying these covariations by means of techniques such as factor analysis will, in turn, indicate the number and the nature of functional response patterns and, by implication, the number and nature of sources of intraindividual variability. Combining this 'single-subject' approach with 'group design' rationale, one can conduct multiple P-technique studies using a common set of variables and determine the extent to which intraindividual variability patterns obtained by individual P-technique analyses are consistent across multiple individuals (Nesselroade & Ford, 1985; Zevon & Tellegen, 1982). A simple version of the data box identifying P-technique data is presented in Figure 3.2.

P-technique has not been without its critics (e.g., Holtzman, 1963; Molenaar, 1985; Wohlwill, 1973). The major criticisms have tended to focus on the fact that in computing intercorrelations among measures, P-technique does not take account of serial relationships in the data. Rather, the string of observations is treated as if each occasion was completely independent of all other occasions. Recent proposals by McArdle (1982) and Molenaar (1985) have provided more sophisticated analytical procedures to rectify the deficiencies of conventional factor analysis of P-technique data. The major point is that the systematic study of intraindividual variability by P-technique and its variations does have a considerable history and the substantive findings (for reviews see Jones & Nesselroade, in preparation; Luborsky & Mintz, 1972) indicate that observed intraindividual variability is not 'noise', but structured, coherent, patterned change.

In summary, we have argued that an individual differences orientation

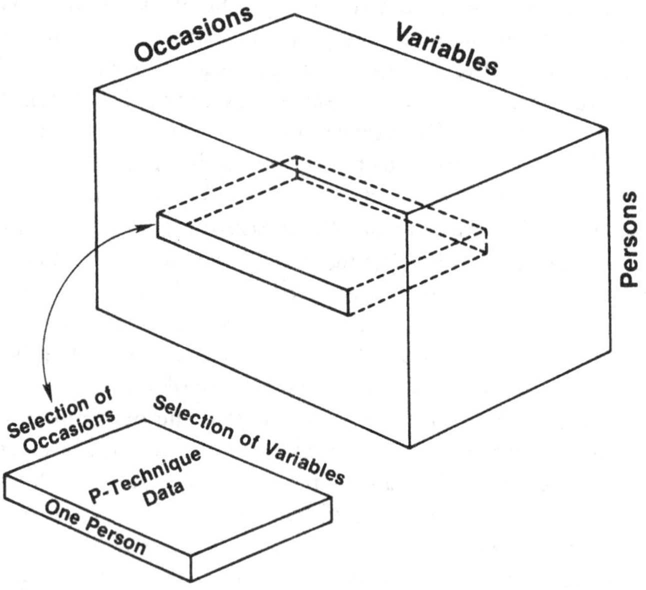

Figure 3.2. The three-dimensional data box highlighting the slice of data used in P-technique studies.

to classifying, predicting, and explaining behavioral and psychological phenomena needs to incorporate a concern for intraindividual variability into the development of measuring instruments, design of experiments, and analysis of data. We have tried to accomplish some of these objectives in an examination of depression in elderly adults in a study to which we now turn.

THE CORNWALL MANOR STUDY

Purpose

The Cornwall Manor study was undertaken to gain information concerning both the stability and the magnitude and nature of short-term intraindividual variability on a wide variety of measures in a sample of elderly adults. Our chief substantive concern had to do with the concept of resiliency in older adults in relation to their capacity for dealing with challenging life events. We did not design the study to test specific hypotheses but rather focused on acquiring descriptive information that might subsequently be used to articulate testable hypotheses concerning stability and change.

Methods and procedures

Sample. The participants in the Cornwall Manor study were volunteers residing at Cornwall Manor at the time of testing. Cornwall Manor is a comprehensive retirement community affiliated with the Methodist Church and located in south central Pennsylvania near Hershey. The mean age of the sample, which consisted of 57 elderly individuals (18 males; 39 females), was approximately 78 years.

Design. The research design included two groups of participants: a multiple-occasion longitudinal group and a two-occasion panel. Participants were not randomly assigned to groups because of potential scheduling and time conflicts. The longitudinal group, hereafter called the *treatment group* ($N = 32$), was originally scheduled for 25 *weekly* measurements designed to span 28 calendar weeks. During the core of data collection, this was shortened to 23 weekly measurements. Because of holidays, the 23 weeks of assessment actually spanned 25 calendar weeks. The panel group, hereafter called the *control* group ($N = 25$), was measured twice: at the beginning, and at the end of the 23 weeks of treatment group measurement. The design is presented schematically in Figure 3.3.

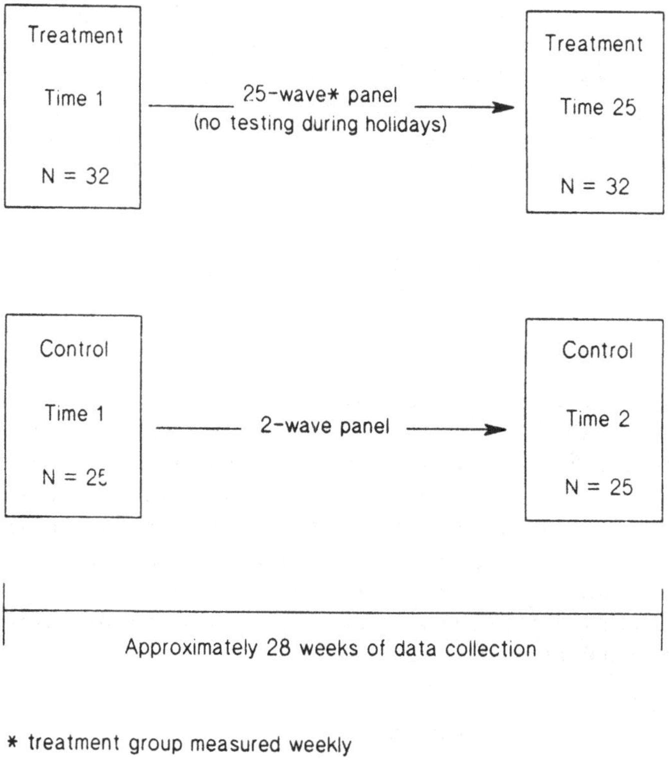

Figure 3.3. Research design implemented in the Cornwall Manor study.

Measurement variables. Measurement foci included biomedical, cognitive, mood/state, attitudinal, and physical function variables. Many of the measures are part of a test battery currently being developed under the auspices of the MacArthur Foundation Research Program on Successful Aging. Other variables were taken from a survey instrument ('Americans' Changing Lives') being used to study productive behaviors in a national probability sample of adults (Herzog, Kahn, Morgan, Jackson & Antonucci, 1989). A few additional measures were included by the investigators to measure aspects of cognition and mood/state.

The interview schedule, which included the depressed mood items, was administered in a standardized format by means of lap-top computers running a program prepared specifically for administering this battery. The program provided for updating information, branching, and cueing the testers when appropriate (Mullen, Orbuch, Featherman & Nesselroade, 1988).

Table 3.1. CES-D item stability coefficients separately by group. (Correlation between time 1 and time 23 scores)

Item	Treatment group	Control group
Felt depressed	0.01	0.51
Everything an effort	0.34	0.20
Sleep restless	0.53	0.67
Felt happy	0.52	0.20
Felt lonely	0.67	0.38
People unfriendly	0.70	[a]
Enjoyed life	0.11	[a]
Poor appetite	0.25	0.48
Felt sad	0.30	0.64
Felt people disliked me	0.47	[a]
Couldn't get going	0.27	0.61

[a] Insufficient variance at one or both time-points to compute correlation.

For our purpose, we will focus on one instrument: The Center for Epidemiological Studies Depression Scale (CES-D; Radloff, 1977). The version used in the present study consisted of 11 items. The parent scale from which these 11 items were taken contains 20 items. The items used are listed in Table 3.1. Item responses were self-reported on a three-point answer format. In cross-sectional work (e.g., Berkman *et al.*, 1986) the items tend to factor into four factors that are identified as: (1) negative affect; (2) somatic and retarded activity; (3) positive affect; and (4) interpersonal relations.

Procedure. Participants in the *treatment* group were assigned to one of two subgroups: (1) those tested on Monday, Wednesday, Friday; and (2) those tested on Tuesday, Thursday, Saturday. Weekly testings remained within these boundaries but the day varied from one week to the next. For example, members of the MWF group were always tested on one of those three days but which of the three was varied over the course of the 23 weeks. Participants were tested in their own living quarters. Interviews averaged 129 minutes for the control group and 123 minutes for the treatment group.

Analysis and results

As was noted above, the present report is focused on the CES-D scale. Before turning to those data, however, we present a brief summary of preliminary findings that bear on interpretation of the CES-D results.

Design effects. First, retention of participants in the study was high. One control group member died before the post-test interview, two withdrew for personal reasons, and one interview failed to record on the computer. Thirty-one of 32 treatment group members completed the entire project. Of the 688 interviews planned for the longitudinal group, only 23 were cancelled. Some 45% of the treatment group completed all interviews.

Second, 150 variables were analyzed for selective volunteering for the two groups comprising the design. There were no more statistically significant differences in means and variances than would be expected by chance and these were scattered across the several different measurement domains.

Third, in a repeated measures design one might expect evidence of practice effects in the treatment group data for those variables on which performance could be improved through learning. Surprisingly, in light of the weekly testing regime, few practice effects were found (Mullen *et al.*, 1988*a*). Nevertheless, a greater use of extreme values manifested as increased variance in the last occasion of measurement was found for some few questions and scales in the interview protocol. Some evidence for the opposite effect – a reduction in last occasion variance – was found for a few items as well. None of these design effects, however, was grouped systematically into domains.

Item stability coefficients. Responses to individual items on the first and final testings for each group were correlated. These correlations (stability coefficients) are presented in Table 3.1. Many of the items show a relatively low degree of stability in interindividual differences over the approximately 25-week interval involved. This does not necessarily mean, however, that the responses are random. Rather, it invites further analyses to ascertain the extent to which the changes are coherent and systematic rather than 'noise'. These analyses are currently being designed using methods and software developed by Milsap and Meredith (1988).

Variability. Additional information concerning the magnitude of intraindividual variability and interindividual differences on the CES-D items is presented in Table 3.2. To obtain this information we identified for each CES-D item the subset of individuals in the treatment group whose responses showed any variation over the 25 weeks of measurement. An intraindividual variability score was obtained for each such individual on each item by calculating the *variance* in his or her weekly responses to that item. For these very same persons, we took the first occasion responses only and computed the variance over persons in the usual way as a measure of interindividual

Table 3.2. CES-D item variances

Item	[a]Intraindividual variability (weeks 1–25)	[b]Interindividual differences	
		First occasion	Last occasion
Felt depressed	0.22 (14)[c]	0.17	0.20
Everything an effort	0.20 (22)	0.34	0.34
Sleep restless	0.22 (24)	0.40	0.41
Felt happy	0.16 (16)	0.11	0.23
Felt lonely	0.15 (11)	0.20	0.23
People unfriendly	0.08 (6)	0.00	0.14
Enjoyed life	0.21 (14)	0.00	0.24
Poor appetite	0.17 (11)	0.43	0.38
Felt sad	0.15 (17)	0.10	0.21
Felt people disliked me	0.10 (7)	0.24	0.20
Couldn't get going	0.18 (20)	0.33	0.25

[a] Intraindividual variability was computed separately for each individual over their weekly measurements. Column entries are averages over people.
[b] Interindividual differences variances were computed on same individuals as are reflected in column 1 using their first and last measurements.
[c] The number of cases on which mean intraindividual variability is computed. Responses of the rest of the treatment group did not vary over time on the item.

differences. Similarly, the last occasion responses of these same persons were used to compute a second estimate of interindividual differences variance for each item. Thus, in Table 3.2 we are comparing intraindividual variability and interindividual differences information from the same subset of individuals. The rationale for analyzing the data in this manner involves a reluctance to combine distinctly different response patterns (varying responses versus constant responses) and interpreting the average as an adequate representation of what actually transpired. Instead, we have recognized a 'two-process' model of responding that is somewhat analogous to the distinction of 'movers' versus 'stayers' in mobility research. Whether this distinction between 'varying and constant responders' applies only at the level of measurement instrument sensitivity or more fundamentally is a question that we are unable to address with our current data. Column 1 of Table 3.2 contains the intraindividual variabilities computed separately for each individual and then averaged across persons. We note explicitly in the table the number of individuals reflected in these averages. Columns 2 and 3 contain the interindividual differences variances at the first and last occasions of measurement, respectively.

The magnitude of the intraindividual variabilities (column 1) tends to run about half or more of the magnitude of the individual differences variances (columns 2 and 3). The magnitude of these item variabilities should be construed in light of the model that underlies the study. Simply put, at time t participant i's observed score (X_{it}) is composed of three components: (1) a stable, 'trait-like' component (T_i); (2) a labile, 'state-like' component (S_{it}); and (3) an error of measurement (e_{it}). Thus,

$$X_{it} = T_i + S_{it} + e_{it}. \tag{1}$$

From this simple model, it follows that the individual differences variance at time $t[\mathrm{Var}(X)]$ can be represented as:

$$\begin{aligned}\mathrm{Var}(X_t) = {} & \mathrm{Var}(T) + \mathrm{Var}(S_t) + \mathrm{Var}(e_t) \\ & + 2\,\mathrm{Cov}(T, S_t) + 2\,\mathrm{Cov}(T, e_t) + 2\,\mathrm{Cov}(S_t, e_t).\end{aligned} \tag{2}$$

Under classical test theory principles, it does not seem unreasonable to assume that the final two covariance terms are zero. Deleting them, we have:

$$\mathrm{Var}(X_t) = \mathrm{Var}(T) + \mathrm{Var}(S_t) + \mathrm{Var}(e_t) + 2\,\mathrm{Cov}(T, S_t). \tag{3}$$

In other words, the interindividual differences variance at any occasion (columns 2 and 3) is composed of trait variance (i.e., a more or less permanent component of between-person differences), state variance (i.e., a more or less transient component of between-person differences), error variance, and twice the trait/state covariance. By contrast, the average intraindividual variabilities in CES-D scores (column 1) provide an estimate of the sum of state and error variation. The fact that $\mathrm{Var}(S_t) + \mathrm{Var}(e_t)$ tends to be half or more of the estimates representing a combination of trait, state, error, and trait/state covariance suggests by subtraction that, rather than being trivially small, the state variation on the depression items is at least of an order of magnitude comparable to what can be ascribed to trait variation. The outcome of decomposing interindividual differences into such components has critical implications for the measurement, design, and analysis activities of students of behavior as has been pointed out by Steyer (1987) and Wittmann (1988). We will consider some of them in closing.

DISCUSSION AND CONCLUSIONS

The concepts and empirical data reviewed here offer considerable support for the recognition of intraindividual variability as a salient component of the individual's attributes. What are some of the key implications of the presence of intraindividual variability in dimensions of interest to behavioral and social scientists?

Significance of change patterns

The evidence for coherent short-term changes in the self-reported depression scores for elderly adults has several important implications. These results suggest that we need to rethink not only our notions of the nature of depression but also the ways depression is assessed. For example, measuring important attributes once or even twice and 'pigeonholing' an individual on that basis is not only misleading but, as Cattell (1966*b*) argued, may even be morally wrong. If, as these and other data suggest, with some concepts we are dealing with considerably more labile phenomena than traditional individual differences notions have implied, this should be reflected in the representations of behavior and behavior change that we attempt to construct. Measurement approaches that feature stability and only gradual change are not adequate to the task and need to be augmented with others that are appropriate for dealing with short-term changes and intraindividual variability.

Rather than surrender to a view of more or less chaotic change, however, we need to find ways to determine the regularities and invariances that must surely exist even though they may have to be sought at a more abstract level than we have typically chosen to look for them. For example, stable individual differences may be found in aspects of intraindividual variability rather than in estimates of true scores in the classical test theory sense. Cattell's concept of *liability* or *proneness* to manifest a given level of state depending on circumstances is a useful example of seeking orderliness and predictability in change (Cattell, 1979).

Models of development change

From a more general perspective, the concepts and findings discussed here support the desirability of seeking alternatives to the classical notion of a relatively fixed, true score as the basis for classifying individuals on psychological attributes and even as the basis for plotting long-term developmental change. An alternative that seems worth pursuing is the use of intraindividual variability as a base condition for characterizing the individual (Nesselroade, 1990). This has important implications not only for assessment and classification but also for studying more 'dynamic' phenomena such as development and aging.

For example, recognizing a base condition of intraindividual variability provides a potentially important adjunct to the conceptualization of plasticity (Baltes, 1987; Lerner, 1984) in development (Nesselroade, 1990). Intraindividual variation as a base condition means that at least some rudimentary plasticity is given. Thus, rather than our having to account for the origin of plasticity, intraindividual variability signifies something already there to be amplified by the 'slings and arrows of outrageous fortune'. The idea that life experience helps to shape and mold the individual is commonly held but with intraindividual variability rather than a fixed true score as a given condition of the organism, somewhat different causal mechanisms can be entertained and tested.

In a related vein, intraindividual variability can also serve as a basis for formulating key aging concepts such as resilience (Rowe & Kahn, 1987). Why, for instance, do two older persons rebound in different ways to what is ostensibly the same traumatic event such as a hip fracture or loss of a spouse? to answer such questions fully, it will be necessary to apprehend the nature of intraindividual variability as well as stable, interindividual differences. The individual's 'central tendency' is no doubt part of the picture but information concerning intraindividual variability should provide even more of it.

Longitudinal research decision

Finally, what are the implications of intraindividual variability concepts and findings for the conduct of longitudinal studies? They can be examined around the following contrast: interindividual differences in intraindividual variability versus intraindividual variability in interindividual differences. Intraindividual variability is obviously a longitudinal phenomenon. Assessment of the state variety of intraindividual variability on which we have primarily focused here implies short-term longitudinal measurement. However, developmentalists who are interested in changes in patterns of intraindividual variability would need to track intraindividual variability parameters over longer longitudinal spans. Thus, incorporating 'bursts' of short-term repeated measurements (to provide intraindividual variability scores) into each of the more separated measurement occasions of traditional longitudinal research offers a way to apprehend both interindividual differences and systematic changes in intraindividual variability.

Conversely, for students of interindividual differences, the measurements obtained on a given measurement occasion are confounded by intraindividual variability. Unconfounding interindividual differences and intraindividual variability at each occasion of measurement should be a valuable aid to developing representations of both stability and change patterns. To be able to accomplish this requires designing studies to provide estimates of intraindividual variability at a given occasion of measurement. This also seems to call for some means for measuring intraindividual variability characteristics such as 'bursts' of repeated measures when assessment is undertaken.

In sum, to the extent that *intraindividual variability* (state) and stable *interindividual differences* (trait) are confounded in one's measurements, measurement schemes and research designs should provide the means for disentangling them, just as theoretical conceptions should allow for integrating them. This suggests the need for critical refinements in the way we design and conduct empirical studies; whether they are cross-sectional or longitudinal in nature.

REFERENCES

Allen, B. P. & Potkay, C. R. (1981). On the arbitrary distinction between states and traits. *Journal of Personality and Social Psychology, 41,* 906–928.

Allport, G. W. (1937). *Personality: A psychological interpretation.* New York: Henry Holt.

Baltes, P. B. (1987). Theoretical propositions of life-span developmental psychology: On the dynamics between growth and decline. *Developmental Psychology, 23,* 611–626.

Bereiter, C. (1963). Some persisting dilemmas in the measurement of change. In C. W. Harris (ed.), *Problems in measuring change.* Madison, WI: University of Wisconsin Press.

Berkman, L. R., Berkman, C. S., Kasl, S., Freeman, D. H., Jr., Leo, L., Ostfeld, A. M., Cornoni-Huntley, J. & Brody, J. A. (1986). Depressive symptoms in relation to physical health and functioning in the elderly. *American Journal of Epidemiology, 124,* 372–388.

Block, J. (1977). Advancing the psychology of personality: Paradigmatic shift or improving the quality of research. In D. Magnusson & N. S. Endler (eds.), *Personality at the crossroads: Current issues in interactional psychology.* Hillsdale, NJ: Lawrence Erlbaum.

Cattell, R. B. (1946). *Description and measurement of personality.* New York: World Book Co.

Cattell, R. B. (1952). The three basic factor analytic designs – their interrelationships and derivatives. *Psychological Bulletin, 49,* 267–283.

Cattell, R. B. (1963). The structuring of change by P- and incremental-R techniques. In C. W. Harris (ed.), *Problems in measuring change.* Madison, WI: University of Wisconsin Press.

Cattell, R. B. (1966*a*). The data box: Its ordering of total resources in terms of possible relational systems. In R. B. Cattell (ed.), *Handbook of multivariate experimental psychology.* Chicago: Rand McNally.

Cattell, R. B. (1966*b*). Patterns of change: Measurement in relation to state-dimension, trait change, lability, and process concepts. In R. B. Cattell (ed.), *Handbook of multivariate experimental psychology.* Chicago: Rand McNally.

Cattell, R. B. (1973). *Mood and personality by questionnaire.* San Francisco: Jossey-Bass.

Cattell, R. B. (1979). *Personality and learning theory: Vol. 1 The structure of personality in its environment.* New York: Springer Publishing Company.

Cattell, R. B. & Scheier, I. H. (1961). *The meaning and measurement of neuroticism and anxiety.* New York: Ronald Press.

Cattell, R. B., Cattell, A. K. S. & Rhymer, R. M. (1947). P-technique demonstrated in determining psycho-physical source traits in a normal individual. *Psychometrika, 12,* 267–288.

Costa, P. T. Jr & McCrae, R. R. (1980). Still stable after all these years: Personality as a key to some issues in adulthood and old age. In P. B. Baltes & O. G. Brim, Jr (eds.), *Life-span development and behavior* (Vol. 3). New York: Academic Press.

Curran, J. P. & Cattell, R. B. (1976). *Handbook for the 8-state battery.* Champaign, IL: Institute for Personality and Ability Testing.

Eysenck, H. J. (1983). Cicero and the state-trait theory of anxiety: Another case of delayed recognition. *American Psychologist, 38,* 114.

Featherman, D. L. (1979). Individual development and aging as a population process. In J. R. Nesselroade & A. von Eye (eds.), *Individual development and social change: Explanatory analysis.* New York: Academic Press.

Featherman, D. L. & Petersen, T. (1986). Markers of aging: Modeling the clocks that time us. *Research on Aging, 8,* 339–365.

Fiske, D. W. & Rice, L. (1955). Intra-individual response variability. *Psychological Bulletin, 52,* 217–250.

Goldstein, H. (1979). *The design and analysis of longitudinal studies.* New York: Academic Press.

Gulliksen, H. (1950). *Theory of mental tests.* New York: Wiley.

Herzog, A. R., Kahn, R. L., Morgan, J. N., Jackson, J. F. & Antonucci, T. C. (1989). Age differences in productive activities. *Journal of Gerontology, 44,* S129–S138.

Holtzman, W. H. (1963). Statistical models for the study of change in the single case. In C. W. Harris (ed.), *Problems in measuring change.* Madison, WI: University of Wisconsin Press.

Horn, J. L. (1966). Short period fluctuations in intelligence. Final Report, NSG-518, University of Denver.

Jones, C. J. & Nesselroade, J. R. (in preparation). Review of P-technique studies completed since 1970.

Lerner, R. M. (1984). *On the nature of human plasticity.* New York: Cambridge University Press.

Luborsky, L. & Mintz, J. (1972). The contribution of P-technique to personality, psychotherapy, and psychosomatic research. In R. M. Dreger (ed.), *Multivariate personality research: Contributions to the understanding of personality in honor of Raymond B. Cattell.* Baton Rouge, LA: Claitor's Publishing Division.

Magnusson, D. (1980). Trait–state anxiety: A note on conceptual and empirical relationships. *Personality and Individual Differences, 1,* 215–217.

Magnusson, D. & Endler, N. S. (eds.) (1977). *Personality at the crossroads: Current issues and future prospects.* Hillsdale, NJ: Lawrence Erlbaum Associates.

McArdle, J. J. (1982). Structural equation modeling of an individual system:

Preliminary results from 'A case study of episodic alcoholism'. Unpublished manuscript, Psychology Department, University of Denver.

Milsap, R. E. & Meredith, W. (1988). Component analysis in multivariate aging research. Unpublished manuscript, Baruch College, City University of New York.

Mischel, W. (1968). *Personality and assessment.* New York: John Wiley.

Molenaar, P. C. M. (1985). A dynamic factor model for the analysis of multivariate time series. *Psychometrika, 50,* 181–202.

Mullen, J. A., Orbuch, T. L. & Featherman, D. L. (1988*a*). Change and stability in the CES-D depression score over time in an elderly sample. Paper presented at the annual meeting of the Gerontological Society of America, San Francisco, November.

Mullen, J. A., Orbuch, T. L., Featherman, D. L. & Nesselroade, J. R. (1988*b*). Feasibility of a single-object, replicated time series design with an elderly population. Unpublished manuscript, Institute on Aging, University of Wisconsin-Madison.

Nesselroade, J. R. (1988). Some implications of the trait-state distinction for the study of development and change: The case of personality. In P. B. Baltes, D. L. Featherman & R. M. Lerner (eds.), *Life-span development and behavior,* Vol. 8. Hillsdale, NJ: Lawrence Erlbaum.

Nesselroade, J. R. (1990). *The warp and the woof of the developmental fabric.* Paper presented at a conference to honor the late Joachim F. Wohlwill, The Pennsylvania State University, University Park, PA.

Nesselroade, J. R. & Baltes, P. B. (eds.). (1979). *Longitudinal research in the study of behavior and development.* New York: Academic Press.

Nesselroade, J. R. & Ford, D. H. (1985). P-technique comes of age: Multivariate, replicated, single-subject designs for research on older adults. *Research on Aging, 7,* 46–80.

Radloff, L. S. (1977). The CES-D scale: A self-report depression scale for research in the general population. *Applied Psychological Measurement, 3,* 385–401.

Rowe, J. W. & Kahn, R. L. (1987). Human aging: Usual and successful. *Science, 237,* 143–149.

Schaie, K. W., Campbell, R. T., Meredith, W. & Rawlings, S. C. (eds.) (1988). *Methodological issues in aging research.* New York: Springer.

Singer, J. L. & Singer, D. G. (1972). Personality. *Annual Review of Psychology, 23,* 375–412.

Spearman, C. (1904). General intelligence, objectively determined and measured. *American Journal of Psychology, 15,* 201–293.

Spielberger, C. D., Gorsuch, R. L. & Lushene, R. (1969). *The state-trait anxiety inventory (STAI) test manual, form x.* Palo Alto, CA: Consulting Psychologists Press.

Steyer, R. (1987). Konsistenz und Spezifizität: Definition weier zentraler Begriffe der Differentiellen Psychologie und ein einfaches Modell zu ihrer Identifikation. *Zeitschrift fuer Differentielle und Diagnostische Psychologie, 8,* 245–258.

Watson, D. & Tellegen, A. (1985). Toward a consensual structure of mood. *Psychological Bulletin, 98,* 219–235.

Wittmann, W. W. (1988). Multivariate reliability theory: Principles of symmetry and successful validation strategies. In J. R. Nesselroade & R. B. Cattell (eds.), *Handbook of multivariate experimental psychology*. New York: Plenum.

Wohlwill, J. F. (1973). *The study of behavioral development*. New York: Academic Press.

Zevon, M. A. & Tellegen, A. (1982). The structure of mood change: An idiographic/nomothetic analysis. *Journal of Personality and Social Psychology, 43*, 111–122.

Zuckerman, M. (1983). The distinction between trait and state scales is not arbitrary: Comment on Allen and Potkay's 'On the arbitrary distinction between traits and states.' *Journal of Personality and Social Psychology, 44*, 1083–1086.

ACKNOWLEDGEMENTS

The research reported here and participation in the conference involved in the production of this volume was supported by the MacArthur Foundation Research Program on Successful Aging (MFRPSA). We deeply appreciate the stimulating interactions and discussions we have had with our MFRPSA colleagues concerning the issues discussed herein. We are also grateful to Julia Mullen, Terri Orbuch, and Joe Donato for their help in conducting the Cornwall Manor study.

4 Now you see it, now you don't – some considerations on multiple regression

GEORGE W. BROWN, TIRRIL O. HARRIS AND LOUISE LEMYRE

There is always a temptation to shrink from the difficult task of grounding identifying assumptions in empirical and theoretical knowledge and to select them instead on grounds of statistical convenience or simplicity. This is a temptation that is worth resisting if we wish to arrive at a real understanding of the phenomena we are studying. In this as in other decisions associated with our statistical methods, it is a snare and a delusion to seek out 'automatic' techniques that can be applied without careful consideration or that are neutral with respect to the substance of our theories. It is not enough to learn the etiquette book. The reason (or lack of reason) for its rules must be understood as well.

Herbert A. Simon (1979)

STATISTICS AND THE ANALYSIS OF SURVEY MATERIAL

It may be useful to begin with a small amount of history. This chapter derives from a series of seminars held in London to stimulate discussion of research issues in social psychiatry and was deliberately couched in somewhat provocative terms (hence its title). In a longer view it relates to a certain lingering skepticism about the usefulness of complex multivariate statistics – at least on the part of the first two of us. To be provocative: in our own field of social psychiatry we know of no important findings whose dissemination required such statistics; we suspect that most discoveries have not owed their origin to such statistics, and the statistics may at times actually have prevented important insights. Finally there is a danger that in an essentially multidisciplinary field they will keep many from comprehending potentially significant results or from viewing them sufficiently critically. Something of this general unease was conveyed by one of us in an earlier seminar in the present series in the context of discussing path analysis:

> In practice there has been a tendency to use it to test a limited range of hypotheses rather than to come to terms with the plethora of possibilities inherent in a complex data set. This practice is worrying and runs counter to the spirit of the Durkheim–Lazarsfeld tradition of analysis and often appears to

reflect a misunderstanding of the delicate balance between getting and testing ideas, between the imaginative and the critical in research (Medawar, 1969). There is an element of this interplay in path analysis in the sense that it might well reveal that certain paths can be excluded, but the possibilities for exploration are limited and I doubt whether its use alone will usually have the necessary depth of contact with material to provide an effective mode of analysis. Path coefficients obtained more or less routinely from a computer-based programme are no substitute for getting to know material by puzzling over it in its innumerable manifestations for months, if not years. It does not, for example, supply the all-important partial tables of the traditional Lazarsfeldian approach. Given the flawed measures, the emphasis on 'factors' and the primitive state of knowledge in most fields of inquiry, path analysis is probably best seen primarily as an aid to exploring material and as providing a useful method of summarizing the results of a broader and more complex analysis.

(Brown, 1989: 308)

In general we are impressed by the ease with which significant effects are easily missed even when working close to data in tabular or diagrammatic form, and how because of this it is highly desirable for a worker to give him or herself the opportunity of arriving at the same insight from as many different directions as possible. And this may only come at times from muddling through data, moving from one thing to another as ideas occur, and reworking analyses over and over again as new factors emerge.

However, we are equally impressed by the elegance and succinctness of a regression analysis done well, when the author knows his or her data thoroughly and has clearly looked at the material in many ways and explored in depth possible counter interpretations of the core results of the multivariate analysis. The perspective we espouse is then one of multi-methods: and the reader should be notified early on that our final somewhat critical conclusion relates far more to shortcomings in analysis than in the technique of multiple regression itself. In this spirit we decided to take a critical finding from our own research dealing with the aetiology of depression and ask what the likely consequences would have been if instead of following the traditional, basically tabular, methods of survey analysis we had employed multiple regression. We had, in fact, three questions:

1. whether we would have arrived at our original conclusions about the aetiology of depression (one that has informed a good deal of our research over the last 10 years) if we had used (as many have advised) multiple regression techniques;
2. whether, even if we had stuck to our traditional methods, we would have gained additional insights by using such techniques as well;
3. whether under such circumstances there was a chance of being led astray about what was going on.

A second issue emerged more prominently as the exercise progressed. We had held (perhaps with more uncertainty) equally unfashionable views about another topic: the advantages that accrued from seeing psychiatric disorder in categorical rather than continuous terms. The choice between the two perspectives cannot be reduced to questions about the fundamental nature of phenomena such as depression. We have been ready enough to recognize that the latter appear to be continuous – and, indeed, have argued that the distinction between 'psychotic' and 'neurotic' depression might best be seen in these terms. (We hasten to add that this is hardly an original view.) However, this is by no means the same as concluding that it is useful to *analyze* depression in such terms. Effective theory will not necessarily emerge from such verisimilitude: despite the apparent continuous nature of depression it may only be possible for certain insights to emerge when its apparent continuous nature is arbitrarily divided into categories. Arbitrary here does not mean that the categorization is unreliable, nor that some intuitive feel about the relevance of the divisions is missing. It merely means that there is no obvious justified 'break' in the continuity of the phenomenon. Justification therefore must come from its usefulness, theoretically and practically. Multiple regression, of course, encourages us to see depressive phenomena in continuous terms because of the potential increase in predictive power of continuous measures and the issue is an inevitable backdrop to the present exercise. The contrasting advantages of using categorical measures expressed as dummy variables in multiple regression are much less often recognized. There is, for example, no problem in using unstandardized regression coefficients in this way to obtain a direct sense of the relative importance of independent variables. This is because they are comparable in the sense of scales reflecting presence or absence (Achen, 1982: 70–1): we are simply asking whether the presence of X has a greater impact than the presence of W upon factor Y. This is non-controversial. The basic problem concerns the evaluation of the different results that can emerge in using a continuous measure as against a categorical measure as the dependent variable. Not only is there some dispute as to whether such a procedure is statistically viable (Hellevik, 1984; Schroeder, Sjoquist & Stephan, 1986), but, as will emerge, the picture presented seems to change even within the same data set.

THE BASIC RESULT IN CATEGORICAL TERMS

The aetiological model of depression to be explored was derived from research which approached the issue in the spirit of giving feed-back to clinicians about the psychosocial origins of that disorder. Like clinicians, it therefore adopted a categorical approach. The early research

Table 4.1. *Basic vulnerability result: vulnerability factor, presence of a provoking agent and onset of caseness depression (303 Islington women excluding cases of depression at first interview)*

Provoking agent	Vulnerability Yes	Vulnerability No	
	Percentage onset case		
Yes	*29* (28/95)	*4* (2/55)	$p < 0.001$*
No	*2* (1/56)	*1* (1/97)	NS

* Significance level of at least 0.05.
NS, Not significant.

established that certain *provoking agents* determine when an episode of depression will take place. Most significant are severely threatening events, usually involving a loss or disappointment, although major ongoing difficulties can also play a role (Brown & Harris, 1978*a*; Brown, Bifulco & Harris, 1987). At a conservative estimate about 80% of episodes of depression in the general population are brought about by such an event or difficulty. However, the chance of such an event bringing about a depressive disorder appears to be considerably influenced by the presence of *vulnerability* factors, such as lack of support. In the original enquiry carried out in Camberwell in South London we concluded that lack of an intimate tie with a husband, having three or more children under 14 living at home, and loss of mother before 11 act as vulnerability factors for women – that is, that they increased risk of depression only in the presence of a provoking agent (Brown & Harris, 1978*a*; 181). (Lack of employment only related to increased risk in the presence of other vulnerability factors.)

Table 4.1 illustrates this effect in terms of a contingency table in which the proportions experiencing the dependent variable are expressed in terms of the four possible combinations of two dichotomous independent variables. The data are drawn from a recent longitudinal study in Islington where the index of vulnerability is based on measures of core relationships made at the time of first contact with the women involved – that is, before the occurrence of any severe events (which made up the great majority of the provoking agents) and before any onset of depression. The index representing vulnerability (negative elements in core relationships) was derived from an analysis of 70 measures dealing with negative interaction with husband, lack of primary quality in the relationship with husband, security-diminishing characteristics of housewife role (a measure largely reflecting shortcomings in the practical and financial help provided by husband) and negative interaction with children (see Brown, Bifulco & Andrews, 1990 for details).

As already intimated, some understanding of the measure of depression used in the enquiry is important for our argument.

In the last 20 years, a number of standardized clinical-type interviews have been developed, using questions aimed to establish the presence of symptoms of a type and severity typically encountered in out-patient and hospital practice. Throughout our research we have used a shortened version of the Present State Examination (PSE) to collect material about basic symptomatology (Wing, Cooper & Sartorius, 1974). There is also in common use the *Schizophrenia and Affective Disorder Schedule* (SADS) (Endicott & Spitzer, 1978), and the *Clinical Interview Schedule* (Goldberg *et al.*, 1970). While each use somewhat different criteria for the inclusion of symptoms, they agree broadly, at a symptomatic level, on the range and severity of symptoms judged to be of psychiatric relevance.

The PSE was used, as designed, to collect symptoms for one month, and its use extended to cover the 12 months before interview in order not to miss the onset of cases earlier in the year, which are crucial for the study of the aetiological role of life events and difficulties (Brown & Harris, 1978*a*). The interviewer dated the onset as accurately as possible within the year, if necessary using events such as move of house as anchor points.

Interviewers, who were permanent members of the research team, were trained in the use and administration of the shortened version of the ninth edition of the Present State Examination (Wing *et al.*, 1974). Although initially designed to be administered by clinicians, there is now extensive evidence to support its use in social surveys by trained lay interviewers (see, e.g. Cooper *et al.*, 1977; Wing, Henderson & Winckle, 1977). Details of the clinical interview, as well as basic information on psychiatric conditions likely to be encountered in community surveys of this kind and on the identification and training and its use is given in Brown, Craig & Harris (1985).

The establishment of an acceptable caseness threshold is always the crux of plausibility in epidemiological psychiatric research using a categorical approach. The threshold used in our surveys has aimed to reflect current psychiatric practice; it was thus deliberately designed to contrast 'cases', who would have syndromes comparable to those of women seen in outpatient clinics, with 'borderline cases'. The latter have symptoms that are not sufficiently typical, frequent, or intense to be rated as cases, but still are more than odd isolated symptoms. There are also women with psychiatric symptoms such as fatigue, sleep disorder, and nervous tension which are not sufficient to warrant even a borderline case rating. The original caseness threshold was established by two psychiatrists (John Cooper and John Copeland) when research began in 1969, but essential to the whole procedure has been the development of reference examples of cases and borderline cases for different diagnostic groups. In the general population, cases of depression and anxiety or phobic states are much the most frequent, but there are also categories for obsessional, tension, alcoholic, and drug-dependent conditions. This diagnostic system, which can now be applied using a simple computer algorithm in so far as it involves depressive and anxiety/phobic conditions, has been described extensively elsewhere, and has been shown to have good inter-rater reliability; there is also good evidence for its construct validity in the context of aetiological research (Brown & Harris, 1978*a*; Finlay-Jones *et al.*, 1980; Finlay-Jones and Brown, 1981; Brown & Prudo, 1981; Prudo, Brown, Harris & Dowland, 1981).

The following checklist has been shown statistically to underlie the clinical criteria for depression (Finlay-Jones *et al.*, 1980) and, as will be seen, has been emphasized in the present exercise.

For the diagnosis of a *case of depression*, both A and B must be present:

(A) depressed mood;
(B) four or more of the following symptoms: hopelessness, suicidal plans or attempts, weight loss, early waking, delayed sleep, poor concentration, neglect due to brooding, loss of interest, self-depreciation, and anergia.

In practice, many other symptoms covered by the PSE are also to be found present – on average about 19 in total.

The two criteria for the diagnosis of a *borderline case of depression* are:

(A) depressed mood;
(B) between one and three of the symptoms listed above.

Major syndromes are treated non-hierarchically. This permits an anxiety state to be rated separately from a depressive disorder and allows a subject to be characterized by separate diagnoses at different levels of severity – for example, case depression: borderline case anxiety. At this point we should perhaps state again that the divisions we have used are essentially arbitrary in the sense that the range of severity of the phenomonon appears to be continuous. Justification for the divisions must depend on what follows from making them.

Since we were concerned with the onset of a new caseness depressive condition Table 4.1 excludes all women suffering from such a condition at the time of first interview (50 women) and includes only the 303 women followed up at a second interview one year later. A total of 32

Table 4.2. *Vulnerability factor, presence of a provoking agent and onset of borderline caseness of depression (271 Islington women excluding cases of depression at first interview and onsets in follow-up years)*

Provoking agent	Vulnerability		
	Yes	No	
	Percentage onset borderline case		
Yes	*22* (15/67)	*15* (8/53)	NS
No	*2* (1/55)	*3* (3/96)	NS

Cases (shown in Table 4.1) are excluded from the denominators.

of the 303 women developed caseness of depression at some time in the follow-up year and, as can be seen, 30 of the 32 had experienced a provoking agent before onset (29 a severe event and 1 a major difficulty only).

We will concentrate on this basic result concerning onset of caseness. However, we will also refer to a second result that has now been replicated in several studies and begins to provide further evidence for the kind of justification we called for earlier for approaching depression in such categorical terms. Table 4.2 shows that the vulnerability effect does not occur for those developing a borderline case depressive condition: see the top row of Table 4.2 (women developing case conditions are excluded). Perhaps the most plausible interpretation is that women are not entirely protected from depression by the lack of vulnerability – but, given the presence of a provoking agent, they are likely to develop a milder, borderline case, rather than case condition, thus accounting for the high rate of the milder borderline conditions where there is a provoking agent but no vulnerability (17% in Table 4.2).

INTERACTIVE EFFECTS

There has been a good deal of controversy over the last 10 years about the analysis of the kind of interactive effect shown in Table 4.1, and some brief reference to it is perhaps in order. The controversy originated from two papers written by members of the MRC Social Psychiatry Research Unit about the basic results of the original Camberwell enquiry (Tennant & Bebbington, 1978; Bebbington, 1980). (See also our replies: Brown & Harris, 1978*b*; 1980.) No-one involved in the debate has questioned the usefulness of dealing with depression in categorical terms. The key issue is whether lack of support (or any other 'vulnerability' factor) has an independent effect or only increases risk of depression in the presence of a provoking agent. Tennant and Bebbington concluded on the basis of our material that 'the social variables involved do not segregate into "vulnerability factors" and "provoking agents". Both categories of variables affect the risk of disorder independently of the other' (Tennant & Bebbington, 1978: 574); and that 'vulnerability factors have an effect somewhat similar to the separate provoking effect of life events' (p. 573). In other words they assert that vulnerability factors act statistically as provoking agents.

One problem with Tennant & Bebbington's criticism is their failure to appreciate that certain assumptions about the world are typically already built into statistical techniques; whether or not it is reasonable to go along with these assumptions cannot then be settled by statistical arguments depending on these very assumptions. Different statistical procedures handle interactive effects differently. It has been traditional in the social sciences to see the kind of result illustrated in Table 4.1 in terms of so-called additive interaction. Very briefly this requires first calculating the independent contributions of the two main variables. Thus in Table 4.1 the independent effect of the provoking agent is 4% (the effect of the provoking agent when vulnerability is not present) minus 1% (the expected rate of depression without either the provoking agent *or* vulnerability factor). Following the same logic the independent effect of the vulnerability factor is 2%–1%. It follows that the excess or interactive effect of provoking agent *and* vulnerability factor when occurring together is 24%: i.e., $29 - ((4 - 1) + ((2 - 1) + 1)$, the final 1% relating to the expected rate when neither factor is present. This is quite sufficient to establish the presence of a vulnerability effect. (It also follows exactly the procedure for establishing regression coefficients where there is a dichotomous dependent variable expressed, as for caseness, in terms of a proportion as in Table 4.1: Hellevik, 1984.)

However, there is an alternative way of considering interaction in which effects are multiplied rather than added – not to be confused with the multiplication of dummy independent variables in multiple regression (see Brown & Harris, 1986*a*: 151–2). The problem is that the two approaches can give quite different answers concerning the presence of interactive effects, and in the Camberwell material (but not in the present data) this multiplicative approach showed a complete absence of interaction and thereby lack of support for a distinctive vulnerability effect.

The original paper by Tennant & Bebbington failed to recognize that the ordinary log-linear approach they employed reflects only multiplicative effects. Everitt & Smith (1979) have confirmed that if alternative linear modeling methods based on an additive approach developed by Grizzle, Stamler and Koch (GSK) are used, interaction is present in the original Camberwell data (see also Swafford, 1980). They state that the choice between models using the two different types of interaction cannot be settled in statistical terms, but none the less show a preference for a multiplicative approach. However, recent opinion in epidemiology has emphasized how much information can be lost by ignoring additive interaction (Rothman, 1974, 1976, 1978; Blot & Day, 1978).

Elsewhere we have given what we believe are reasonably convincing pragmatic reasons for preferring an additive approach (Brown & Harris, 1986*a*: 153–154). Given the presence of such interaction the application of separate chi-square tests to the two parts of the data (as in Table 4.1) is appropriate. However, we recognize that there is no satisfactory way of finally settling on the appropriate mode of analysis by such arguments and we have therefore also presented more *theoretically* based reasons for preferring an additive model (see Brown & Harris, 1986*a*: 154–157; and Brown, 1986).

THE BASIC RESULT IN CONTINUOUS TERMS

Implicit in our presentation so far has been the assumption, noted earlier, that it is appropriate to see depression (and, for that matter, the variables involved in its onset) in categorical terms. But since we wished to explore the implications of dealing with depression in continuous terms, we developed a straightforward continuous scale of depression based on the count of PSE symptoms. But this immediately confronted us with a diagnostic decision about the particular PSE symptoms which, not being relevant for depression, should be ignored in such a procedure. We proceeded by adding to the 11 core PSE symptoms of depression presented earlier further PSE symptoms of depression, usually quite rare, together with symptoms largely dealing with tension and worry: widely used in scales such as that of the Hamilton Rating Scale (Hamilton, 1960) and the Beck Depression Inventory (Beck *et al.*, 1961). These extra symptoms were (a) inefficient thinking, morning depression, social withdrawal, lack of self-confidence, ideas of reference, guilty ideas of reference, pathological guilt, depressive delusions, delusions of reference, loss of libido, and (b) worrying, hypochondriasis, headaches (tension pains), tiredness/exhaustion, muscular tension, restlessness, nervous tension, premenstrual exacerbation and irritability.

Table 4.3 is a straightforward contingency table and shows that, once the vulnerability factor is controlled and those not at risk (because of their chronicity) are excluded, there is at best a small (and non-significant) trend for those with a higher initial symptom score to

Table 4.3. *Initial symptom score, vulnerability factor, and onset of depression at caseness level (150 Islington women with a provoking agent excluding cases at first interview)*[a]

Clinical data: continuous time 1 and categorical time 2

High vulnerability ($N = 95$)					Low vulnerability ($N = 55$)				
Initial symptom score					Initial symptom score				
0–1	2–3	4–5	6–8	9+	0–1	2–3	4–5	6–8	9+
Percentage onset case					Percentage onset case				
11	*34*	*36*	*32*	*36*	*0*	*29*	*0*	*0*	*0*
(2/19)	(10/29)	(5/14)	(6/19)	(5/14)	(0/27)	(2/7)	(0/10)	(0/8)	(0/3)
		gamma = 0.23, NS					NS		

[a] Women without a provoking agent not included since only 2/153 developed onset.

Table 4.4. *Basic vulnerability result: initial symptom score, vulnerability factor, presence of provoking agent and final symptom score (303 Islington women excluding cases of depression at first interview)*

Clinical data: continuous time 1 and time 2

Overall linear multiple regression – forced entry		Beta	Significance
1.	Initial symptom score (S)	0.45	0.000*
2.	Vulnerability (V)	0.09	0.251
3.	Provoking agent (P)	0.18	0.015*
	1×2 $S \times V$	−0.02	0.830
	1×3 $S \times P$	0.02	0.811
	2×3 $V \times P$	0.12	0.160
	($R^2 = 0.42$)		

R^2 Adjusted coefficient of multiple determination.
* Significance level of at least 0.05.

experience more later onsets of caseness of depression. The implication of this result will be clear as we proceed.

Table 4.4 is crucial for our argument. It is an attempt to reproduce the basic result of Table 4.1 using multiple regression with the continuous measure of depression. It is normal practice in such analyses to include, as we have done here, the symptom score at first interview as a control factor. Material has been entered in an hierarchical (forced entry) manner in which the three main effects have been entered together with the three two-way interaction terms. The equivalent control was less complicated in the categorical analysis already shown in

Table 4.5. *Continuous score at both time 1 and time 2, initial symptom score, vulnerability factor, and onset of depression (150 Islington women with a provoking agent excluding cases of depression at first interview)*

Time 2 Symptom score	High vulnerability ($N = 95$) Initial symptom score 0–1	2–3	4–5	6–8	9+	Low vulnerability ($N = 55$) Initial symptom score 0–1	2–3	4–5	6–8	9+
0–1	8	3	1	2	0	11	0	2	1	0
2–3	4	10	2	2	1	9	3	1	0	0
4–5	3	1	4	0	0	4	0	3	4	1
6–8	2(1)	3	2	6	1	3	2	1	1	1
9+	2(1)	12(10)	5(5)	9(6)	12(5)	0	2(2)	3	2	1
	gamma 0.56 $\chi^2 = 16$ d.f., $p < 0.001$					gamma 0.63 $\chi^2 = 16$ d.f., $p < 0.05$				

Figures in brackets represent onset cases during follow-up – categorical variable.

Table 4.3, merely involving the omission of cases at time 1, i.e. those rated '1' on the dichotomous dependent variable of caseness of depression. Of course, with the more wide-ranging dependent variable provided by the continuous score, such a control must involve more than this. Therefore, in Table 4.4, not only have all cases of depression at first interview been excluded but the continuous score of depression at time 1 has also been entered in the regression.

Two results shown are surprising in the light of the earlier categorical analysis. First, the beta weight for the interaction between provoking agent and vulnerability factor is small and falls far short of significance. Second, the beta weight for initial symptoms far exceeds that of the only other factor of statistical significance, provoking agent: 0.45 versus 0.18.

The apparent importance of initial symptoms is, of course, in direct conflict with the earlier result using caseness which showed at best a small trend for initial continuous score to relate to caseness of depression in the follow-up period (Table 4.3). The most plausible explanation is that the continuous measure, unlike that of caseness, is essentially one of well-being rather than depression, the high beta weight for initial symptoms merely reflecting the ability of absence of symptoms at time 1 to predict the same at time 2. The beta weight is high because there is considerable variability of the score, both at time 1 and time 2, and the high resulting variances are bound to be reflected in any measure (like standardized beta coefficients) that are based on variance explained. Table 4.5, repeating Table 4.3 but using the continuous scores at both times, shows how this has happened. Not

Table 4.6. *Basic vulnerability result: initial symptom score, vulnerability factor, presence of provoking agent, and final symptom score (303 Islington women excluding cases of depression at first interview)*

Clinical data: continuous time 1 and time 2

Stepwise multiple regression entering the terms used in Table 4.4	Beta	Significance
Initial symptom score (S)	0.47	0.000*
Provoking agent (P)	0.16	0.007*
Vulnerability × provoking agent ($V \times P$)	0.19	0.002*
($R^2 = 0.431$)		

only is the degree of association between time 1 and time 2 scores markedly increased over Table 4.3, but the single most populated cell is clearly that where scores are 0–1 in both time periods ($N = 19$ for both vulnerability groups combined); in other words, one of the prime functions in Table 4.5 is the prediction of marked well-being at time 2 by marked well-being at time 1. If we return to the basic result shown in Table 4.4, it is easy to fall into the trap of believing that we see reflected the relative importance of psychiatric and psychosocial factors in determining *clinically relevant depression*, and, indeed, this appears to be the most usual interpretation in the literature of such a patterning of results (see, e.g., Warheit, 1979).

The reason why the analysis so singularly fails to reflect interaction is, however, less obvious, and we will delay discussion of this surprising result. None the less, it should be noted that when, instead of a conventional hierarchical (forced-entry) approach, stepwise linear regression is used which allows effects to emerge in order of their importance, some indication of an interactive effect does appear (Table 4.6). However, it is essential here to distinguish between an exploratory and a confirmatory analysis. It will be recalled that one of our questions is how far we would have been likely to uncover the basic vulnerability result by using a multiple regression approach. The answer is that it would appear unlikely. In the first place, many would take the position that, without a prior result indicating such an interactive effect, it would be inappropriate to utilize the kind of non-hierarchical approach resulting from this latter stepwise analysis. And it would thus have been very unlikely to have been run in the light of the negative forced entry results shown in Table 4.4, where no inkling of an interactive effect

Table 4.7. *Basic vulnerability result: initial symptom score, vulnerability factor, presence of a provoking agent and onset of caseness depression (303 Islington women excluding cases of depression at first interview)*

Clinical data: continuous time 1 and categorical time 2

Overall linear multiple regression – forced entry		
1. Initial symptom score (*S*)	0.15	0.175
2. Vulnerability (*V*)	0.04	0.659
3. Provoking agent (*P*)	0.03	0.729
1 × 2 *S* × *V*	0.05	0.742
1 × 3 *S* × *V*	−0.05	0.660
2 × 3 *V* × *P*	0.38	0.000*
($R^2 = 0.17$)		

emerged. (It should perhaps be added that even if the initial symptom scale is omitted from the regression an interactive effect still does not emerge.) At this point therefore we conclude that the vulnerability effect clearly shown in Table 4.1 would have been missed in any exploratory analysis using multiple regression with a continuous rather than a categorical measure of depression; and that even if someone set out initially with such a result in mind they might well still have reached a negative conclusion – this time about its replicability.

Before seeking reasons for the failure of the multiple regression analysis to reveal interaction, it is important to note that even when symptoms at time 1 are measured by the same continuous score, if the dichotomous case versus non-case measure of depression is used for psychiatric status at time 2 (the dependent variable) a strong interactive effect does emerge using the forced-entry approach. Moreover the effect of initial symptom score is low and non-significant (Table 4.7). These are exactly the results that would be expected since such a binary multiple regression arrives at exactly the same estimates of main effects and interaction as the use of more traditional methods of analysing the proportions via the contingency table (Hellevik, 1984).

The problem therefore does not appear to be one of using multiple regression as such, but of using it with a *continuous* measure of depression as the dependent variable. However, using multiple regression with a dichotomous categorical outcome measure does not entirely replicate the basic vulnerability finding of Table 4.1. When borderline caseness is also included as part of a trichotomous categorical outcome variable, the beta weights of the dichotomous analysis remain practically identical. (They are so close to those in Table 4.7 that no further table has been given.) In other words we would still have missed the fact that borderline case conditions are not involved in vulnerability (Table 4.2).

Table 4.8. *Basic vulnerability result: initial symptom score, vulnerability factor, presence of a provoking agent, and final symptom score (353 Islington women including cases of depression at first interview)*

Clinical data: continuous time 1 and time 2

1. Initial symptom score (S)	0.78	0.000*
2. Vulnerability (V)	0.11	0.071
3. Provoking agent (P)	0.16	0.007*
1 × 2 $S \times V$	−0.15	0.073
1 × 3 $S \times P$	−0.05	0.561
2 × 3 $V \times P$	0.09	0.236
($R^2 = 0.58$)		

In terms of a wider perspective we believe it essential to be in a position to pick up such 'discontinuities', particularly when, as in this case, the result appears to be replicable (Brown & Harris, 1986*b*). As already noted, it is unnecessary in the light of the discontinuity involved in the case/borderline case/normal distinctions to assert anything about the underlying nature of the phenomenon – only that it is useful to treat the apparent continuum categorically. If the possibility of this kind of discontinuity is accepted, it will be necessary to do more than examine the coefficients of a regression analysis; the data will need to be examined specifically for such thresholds between categories in order to identify the cut-point at which the change in quantity becomes the change in quality.

One further point needs to be made about the use of continuous symptom scores. Most multiple regression studies would probably not have excluded altogether the cases of depression at the time of first interview as we did here. These would be included despite the fact that, unless they recovered early in the follow-up period, they would not be at risk for a further onset at a caseness level; but this would be justified by the general notion that in entering initial symptom score into the regression such a problem would be 'controlled for'. If the 50 who have initial caseness of depression are included in this way, findings of the earlier analysis (Table 4.4) are, if anything, exaggerated with the beta weight of initial symptom score almost doubling (0.78 versus 0.48) and again there is a failure of any interaction to emerge (Table 4.8). A re-examination of Table 4.5 on the larger population including those depressed at time 1 illuminates this. Not only is the range of scores yet further increased (several scored 21 at time 1), but the 50 cases introduce further stability to the correlation of scores between the two periods. Of the 50 only 10 had changed score by more than 2 points (8 improving and 2 worsening).

In many ways, these conclusions concerning the inclusion of those with initial caseness of depression will not surprise habitues of multiple regression. There is a whole literature describing how time-series analyses (repeated observations on the same item through time) are more likely than cross-sectional analyses (unique observations on different items at the same point in time) to give misleading importance to the variables measured more than once (Ostrom, 1978; Lewis-Beck, 1980). The low autocorrelation assumption of multiple regression requires that error for an observation at an earlier time is not related to errors for an observation at a later time and clearly this is untenable – the unmeasured forces accounting for symptom score at time 2 are not independent of the unmeasured forces influencing it at time 1.

One way of coping with this problem is to adopt a different method of controlling for initial symptoms. Instead of regressing the independent variables upon symptom score at time 2, a differential score can be calculated to indicate the degree and direction of changes in scores between the two times. When this is done for this data set, the key effect (the interaction between provoking agent and vulnerability factor) still fails to emege as statistically significant.

Therefore at this point our main conclusions are that forced-entry multiple regression, when using standardized beta coefficients, fails to produce evidence for the critical vulnerability effect; and that moreover it gives misleading weight (in the light of Table 4.3) to the relative importance of initial symptom score in predicting phenomena of clinical importance (as opposed to less substantial variations in mood). Table 4.9 summarizes material in the earlier tables in terms of initial symptom score and the vulnerability factor, although it would hold equally for provoking agent.

One possible objection to the analysis so far is our use of standardized regression coefficients to reflect causal effects and thus the relative importance of particular factors. In doing so, of course, we reflect a great deal of current practice in the social sciences where the distinction between prediction and explanation is often blurred. Achen (1982) is particularly critical of this usage. He points out how such measures (all depending on variance explained) have 'doubtful meaning but great rhetorical value': p. 59). Their value is highly dependent on the tightness of the grouping of the variables involved and this by no means reflects the 'strength' of the underlying relationship. The example he discusses illustrates how the R^2 of two regressions coefficients can be totally at odds with an actual measure of 'level of importance' based on the unstandardized coefficients. He points out that such an index of relative importance has the attractive property that, when the contributions of the independent variable to be contrasted are added, together with the intercept, the result is precisely the mean of the dependent variable (Achen, 1982: 72).

Table 4.9. *Relative size beta weights of initial symptom score and vulnerability factor in terms of various outcome measures (150 Islington women with a provoking agent)*

Clinical data: various

	A. Outcome: (categorical)		B. Outcome: caseness and borderline caseness (categorical)		C. Outcome: symptom score (continuous)	
	Beta	Sig.	Beta	Sig.	Beta	Sig.
1. Initial symptom score (150 women excluding cases at first interview)	0.10	0.206	0.14	0.092	0.45	0.000*
2. Vulnerability	0.29	0.000*	0.28	0.001*	0.18	0.013*
Ratios 1/2	0.35		0.48		2.49	

	D. outcome: symptom score (continuous)	
	Beta	Sig.
1. Initial symptom score (189 women including cases at first interview)	0.64	0.000*
2. Vulnerability	0.11	0.047*
Ratio 1/2	5.82	

As it happens, this does not appear to explain the difference in relative importance of the clinical and social measures in the results so far presented. For example, in Table 4.4 the ratio of the two beta coefficients of initial symptom score and provoking agent is 2.04, whereas if Achen's level of importance measure is used this ratio is still much the same at 2.24.

There are other complexities which we will not pursue (e.g., whether non-significant interaction factors should be ignored). However, we trust we have conveyed that the issue of the relative importance of various factors needs to be argued carefully. Given the point made earlier about the continuous clinical measures reflecting well-being, multiple regression as a technique appears to place misleading weight in the present instance on clinical as against social phenomena.

So far we have placed a good deal of weight upon more mathematical considerations, as a possible explanation of the discrepant findings about the presence of an interaction effect. However we also wondered whether there might not be more substantive issues of measurement involved. For example, could another continuous score better capture the essence of depression?

OTHER CONTINUOUS MEASURES OF DEPRESSION

So far for the continuous depression score we have used quite a *general* measure because it appears to reflect other current measures reasonably well. The score ranged from 0 to 13 PSE symptoms at time 1 (excluding cases at first interview) with a mean of 2.78. But symptoms such as tension and lack of energy can exist in the absence of a core depressive condition and could therefore represent 'noise' as far as a measure of depression is concerned. We therefore examined the consequences of using a continuous measure that followed more closely our own definition of depression, taking account of depressed mood and only the 10 other symptoms of depression listed when the categorical measure was outlined earlier. (This shortened measure of core symptoms will be referred to as symptom score B.) The score at time 1 now only ranged from 0 to 7 (excluding cases at first interview) with a mean of 0.67.

With this less dispersed measure the interactive effect of provoking agent and vulnerability factor emerges clearly with a forced-entry multiple regression (Table 4.10). The beta coefficient for initial symptoms is of much the same order as before (Tables 4.10 and 4.4). None the less in the light of our earlier argument it is still doubtful whether the relative size of the beta weights for initial symptom score (0.53) and interaction between provoking agent and vulnerability factor (0.37) should be accepted as reflecting their relative importance. Interestingly enough when the cases at first interview are included, although the beta coefficient for initial symptoms is particularly high, the interaction between provoking agent and vulnerability factor is still the second most important effect (Table 4.11).

Thus conclusions reached with score B are radically different from those with the first continuous measure. Results follow much more closely the original findings based on the categorical measure of caseness. The best-fitting model would include the interaction between provoking agent and vulnerability. There is one further consistency: if a

Table 4.10. *Basic vulnerability result: initial symptom score B, vulnerability factor, presence of a provoking agent, and final symptom score B (303 Islington women excluding cases of depression at first interview)*

Clinical data: coninuous time 1 and time 2

Overall linear multiple regression – forced entry	Beta	Significance
1. Initial symptom score B (*S*)	0.53	0.000*
2. Vulnerability (*V*)	−0.01	0.875
3. Provoking agent (*P*)	0.09	0.237
1 × 2 $S \times V$	−0.09	0.387
1 × 3 $S \times P$	−0.18	0.100
2 × 3 $V \times P$	0.37	0.000*
($R^2 = 0.303$)		

Table 4.11. *Basic vulnerability result: initial symptom score B, vulnerability factor, presence of a provoking agent, and final symptom score B (353 Islington women including cases of depression at first interview)*

Clinical data: continuous time 1 and time 2

Overall linear multiple regression – forced entry	Beta	Significance
1. Initial symptom score B (*S*)	0.91	0.000*
2. Vulnerability (*V*)	0.04	0.561
3. Provoking agent (*P*)	0.08	0.195
1 × 2 $S \times V$	−0.36	0.001*
1 × 3 $S \times P$	−0.12	0.271
2 × 3 $V \times P$	0.27	0.001*
($R^2 = 0.46$)		

tabular approach is used for initial symptoms (as earlier in Table 4.3) there is now a better case to be made that they are of some significance (Table 4.12). The relationship of initial symptom score and caseness of depression now reaches statistical significance. (We had in fact in an earlier analysis recognized the importance of a chronic borderline case condition of either depression *or* anxiety as a factor predicting subsequent onset of case depression and explored this using logistic regression: see Brown *et al.*, 1986).

The reasons for these dramatic changes, following the changes in the scale used, are by no means clear. It seems likely that the longer

Table 4.12. *Initial symptom score B, vulnerability factor, and onset of depression at caseness level (150 Islington women with a provoking agent excluding cases of depression at first interview)*

Clinical data: continuous time 1 and categorical time 2

High vulnerability ($N = 95$)					Low vulnerability ($N = 55$)				
Initial symptom score B					Initial symptom score B				
0	1	2	3	4+	0	1	2	3	4+
Percentage onset case					Percentage onset case				
15	*57*	*31*	*20*	*36*	*3*	*10*	*0*	*0*	*0*
(6/40)	(12/21)	(4/13)	(2/10)	(4/11)	(1/34)	(1/10)	(0/8)	(0/2)	(0/1)
	40 (22/55)					*5* (1/21)			
	gamma = 0.31, $p < 0.02$, 4 d.f.					NS			

Table 4.13. *Basic vulnerability result: initial ID (Index of Definition), vulnerability factor, presence of a provoking agent and final ID (303 Islington women excluding cases of depression at first interview)*

Clinical data: continuous time 1 and 2

Overall linear multiple regression – forced entry	Beta	Significance
1. Initial symptom ID (S)	0.44	0.000
2. Vulnerability (V)	0.08	0.538
3. Provoking agent (P)	0.34	0.006
1×2 $S \times V$	0.06	0.679
1×3 $S \times P$	−0.15	0.307
2×3 $V \times P$	0.06	0.539
	($R^2 = 0.36$)	

measure had greater variability owing to the inclusion of non-depressive symptoms and this in some manner swamped the interactive effect of provoking agent and vulnerability factor. In order to investigate this we looked at a third continuous measure of symptoms – the Index of Definition of the PSE (or ID) – which has been used in multiple regression analyses (see, e.g., Tennant, Bebbington & Hurry, 1982). This is an algorithm developed for the PSE to reflect the chances of a symptom picture reflecting a psychiatric case of any kind, not only of depression; it has a more modest range of scale points than the total PSE score which has been usually employed, running from 1 (no disorder) to 8 (most definite caseness). Table 4.13 shows that with this third measure the interactive effect does not emerge as significant in a

Table 4.14. *Initial symptoms with score B by Index of Definition: women in Islington followed up, excluding cases of depression (N = 303)*

		Score B (Low) 0	1	2	3	4	5–7	Total
(Index of definition)	(Low) 1	55						55
	2	83	15	5				103
	3	38	24	10	1			73
	4	8	10	11	7	0	1	37
	5	5	2	8	6	5	5[a]	31
	6	0	0	0	0	1	3[b]	4
Total		189	51	34	14	6	9	

[a] on score B 5 = 3 and 6 = 2.
[b] on score B 5 = 1, 6 = 1 and 7 = 1.

multiple regression despite the apparent similarity of ID to score B in terms of distribution.

At time 1 the distribution of ID is: 1 & 2:158, 3:73, 4:37, 5:31, and 6:4; and for score B: 0:189, 1:51, 2:34, 3:14, 4:6, 5:5, 6:3 and 7:1 (see marginal totals in Table 4.14). A further look at the two scores, however, in Table 4.14 suggests that they are picking up different phenomena: there were many more scoring low on score B and high on ID than high on Score B and low on ID. This is not surprising, given our knowledge that the ID level picks up conditions other than depression while score B is designed to mimic the Bedford College depressive caseness criterion. It suggests that the non-emergence of the interactive effect between provoking agent and vulnerability may result from the introduction of these other conditions into the continuous scale which therefore fails to reflect a dimension of pure depression. This introduction of 'noise' may be even more important in explaining the failure of the original continuous score to reflect interaction (Table 4.4) than our earlier speculations concerning the fact it tended to reflect well-being with a consequent relative neglect of depressive disorder as such.

SUMMARY AND CONCLUSIONS

In the light of the basic findings using categorical measures of depression (Tables 4.1 and 4.2) we find it difficult to give much weight to the results of the initial forced entry multiple regression analysis using a continuous measure of depression (Table 4.4). The most likely reason for the failure to find an interactive effect between provoking agent and vulnerability factor in predicting subsequent depression is that the general and continuous symptom measure includes too much that is strictly unrelated to depression. There is already evidence that the vulnerability model involving provoking agent and support does not hold for the onset of anxiety conditions (Finlay-Jones, 1989), and for this reason we had deliberately omitted a count of anxiety symptoms from this larger continuous measure. But it will also follow that the effect is likely to be attenuated by the inclusion of the tension conditions that form the bulk of other diagnoses (Brown, Craig & Harris, 1985). However, it is also possible that the lack of an interactive effect relates to the greater variability inherent in the general scales and this in some way influences the standardized coefficients that reflect variance. It is of interest here to note the result of using the third psychiatric measure, the Index of Definition (ID), which, although resembling score B in variability, did not identify the key interactive effect as significant, thus resembling the longer score. This suggests that the failure of the general scales may be more related to the nature of the symptoms they combine, which introduces noise into the dimension of pure depression, rather than to the distribution of the scores as such.

A second reason to doubt the initial forced-entry regression analysis is that the preeminent importance given to the continuous initial symptom score compared with that of the established social aetiological factors (Table 4.4) runs quite counter to the, at best modest and non-significant, association between initial symptom score and onset of *caseness* of depression (Table 4.3). Here the high beta weight almost certainly reflects the ability to predict well-being at one point in time on the basis of well-being at an earlier point. In short it would be misleading to see such a measure as crucially focusing upon *clinically* relevant psychiatric phenomena.

We have therefore been forced to the conclusion that the use of multiple regression as the sole technique with the original long clinical measure would have failed to reveal the basic interactive effect necessary for the vulnerability result and may well have led to quite erroneous conclusions about the relative importance of subclinical conditions and social factors in predicting future depression. This most clearly holds for any study not setting out with a particular hypothesis about the vulnerability effect. However, even if multiple regression had been used in a study specifically designed to replicate the earlier findings, it might well have led to the conclusion that there was no replication. It is true that a stepwise approach to regression would have been able to reveal some evidence for the relevant interaction effect (Table 4.6); however, this might well not have been carried out, given the negative results of the forced entry, and some would question the status of such a non-hierarchical approach when the initial findings, involving the 'main effects', were negative.

Finally, the common practice of including all depressive conditions (whether or not they had at first interview reached caseness of depression in our terms) would only have compounded these problems (Table 4.8).

Despite these difficulties, when the long version of the continuous clinical measure was used as a control measure (for state at time 1) and a categorical measure of caseness used as the outcome measure, the expected interactive effect clearly emerged as the only effect of statistical significance: i.e., initial symptom score did not relate to outcome (Table 4.7). This, as already noted, is expected from the fact that multiple regression when used with a dichotomous dependent variation parallels the results of more traditional analyses in terms of differences in proportions (Hellevik, 1984). However, even this result has the shortcoming that it cannot reveal that onsets of borderline case conditions do not reflect a vulnerability effect (Table 4.2).

This initial largely negative exercise with multiple regression led us to reconsider our continuous measure of depression (which included strictly non-depressive symptoms such as worry, tiredness and muscular tension) as it seemed unlikely that the negative results could be solely attributed to the use of multiple regression as such. The use of a shortened measure of depression (score B) in fact produced a radically different set of findings. The expected interactive effect clearly emerged (Table 4.10). The trouble is that there is no reason to believe that such an instrument would be the measure of choice for those wedded to a regression approach. It needs to be borne in mind that the shortened scale, using only 11 core symptoms of depression, was derived from our 'categorical' measure of depression. Moreover, the results dealing with the shortened version still leave obscure the question of the relative importance of initial symptoms and social factors in predicting subsequent depression. We believe it therefore would be highly misleading to take literally the relative importance of the relevant beta weights when using score B (Table 4.10).

The issues here are complex, and perhaps it is sufficient to state our belief that the contribution of symptoms falling short of caseness is best explored by traditional tabular analyses and this followed up by logistic regression using categorical measures of clinical state. For example, a straightforward tabulation makes clear that the predictive importance of symptoms at time 1 (once cases of depression are excluded) appears to involve all diagnostic conditions, particularly of anxiety, as long as they are chronic (Brown *et al.*, 1986: Tables 2 and 3). However, their importance appears to be related to their correlation with ongoing difficulties: chronic subclinical symptoms present at the time of first interview are entirely unrelated to subsequent development of caseness depression once such background difficulties and the severe events (to which they often lead) are taken into account (Brown *et al.*, 1986). In other words we are not rejecting multivariate techniques as such – but advocating their use in parallel with more traditional methods.

It is perhaps in order here to cite just one more result since it further underlines the importance of a categorical approach. In an exercise, not so far reported, the original continuous measure (which did not produce an interactive effect) was used as a dichotomy. The cut-point used defined 21% of the sample as 'cases' of depression in the follow-up year (63/303) once the chronic Bedford College cases were excluded. This did produce a statistically significant interactive effect for provoking agent and vulnerability factor unlike its counterpart analysis with the continuous measure in Table 4.4. This measure of 'caseness' as well as including all 32 onsets of depression included 21 of the 27 onsets of borderline depression. Given the inclusion of the latter (and 10 without an onset of a depressive condition), it would be expected that the beta weight for the interaction between provoking agent and vulnerability factor is somewhat lower than with symptom score B (0.26 versus 0.37: see Table 4.10). The important point is that a measure of depression apparently unsuitable for use as a continuous measure produced the 'correct' result when used as a dichtomy.

In the light of these comments it is interesting to reconsider some of the conclusions often cited in the literature. For example, Akiskal cites two studies as evidence that psychosocial factors 'seem to determine the timing of depressive onsets, rather than their fundamental causes' because the authors found that 'the variance contributed by life stressors was quite modest, compared with that contributed by a personal history of depression' (Akiskal, 1985: 133). One of these studies had carried out an analysis not unlike our Tables 4.8 and 4.11 here, but over a three-year rather than a one-year follow-up period, concluding that time 1 depression scores accounted for more explained variance (both unique and shared) than the other factors, losses (like our provoking agents) and resources (like our vulnerability) (Warheit, 1979). Although most of the 18 items of the depression scale used are relatively specific to depression rather than tension or anxiety, there was still scope for noise to enter the dimension through some of the less specific items such as tiredness and somatic complaints. It is therefore difficult to tell whether the depression score used by Warheit would more resemble the longer one used in Table 4.8 or score B used in Table 4.11 but, as we have argued, his inclusion of 'cases' at time 1 would be bound to have raised the beta coefficient of initial symptom score, and to draw conclusions about the relative causal importance of factors on that basis would be misleading in the way we have outlined. The second study spanned a nine-year follow-up period and examined its series of multiple logistic models twice, once including and once excluding those who were cases at first interview (Kaplan, Roberts, Camacho & Coyne, 1987). The authors comment that it is 'perhaps not surprising' that the strongest predictor of a high level of depressive symptoms in 1974 was a high level in 1965, and in general do not adopt the rather superior attitude towards the variable embodying the psychosocial environment which Akiskal seems to attribute to them. They conclude 'what is most important is that the pattern of depressive symptoms at baseline status... psychosocial factors and physical health problems are major predictors of high levels of depressive symptoms'. They have not, however, given models with interaction terms.

Another analysis often cited in the literature used multiple regression to explore the effects of a number of childhood and adult demographic variables upon adult psychiatric morbidity, measured by the Index of Definition (Tennant *et al.*, 1982). This was a cross-sectional analysis, so the problems arising from the inclusion of initial symptom score, or cases at first interview, do not arise; but another issue raised in our analysis might have some relevance and so is worth airing. This concerns the use of ID rather than a purer measure of depression. The authors themselves address the possibility that the estimate of variance explained by childhood loss and deprivation might have been higher if there had not been, what we have here called 'noise', introduced by their choice of dependent variable, and mention that 'most subjects with "disorder" had depressive syndromes (67%)' (p. 326). However the noise which concerns them is rather different from the noise we focused on here in discussing ID. The very fact that they slip so easily into talking in terms of a dichotomous category (with or without 'disorder') suggests that they are forgetting that the dispersion of ID points 1 to 4 is going to prove just as important for their analysis as the points above the usual threshold taken for caseness – level 5 – which is presumably where they divide those with and without disorder. For us the noise is introduced by the respondents with zero on score B but scores of 2 and above on ID (see Table 4.14). Tennant and colleagues, however, are concerned about the possibility that respondents with 'transient distress responses' might be diluting the true depressions, and suggest that the way to distinguish these would be to determine which were caused by life events rather than to incorporate further symptom criteria to make the distinction. Nevertheless, despite our substantially differing definitions of the noise, Tennant and colleagues are highlighting a similar general issue to the one identified in this chapter: that estimates of a variable's importance occasionally need an upward revision if the variable concerned really specifically affects depression, and the measure used has been the ID.

What is interesting is that all of the three studies just cited have felt the need to utilize categorical measures at some point in the reports, usually in describing how many were depressed or suffered from disorder at a given stage. But then they have gone on to analyse the data using a continuous measure. Finally we should not omit to mention a fourth study which, with concepts similar to those discussed here, did analyze the data twice: once treating depression as an interval variable (CES-D), and once as a dichotomy – with the cut-off at 16 and above (Lin & Ensel, 1984). In neither analysis did they confirm any effect of the interaction between life events (corresponding to our provoking agent) and social support (corresponding to our vulnerability), but this may be the result of their using *change* in CES-D score rather than CES-D score at time 2, and especially change in life event score and change in social support, as the key variables. As will be appreciated, the effect of social support upon depressive onset is not necessarily through a *change* in its amount but more usually through an absolute low level which may be unchanging. Lin & Ensel control for initial symptom score by entering CES-D at time 1 (CES-D1) along with change in life events and change in social support, and find it has a higher beta weight than the latter two, but do not then move on to attribute greater aetiological importance to CES-D1 than to psychosocial factors. This is possibly because the beta weight here is negative as a result of the nature of the dependent variable (change in CES-D score rather than its absolute level at time 2). However another series of analyses of the same data focusing on CES-D2 (Lin & Dean, 1984) does not automatically enter CES-D1 along with the psychosocial variables: this suggests that in general they are considerably less preoccupied with this issue of the relative importance of symptomatological and psychosocial factors than the other authors cited earlier.

To sum up then, we have identified a set of possible analyses which, if reported, could prove genuinely misleading. The origins of these misconceptions may lie as much in substantive issues of measurement as in the use of the regression procedure itself. In other words, the failure to appreciate discontinuities in the aetiological process may arise more from deficiencies in conceptualizing the specific nature of depression as opposed to psychiatric disorder in general, than from the use of continuous scores and the consequent failure to employ categories with boundaries which coincide with this discontinuity. After all, it could be said that specificity is conceptually allied to discontinuity. Yet it could be argued that it is exactly the beguiling accessibility of computerized multiple regression programmes requiring a continuous score for the dependent variable that tempts research workers into the use of dimensions which do not embody the phenomenon they set out to study.

Finally, it has become much clearer to us that the shortcomings of multiple regression in the present instance primarily involve its use in opening up a field of enquiry. It would clearly be possible with the exercise of some ingenuity to replicate and make sense of the basic findings concerning the vulnerability effect in terms of multiple regression as long as we are willing to deal with effects non-hierarchically. If we are forced to draw a conclusion, other than underlining the possible pitfalls of multiple regression as a technique of choice for studying clinically relevant phenomena, it is to emphasize the wisdom of employing a number of approaches in opening up an area of enquiry, and particularly that multivariate statistical techniques should not be seen as replacing traditional methods involving direct 'eyeballing' of data.

ACKNOWLEDGEMENTS

The Islington study was funded by the Medical Research Council London. We are grateful to Laurie Letchford for his tireless help with the computer, to Sue Ross for preparation of the manuscript and to Martin Eales and Andrew Pickles for their comments on an earlier draft.

REFERENCES

Achen, C. H. (1982). Interpreting and using regression. Sage University Paper series on: *Quantitative applications in the Social Sciences*, (eds.) John L. Sullivan & Richard G. Niemi. Sage Pubns.

Akiskal, H. S. (1985). Interaction of biologic and psychologic factors in the origin of depressive disorders. *Acta Psychiatrica Scandinavica, 71*, 131–139.

Bebbington, P. (1980). Causal models and logical inference in epidemiological psychiatry. *British Journal of Psychiatry, 136*, 317–325.

Beck, A. J., Ward, C. H., Mendelson, M., Mock, J. & Erbaugh, J. (1961). An inventory for measuring depression. *Archives of General Psychiatry, 4*, 561–571.

Blot, W. J. & Day, N. E. (1978). Synergism and interaction: are they equivalent? *American Journal of Epidemiology, 110*, 99–100.

Brown, G. W. (1986). Statistical interaction and the role of social factors in the aetiology of clinical depression. *Sociology, 20*, 135–140.

Brown, G. W. (1989*a*). Causal paths, chains and strands. In M. Rutter (ed.), *The power of longitudinal data: Studies of risk and protective factors for psychosocial disorders.* Cambridge University Press.

Brown, G. W., Bifulco, A. & Andrews, B. (1990). Self-esteem and depression III. Aetiological issues. *Social Psychiatry and Psychiatric Epidemiology, 25*, 235–243.

Brown, G. W. & Harris, T. O. (1978*a*). *Social origins of depression: A study of psychiatric disorder in women.* London: Tavistock Publications.
Brown, G. W. & Harris, T. O. (1978*b*). Social origins of depression: A reply. *Psychological Medicine, 8,* 577–588.
Brown, G. W. & Harris, T. O. (1980). Further comments on the vulnerability model. *British Journal of Psychiatry, 137,* 584–585.
Brown, G. W. & Harris, T. O. (1986*a*). Establishing causal links: The Bedford College studies of depression. In H. Katschnig (ed.), *Life events and psychiatric disorders* (pp. 107–187). Cambridge University Press.
Brown, G. W. & Harris, T. O. (1986*b*). Stressor, vulnerability and depression: A question of replication. *Psychological Medicine, 16,* 739–744.
Brown, G. W. & Prudo, R. (1981). Psychiatric disorder in a rural and an urban population. 1. Aetiology of depression. *Psychological Medicine, 11,* 581–599.
Brown, G. W., Craig, T. K. J. & Harris, T. O. (1985). Depression: Distress or disease? Some epidemiological considerations. *British Journal of Psychiatry, 147,* 612–622.
Brown, G. W., Bifulco, A., Harris, T. O. & Bridge, L. (1986). Life stress, chronic subclinical symptoms and vulnerability to clinical depression. *Journal of Affective Disorders, 11,* 1–19.
Brown, G. W., Bifulco, A. & Harris, T. O. (1987). Life events, vulnerability and onset of depression: Some refinements. *British Journal of Psychiatry, 150,* 30–42.
Cooper, J. E., Copeland, J. R. N., Brown, G. W., Harris, T. O. & Gourlay, A. J. (1977). Further studies on interviewer training and inter-rater reliability of the Present State Examination (PSE). *Psychological Medicine, 7,* 517–523.
Endicott, J. & Spitzer, R. L. (1978). A diagnostic interview – The schedule for affective disorders and schizophrenia. *Archives of General Psychiatry, 35,* 837–844.
Everitt, B. S. & Smith, A. M. R. (1979). Interactions in contingency tables: a brief discussion of alternative definitions. *Psychological Medicine, 9,* 581–583.
Finlay-Jones, R. (1989). Anxiety. In G. W. Brown & T. O. Harris (eds.) *Life events and illness.* New York: Guilford Press. London: Unwin Hyman.
Finlay-Jones, R. & Brown, G. W. (1981). Types of stressful life events and the onset of anxiety and depressive disorders. *Psychological Medicine, 11,* 803–815.
Finlay-Jones, R., Brown, G. W., Duncan-Jones, P., Harris, T. O., Murphy, E. & Prudo, R. (1980). Depression and anxiety in the community: Replicating the diagnosis of a case. *Psychological Medicine, 10,* 445–454.
Goldberg, D., Cooper, B., Eastwood, M., Kedward, H. & Shepherd, M. (1970). A standardized psychiatric interview for use in community surveys. *British Journal of Preventive and Social Medicine, 24,* 18–23.
Hamilton, M. (1960). A rating scale for depression. *Journal of Neurology and Neurosurgical Psychiatry, 23,* 56–62.
Hellevik, O. (1984). *Introduction to causal analysis.* London: Allen and Unwin.
Kaplan, G. A., Roberts, R. E., Camacho, T. C. & Coyne, J. C. (1987). Psychosocial predictors of depression. Prospective evidence from the human population laboratory studies. *American Journal of Epidemiology, 125*(2), 206–220.

Lewis-Beck, M. S. (1980). Applied regression – an introduction. Sage University Paper series: *Quantitative applications in the social sciences.* Beverly Hills and London: Sage Pubns.

Lin, N. & Dean, A. (1984). Social support and depression: A panel study. *Social Psychiatry, 19,* 83–91.

Lin, N. & Ensel, W. (1984). Depression-mobility and its social etiology: The role of life events and social support. *Journal of Health and Social Behaviour, 25,* 176–188.

Medawar, P. B. (1969). *Induction and intuition in scientific thought.* London: Methuen.

Ostrom, C. W., Jr (1978). Time series analysis: Regression techniques. Sage University Paper series: *Quantitative applications in the social sciences.* Beverly Hills and London: Sage Pubns.

Prudo, R., Brown, G. W., Harris, T. O. & Dowland, J. (1981). Psychiatric disorder in a rural and an urban population: 2. Sensitivity to loss. *Psychological Medicine, 11,* 601–616.

Rothman, K. J. (1974). Synergy and antagonism in cause-effect relationships. *American Journal of Epidemiology, 99,* 385–388.

Rothman, K. J. (1976). The estimation of synergy or antagonism. *American Journal of Epidemiology, 103,* 506–511.

Rothman, K. J. (1978). Occam's razor pares the choice among statistical models. *American Journal of Epidemiology, 108,* 347–349.

Schroeder, L. D., Sjoquist, D. L. & Stephan, P. E. (1986). Understanding regression analysis – an introductory guide. Sage University Paper series: *Quantitative applications in the social sciences.* Beverly Hills and London: Sage Pubns.

Swafford, M. (1980). Three parametric techniques for contingency table analysis: a nontechnical commentary. *American Sociological Review, 45,* 664–690.

Tennant, C. & Bebbington, P. (1978). The social causation of depression: A critique of the work of Brown and his colleagues. *Psychological Medicine, 8,* 565–575.

Tennant, C., Bebbington, P. & Hurry, J. (1982). Social experiences in childhood and adult psychiatric morbidity: A multiple regression analysis. *Psychological Medicine, 12,* 321–327.

Warheit, G. J. (1979). Life events, coping, stress, and depressive symptomatology. *American Journal of Psychiatry, 136,* 502–507.

Wing, J. K., Cooper, J. E. & Sartorius, N. (1974). *The measurement and classification of psychiatric symptoms: an instruction manual for the Present State Examination and CATEGO Programme.* Cambridge University Press.

Wing, J. K., Henderson, A. S. & Winckle, M. (1977) The rating of symptoms by a psychiatrist and a non-psychiatrist: A study of patients referred from general practice. *Psychological Medicine, 7,* 713–715.

5 Differential development of health in a life-span perspective

LEIV S. BAKKETEIG, PER MAGNUS AND JON MARTIN SUNDET

The area of research suggested in the title covers both descriptive and analytical epidemiology. The challenge for descriptive studies is to demonstrate in a valid and representative manner the variance among individuals or groups of individuals in health-related issues at any one time, and to describe alterations in health status over extended periods of time. This makes it possible to study interindividual variation in longitudinal health patterns. In the analytical studies, the aim is to explain this variation in terms of environmental or genetic exposures. The focus in this presentation is on methods for empirical research in analytic epidemiology. Some alternative designs will briefly be discussed, but the main emphasis will be placed on data linkage studies employing data from a population-based medical birth register in Norway.

The analytical designs can be roughly divided into ecological studies, cross-sectional studies, and longitudinal studies (or cohort studies) of individuals or groups of individuals.

Let us first briefly look at how, in the lack of individual data, ecological approaches have been used to examine differential development of health in a life-span perspective. Mortality has a long tradition for being used as an indicator of health when one has to rely on vital statistics or other routinely collected health data. The relative development of mortality (be it crude, disease specific, or age and sex specific) over time can be of interest to use as the basis for comparison between areas or populations.

In Norway, in the middle of the last century, a theologist, Eilert Sundt, did some highly interesting studies. He described the overall mortality in the country using a clerical administrative basis for defining the geographical areas. 130 years later a medical geographer, Asbjørn Aase, in Trondheim has reproduced Sundt's exercise. The relative mortality in different regions of Norway has not changed too much over this long period (Aase, 1985), with one exception, however: namely parts of western Norway (Bergen and surrounding areas) which have changed dramatically from being among the worst regions to become among the best ones.

This, of course, represents a very crude approach to examining developments of health in different geographical areas over an extremely long time period (3–4 generations). However, this crude look into relative trends might provide useful insights, and clues for further research.

Another Norwegian example is shown in Figure 5.1. Here geographical units (in this case counties) are used to compare adult mortality among males aged 40–69 years with the general living conditions during their childhood, using infant mortality in their home areas at time of birth as an indicator of their childhood living conditions. The curves are strikingly parallel.

This covariation is particularly strong for coronary heart deaths, which has been pursued in separate analyses in the northern part of Norway as part of the cardiovascular disease survey in the county of Finnmark, 1974–5. The question was raised whether poor living

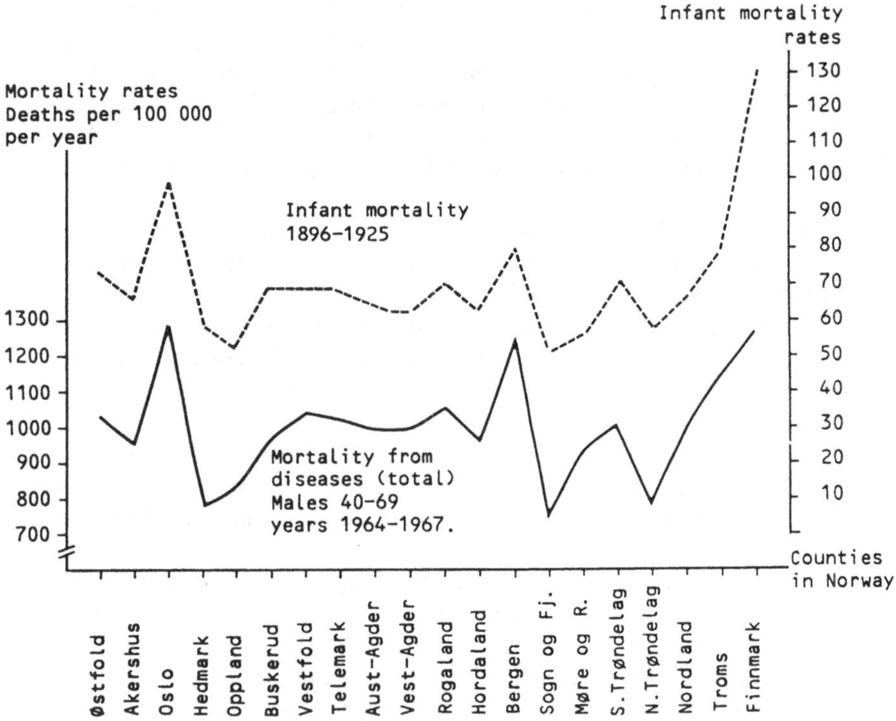

Figure 5.1. General mortality for Norwegian males aged 40–69 years during the time period 1964–7, and the infant mortality around the time of their birth 1896–1925 by county. Forsdahl (1988, personal communication).

conditions during childhood and adolescence are important risk factors for arteriosclerotic heart disease later in life (Forsdahl, 1977, 1978). Also, using a similar approach to the one mentioned above, serum cholesterol for men aged 35–49 years living in the different municipalities of Finnmark county (the northernmost county in Norway) has been compared with the infant mortality around the time of the birth of these men in their home areas. Again, as shown in Figure 5.2, a quite striking covariation emerges.

Of course such relationships as the ones shown here must be interpreted with the greatest caution, and the comparisons are associated with many fallacies which will not be further discussed in this chapter. But the findings might point to issues worth pursuing in further studies. In the Tromsø heart study it became possible to examine this relationship on an individual basis (Arnesen & Forsdahl, 1985). They were able to demonstrate, based on 7405 males and 7247 females, a significant correlation between age-adjusted cholesterol level and their parents' economic conditions during their childhood. Poverty during childhood was positively associated with age-adjusted levels of total cholesterol and negatively associated with body weight. When cholesterol was adjusted for age, body mass index, physical activity, coffee and alcohol consumption, and cigarette smoking, there remained a significant linear correlation with poverty during childhood.

Several later similar correlation studies have indicated that the mixture of early poverty and later affluence could be a leading determinant of degenerative arterial diseases during adulthood (Barker & Osmond, 1986, 1987), although there is still a lot of controversy over these issues

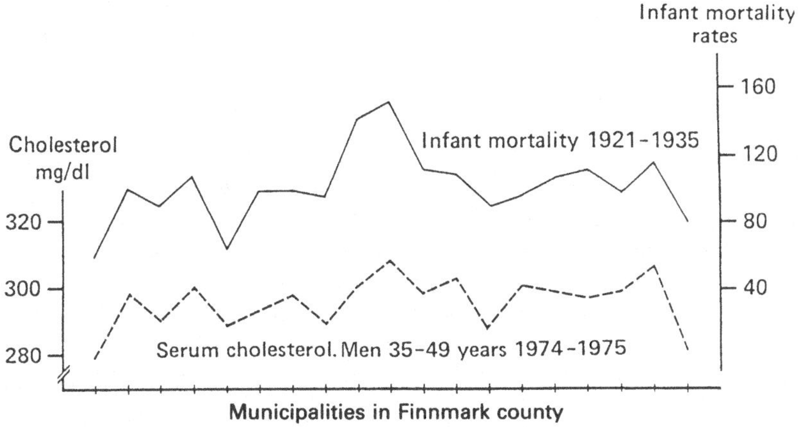

Figure 5.2. Serum cholesterol (mg/dl) for men aged 35–49 years in 1974–5 and the infant mortality at time of their birth 1921–35 by municipality in Finnmark county. Forsdahl (1978).

(Williams, Roberts & Davis, 1979). Infant nutrition has been singled out as a possible mechanism behind the above mentioned correlations (*Lancet*, 1988). However, a great deal of uncertainty still exists as to the other factors which could act as programming mechanisms for long-term effects of infant nutrition as well as for later developments and susceptibility of diseases (Lucas, 1987; Byckling *et al.*, 1985).

Further longitudinal studies are needed to explore some of these relationships between intrauterine, infancy and childhood exposures, and adult morbidity and mortality.

Some longitudinal data analysis approaches will be demonstrated in the following sections of this chapter based on data from the Norwegian Medical Birth Register. This register is based on medical notification of all births in Norway since 1967. The register contains civic and medical information on all live births and fetal deaths aged 16 weeks or more, and some information on their parents.

The infants and their parents are all identified through a unique ID-number (11 digits). Furthermore, the data in the register are constantly updated with survival data provided through a record linkage with the death file kept in the Central Bureau of Statistics.

This updated register facilitates three different types of 'life-span' longitudinal approaches.

1. A complete follow-up of survival through childhood can be provided.
2. The complete reproductive lifetime of women can be examined, based on linkage of successive pregnancies to the same mothers.
3. Generation studies can eventually be carried out as the cohorts of births start to reproduce themselves, regarding the time from conception of a fetus until it reproduces itself as a generation 'life-span'.

CHILDHOOD 'LIFE-SPAN' COHORT STUDY

Let us look at the first approach. Table 5.1 shows the total mortality during the first 15 years of life for births in Norway 1967–71. The births are separated into two groups: illegitimate and legitimate. As the table shows, the illegitimate births had about an 80% increased mortality at birth and shortly thereafter. It is also worth noticing that the relative risk was increased throughout their childhood. This increased risk is even better demonstrated in Table 5.2 where the cumulative survival rates at different ages are shown. From the table it can be derived that at the age of one year the illegitimate children had a cumulative mortality 75% higher than the legitimate ones. And during childhood (from two years onwards) the illegitimate children still had 40% higher mortality. This observation indicates that the factors

Table 5.1. *Stillbirth rates (per thousand births) and childhood mortality rates (per thousand liveborn children) up to 15 years of age according to maternal marital status at time of birth*

	Marital status Married		Unmarried		
	N	Rate	*N*	Rate	Relative risk
Total births	314 813		19 859		
Stillbirths	4337	13.78	486	24.47	1.78
Total live births	310 476		19 373		
Neonatal deaths	2974	9.58	344	17.76	1.85
Postneonatal deaths	1016	3.27	90	4.65	1.42
Deaths 2nd year	345	1.11	19	0.98	0.88
Deaths 3rd year	239	0.77	19	0.98	1.27
Deaths 4th–6th year	507	1.63	48	2.48	1.52
Deaths 7th–9th year	295	0.95	21	1.08	1.14
Deaths 10th–12th year	181	0.58	18	0.93	1.60
Deaths 13th–15th year	195	0.63	13	0.67	1.06
Total deaths among live births	5752	18.53	572	29.53	1.59

associated with their mothers' marital and social status at time of birth play a role in determining their long-term survival chances.

These observations will have to be followed up by specially designed studies aimed at teasing out the factors and mechanisms which underlie such associations.

REPRODUCTIVE 'LIFE-SPAN' COHORT STUDY

As to the second approach, in the study of perinatal events it is desirable to take advantage of the heterogeneity of reproductive careers which exists within the population of childbearing women. Data collected longitudinally on successive pregnancies to the same mother facilitate comparisons between groups of women with contrasting reproductive outcomes (Bakketeig & Hoffman, 1981). The results from such studies are more directly related to understanding different outcomes as they relate to the reproductive careers of individual women. Also such a longitudinal approach will tend to disclose obvious artefact of groupings which are associated with cross-sectional data analyses.

An example is shown in Figure 5.3. The data shown are based on 232 359 women who gave birth to their firstborns (singleborns) during the first five-year period with available register data, 1967–71. By

Table 5.2. *Survival through pregnancy, infancy and childhood of births in Norway 1967–71 by their mothers' marital status at time of birth*[a]

Interval	Legitimate				Illegitimate			
	Alive at start of interval	Dead during interval	$P_{Survival}$	Cumulative $P_{Survival}$	Alive at start of interval	Dead during interval	$P_{Survival}$	Cumulative $P_{Survival}$
16 weeks gest.–birth	314 813	4337	0.9862	0.9862	19 859	486	0.9755	0.9755
Birth–23 hours	310 476	1575	0.9949	0.9812	19 373	186	0.9904	0.9661
1–6 days	308 901	1055	0.9966	0.9778	19 187	119	0.9938	0.9601
7–27 days	307 846	344	0.9989	0.9767	19 068	39	0.9980	0.9581
28–364 days	307 502	1016	0.9967	0.9735	19 029	90	0.9953	0.9536
1–2 years	306 486	345	0.9989	0.9724	18 939	19	0.9990	0.9526
2–15 years	306 141	1417	0.9954	0.9680	18 920	119	0.9937	0.9467

[a] The assumption made here is that all births can be followed up.

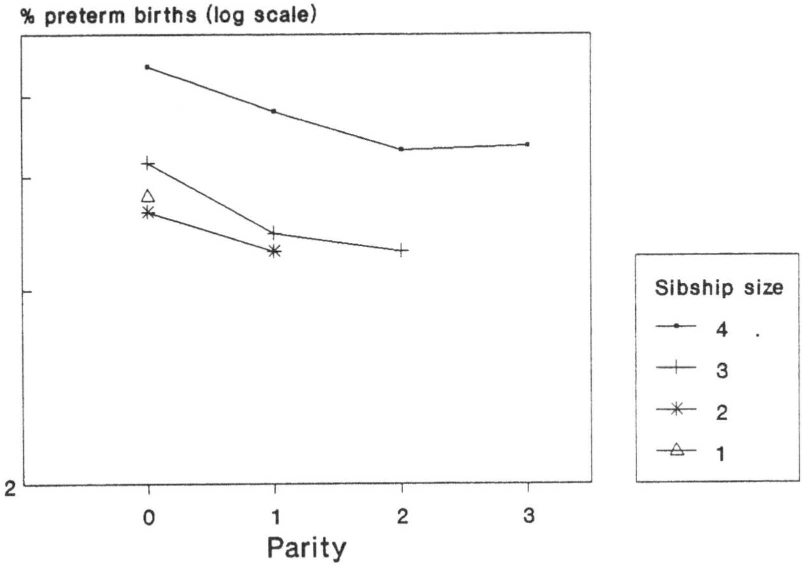

Figure 5.3. Frequency of preterm birth by parity for women grouped by the size of their sibships. (Based on a 15–20 year follow-up of 232 359 women who had their first singleton birth in the five-year period 1967–71.)

following these women during a 15–20 year period (through 1986), one can assume that practically all of them have completed their childbearing period. Thus, we can group the women according to the size of their attained sibships, one to four, and examine a time-related variable such as parity and its association with for example the risk of preterm birth (defined as delivery before 37 completed weeks or 259 days of gestation).

Two features emerge from the figure: first, within each sibship group the risk of preterm birth drops with increasing parity and, secondly, the level of risk increases with the sibship size. This relationship is in contrast to the association between parity and the risk of preterm birth, which emerges when a cross-sectional approach is employed. There one lumps together all first births, all second, all third and all fourth births regardless of which subgroup of mothers to which they belong. And the well-known U-shaped (or J-shaped) curve appears as shown in the superimposed line graph in Figure 5.4. This means that the cross-sectional approach obviously masks the underlying associations between parity and risk of preterm birth, and the U-shaped curve in itself becomes an artefact.

However, the associations demonstrated using the longitudinal approach based on groups of women defined by their attained sibship size do not necessarily disclose the 'true' relationship between parity and the

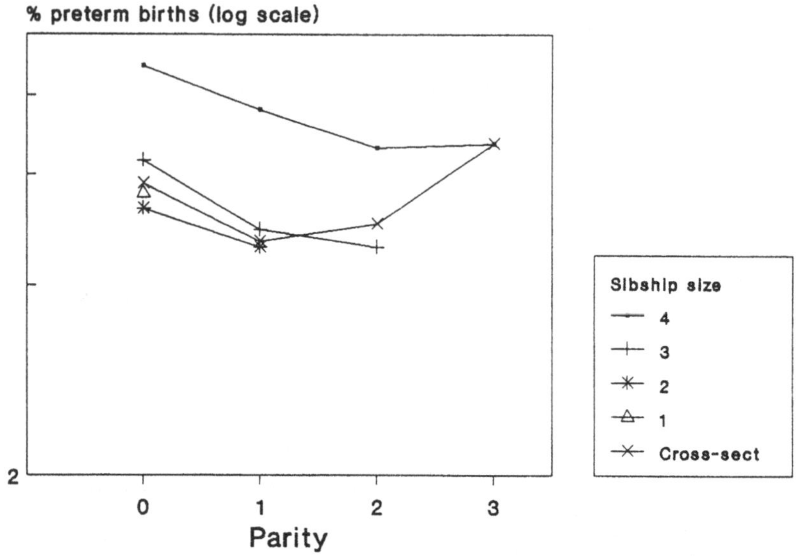

Figure 5.4. Frequency of preterm births by parity comparing a longitudinal and cross-sectional approach to the data analyses. (Based on a 15–20 year follow-up of 232 359 women who had their first singleton birth in the five-year period 1967–71.)

risk of preterm birth. The self-selection for pregnancy which obviously takes place tends to bias the larger sibship groups to have an over-representation of women with adverse pregnancy outcomes. Thus, for example there is a tendency to replace a lost birth, while women are more likely to stop childbearing after a 'success'. But such built-in biases do not fully explain the pattern within sibship groups shown. Thus, for example, by excluding all fetal deaths from the analysis the basic features shown still persist, although the differences in the level of risk between the different sibship size groups become somewhat reduced (Bakketeig & Hoffman, 1981). Also, the downward slope with increasing parity within sibship groups persists after adjusting for the trend of falling mortality rates over the period of observation.

LONGITUDINAL VERSUS CROSS-SECTIONAL FINDINGS

The discrepancy between cross-sectional and longitudinal findings demonstrated here are quite universal. They certainly apply to a whole variety of analyses based on perinatal events and the assessment of risks, for example perinatal mortality and the occurrence of congenital malformations (Bakketeig & Hoffman, 1979).

As mentioned previously, in analytical longitudinal studies one needs to collect data on exposures and potential effects preferably in a rather detailed manner. And this becomes of great importance once one examines variables which vary over time and particularly variables which can be affected by the outcome under study. In such situations findings based on cross-sectional studies might be very misleading indeed. For example, the U-shaped curve which has been demonstrated for the association between mortality (particularly cardiovascular) and alcohol drinking, seems to be produced by this kind of bias, ignoring the dynamic relationship between ill-health and drinking behavior (Shaper, Walker & Wannamethee, 1988). Another example can be found in the study of body weight (body mass index) and general mortality focusing on middle-aged men, where those with the lowest and highest body mass index (BMI) have the highest mortality. However, adding the information on BMI at younger ages it appears that the increased mortality among thin middle-aged men is often due to occult antecedent diseases rather then leanness *per se* and these middle-aged men tended to have lost weight before the weight examination in their middle age. (Rhoads & Kagan, 1983).

GENERATION 'LIFE-SPAN' STUDY

The third approach based on the medical birth register data set refers to generation studies. Let us focus on girls born in 1967 and 1968 who in 1986 and 1987 have delivered a total of 4485 children. The covariation across generations of the variables gestational length and birth weight are studied.

The factors governing the length of gestation are largely unknown. For example, is there a strong genetic component associated with the risk of having a preterm delivery? For the 3663 mother–child pairs where gestational age was known, the correlation in gestational length was 0.043. Among 153 mothers who themselves were preterm (less than 37 weeks gestation), 13 (8.5%) gave birth to preterm children. Among the remaining 3510 pairs where the mother had been born after 37 weeks, 301 (8.6%) preterm children were born in the next generation. Thus, no significant covariation across generations was observed for this variable, suggesting that genetic effects have little influence on the variance.

Birth weight was known in both generations for 4464 mother–child pairs. The correlation coefficient for this variable across generations was 0.198 ($p < 0.001$). The 179 mothers who themselves had a birth weight below 2500 grams, delivered 20 (11.2%) children with low birth weight, whereas 272 (6.4%) children with low birth weight was born of the 4285 mothers with birth weight of 2500 grams or more, yielding a relative risk of 1.76.

The observed covariation between the birth weights of mother and child could be explained by several mechanisms. One mechanism could be underlying covariation between environmental factors across generations, for instance associated with socioeconomic status. Another mechanism could be covariation (between effects in the grandmother and the mother) in natural genetic effects in pregnancy, and a third possibility could be covariation in effects of fetal genes. These alternative mechanisms will be explored in future studies in the birth register based on observed covariations in birth weight between father and child and between members of maternal and paternal halfsibships. Using models developed in the field of quantitative genetics, expectations based on the alternative mechanisms will be compared with the observed patterns of covariation (Magnus, 1984).

RECORD LINKAGE STUDIES

The types of studies mentioned above are based on exploration of the data within the medical birth register. In addition possibilities exist for linking information with other registers. For example, record linkage based on the individual ID number can be made with the cancer register, examining the associations between perinatal conditions and events and later occurrence of cancer. Further, census data can be linked to the medical birth register data and provide valuable information on educational, occupational and social factors, which are lacking in the medical birth register (Arntzen, Magnus & Bakketeig, 1988). Furthermore, a twin register exists in Norway covering twins born since 1895. The medical birth register data can be linked with data from the twin register, for example, studying the birth weight for offspring of birth weight discordant monozygotic female twins (Magnus, Berg & Bjerkedal, 1985).

However, we still lack morbidity data for longitudinal studies: for example, there is a need for data on disorders/handicaps among children which could be related to perinatal events. A register based on information about hospital in-patients might be a valuable source for some of the needed longitudinal health data. A reporting system needed for such a register is underway in Norway.

It should be stressed that even though some valuable health registries do exist in countries such as Norway and some new important data collection systems might appear on the scene in the not-too-distant future, we still need to establish better exposure measurements and even exposure registers. This will turn out to be crucial in future epidemiological research, especially in longitudinal studies.

Also, we stress that register data will definitely need to be supplemented by data obtained retrospectively through special studies, by for example, using population registers as the sampling frame.

CONCLUDING REMARKS

In this chapter we have underlined the importance of longitudinal data analyses and the need for longitudinal information of individual exposure to health hazards as well as health consequences themselves throughout life. We have demonstrated the utilization of a population-based medical birth register in 'life-span' studies (childhood, reproductive and generation 'life-span'). And we have stressed some of the fallacies associated with cross-sectional analyses. Finally, we have underlined the importance of generation studies as such data eventually become available.

Although longitudinal studies based on longitudinally collected data are superior, we will also have to rely on longitudinal studies based on retrospectively collected data.

ACKNOWLEDGEMENT

We want to express our gratitude to professors Asbjørn Aase and Anders Forsdahl for their kind assistance in making data available. Also we thank Mrs Inger Naerbø for highly skilful secretarial assistance.

REFERENCES

Aase, A. (1985). Levekår i velferdsstaten. 3. Gjessing I, In H. Myklebost & H. Solerød (eds.), *Norge 3 Folk og Samfinn* (pp. 216–239). Oslo: Cappelen.

Arnesen, E. & Forsdahl, A. (1985). The Tromsø heart study: coronary risk factors and their associations with living conditions during childhood. *Journal of Epidemiology and Community Health, 39,* 210–214.

Arntzen, A., Magnus, P. & Bakketeig, L. S. (1988). Parental education in relation to foetal death and early infant deaths. *Tidsskrift for Den norske laegeforening, 108,* 3082–3085.

Bakketeig, L. S. & Hoffman, H. J. (1979). Perinatal mortality by birth order within cohorts based on sibship size. *British Medical Journal, 2,* 693–696.

Bakketeig, L. S. & Hoffman, H. J. (1981). Epidemiology of preterm birth: results from a longitudinal study of births in Norway. In M. G. Elder & C. H. Hendricks (eds.), *Preterm labor.* London: Butterworth.

Bakketeig, L. S., Hoffman, H. J. & Harley, E. E. (1979). The tendency to repeat gestational age and birth weight in successive births. *American Journal of Obstetrics and Gynecology, 135,* 1086–1103.

Barker, D. J. P. & Osmond, C. (1986). Infant mortality, childhood nutrition and ischemic heart disease in England and Wales. *The Lancet, 1,* 1077–1081.

Barker, D. J. P. & Osmond, C. (1987). Death rates from stroke in England and Wales predicted from past maternal mortality. *British Medical Journal, 295,* 83–86.

Byckling, T., Åkerblom, H. K., Viikari, J., Louhivouri, K., Uhari, M. & Kasanen, L. *et al.* (1985). Artherosclerosis precursors in Finnish children and adolescents IX Socioeconomic status and risk factors of coronary heart disease. *Acta Paediatrica Scandinavica Suppl., 318,* 155–167.

Forsdahl, A. (1977). Are poor living conditions in children and adolescence an important risk factor for arteriosclerotic heart disease? *British Journal of Preventive and Social Medicine, 31,* 91–95.

Forsdahl, A. (1978). Living conditions in childhood and subsequent development of risk factors for arteriosclerotic heart disease. *Journal of Epidemiology and Community Health, 32,* 34–37.

The Lancet (1988). Editorial: Infant nutrition and cardiovascular diseases. *The Lancet, 1,* 568–569.

Lucas, A. (1987). Diet in early life: evidence for its later effects. Environmental epidemiology, infant nutrition and cardiovascular disease. Medical Research Council Conference Report.

Magnus, P. (1984). Causes of variation in birth weight: A study of offspring of twins. *Clinical Genetics, 25,* 15–24.

Magnus, P., Berg, K. & Bjerkedal, T. (1985). No significant difference in birth weight for offspring of birth weight discordant monozygotic female twins. *Early Human Development, 12,* 55–59.

Rhoads, G. G. & Kagan, A. (1983). The relation of coronary disease, stroke and mortality to weight in youth and in middle age. *The Lancet, 1,* 492–495.

Shaper, A. G., Walker, M. & Wannamethee, H. (1988). Alcohol and mortality in British men: explaining the u-shaped curve. *The Lancet, 2,* 1267–1273.

Williams, D. R., Roberts, S. J. & Davies, T. W. (1979). Deaths from ischemic heart disease and infarct mortality in England and Wales. *Journal of Epidemiology and Community Health, 33,* 199–202.

6 Assessing change in a cohort-longitudinal study with hierarchical data

DAN OLWEUS AND FRANÇOISE D. ALSAKER

The basic research question to be addressed in the present chapter is the following: How do we measure time-related change in a study with a non-experimental design? Or more specifically: How can we document possible effects of an intervention program against bully/victim problems in school when it is not possible to employ an experimental set-up with randomized assignment of observational units to various treatment conditions?

SOME BACKGROUND INFORMATION

Bully/victim problems among children ('mobbing') have been an issue of great concern in Scandinavia for almost two decades (Olweus, 1973, 1986, in preparation). There is a bully/victim problem in a class or a school when a student, repeatedly and over time, is exposed to harassment and attacks from one or several other students (Olweus, 1991). In addition, there should be a certain imbalance in the strength relations: the student who is exposed to the negative actions should have difficulty defending himself or herself and be somewhat helpless against those who harass.

In Norway, bully/victim problems were a matter of general interest and concern in the mass media and among teachers and parents for a number of years, but the school authorities did not engage themselves officially with the phenomenon. A few years ago, a marked change took place.

In late 1982, a newspaper reported that three 10–14 year old boys from the northern part of Norway had committed suicide, in all probability as a consequence of severe bullying by peers. This event aroused a lot of uneasiness and tension in the mass media and the general public. It triggered a chain of reactions the end result of which was a nationwide campaign against bully/victim problems in Norwegian comprehensive schools (grades 1–9), launched by the Ministry of Education in the fall of 1983.

In that context, I was commissioned by the Ministry of Education to conduct two large-scale research projects on bully/victim problems, one of which will be discussed in some detail in the present chapter. Its basic goal was to evaluate the possible effects of the intervention program that we developed in connection with the nationwide campaign (Olweus, 1986; Olweus & Roland, 1983). Since the campaign was nationwide it was not possible to use an experimental strategy with random allocation of units to various treatments. The task thus made it necessary to face the basic question stated in the introductory section: How do we assess time-related change in a non-experimental study for this kind of problem?

GENERAL METHODOLOGICAL CONSIDERATIONS

In this situation an expanded version of what has been called a 'selection cohorts design' (Cook & Campell, 1979; Reichardt, 1979) was chosen. It may also be termed a *cohort-longitudinal design with adjacent or consecutive cohorts.* Approximately 2500 students, originally in grades 4–7, in 112 classes drawn from 42 schools in Bergen, Norway, were followed over a period of two and a half years. The 500–700 boys and girls selected at each grade level were considered to constitute a cohort. A *cohort* can generically be *defined* as an aggregate of individuals who are born, enter or belong to a particular system (such as the school) in a given year or period and who then age together, at least for some time (cf. Rosow, 1978; Ryder, 1965). In the present study, the subjects belonged to a cohort in the sense that they were joined together in distinct classes within a particular grade level and were approximately the same age. The modal age of members in successive cohorts differed by one year (11–14 at Time 1, see below). For convenience, the four cohorts were named Cohorts 4, 5, 6, and 7 (rather than the more complete 'the Grade 4 cohort', 'the Grade 5 cohort', etc.).

The first measurement took place in May 1983 (Time 1), approximately four months before the initiation of the anti-bullying program. New measurements were taken in May 1984 (Time 2) and May 1985 (Time 3).

A cohort-longitudinal design with adjacent cohorts generates what may be described as an incomplete age-cohort matrix (Nesselroade & Baltes, 1984) in which all of the cohorts are measured at the same time points but (necessarily) at different ages. The basic structure of the design is portrayed in Figure 6.1 (with fictitious data which, however, in some measure resemble the data actually obtained) and in Table 6.1. The modal ages of the various cohorts at the three time points are shown in the cells.

Table 6.1. *Design of the cohort-longitudinal study*

	Time 1	Time 2	Time 3
Cohort 4	11	12	13
Cohort 5	12	13	14
Cohort 6	13	14	15
Cohort 7	14	15	16

Note: The modal ages of the subjects at different time points are given in the cells.

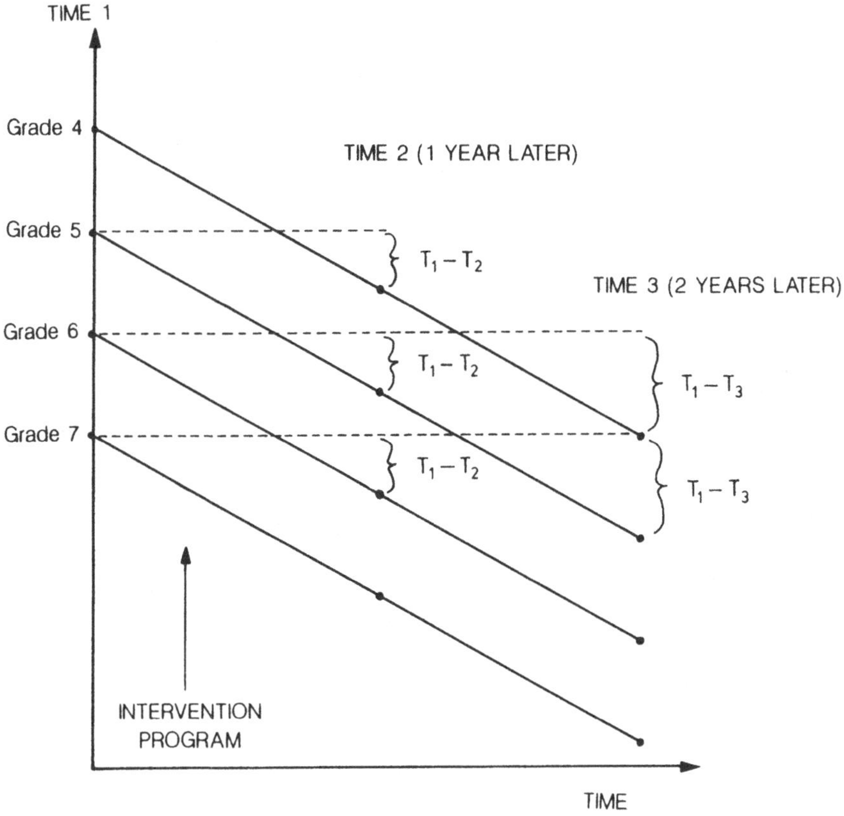

Figure 6.1. Design for evaluation of effects of intervention program. Fictitious data (which to some extent reflect the general trend of the empirical findings).

Since the present study involves several cohorts followed over time it might be thought possible to conduct a straightforward 'cohort analysis' in which the effects of time, age, and cohort and their interactions (and possibly other effects) were unequivocally sorted out. However, there is no simple analytic scheme or combination of schemes that permits unambiguous separation of these effects, as convincingly argued and/or demonstrated by a number of authors (Adam, 1978; Baltes, 1968; Baltes, Cornelius & Nesselroade, 1979; Glenn, 1976; Nesselroade & Baltes, 1974). This is because two kinds of effects are confounded with one another, regardless of how the data are examined: age and time effects in longitudinal (within cohort) trends, age and cohort effects in cross-sectional data for a particular time point, and time and cohort effects for a particular age. Statistical attempts to 'unconfound' these effects mechanically have proven futile and it is now (almost) generally agreed that meaningful disentangling of such effects must rely on theoretical and substantive reasoning and on the making of one or more restricting or simplifying assumptions.

In the present study, the key research question concerns the possible existence of time-related change, in particular effects associated with the operation of the anti-bullying intervention program. In order to evaluate this issue, the strategy of 'time-lagged contrasts between age-equivalent groups' was used. In such an analysis, time of measurement is allowed to vary while age is held constant. More specifically, data collected at Time 1 were used as a base line against which data from Time 2 and Time 3 could be compared (see Figure 6.1). As mentioned, base line data (Time 1) were collected four months before initiation of the intervention program while data obtained at Times 2 and 3 could reflect possible effects of an 8-month and 20-month exposure to the program. To exemplify, the data for Cohort 5 at Time 1 (modal age 12 years) were compared with the Time 2 data for Cohort 4 which at that time had reached the same age as the base line group. The same kind of comparisons were made between Cohort 6 (Time 1) and Cohort 5 (Time 2) and between Cohort 7 (Time 1) and Cohort 6 (Time 2).

Comparisons of data collected at Time 1 and Time 3 permit an assessment of the persistence or possible decline or enhancement of the effects over a longer time span. For these comparisons only data for two of the cohorts could be used as a base line, those of Cohort 6 and Cohort 7, which were contrasted with data collected at Time 3 on Cohort 4 and Cohort 5, respectively. The latter groups had been exposed to the intervention program during approximately 20 months at that time.

The main reason for using time-lagged contrasts between cohorts of the same age, rather than longitudinal comparisons, to evaluate the effects of the intervention program was the fact that there are grounds for expecting changes in bully/victim problems as a function of age (see, e.g., Olweus, 1991). In such a situation, longitudinal comparisons between different time points would reflect both age-related ('maturational') changes and potential effects of the intervention program (and possibly other time-related effects; see below).

However, time-lagged constrasts analysis involves comparison of (at least) two cohorts measured at different time points and, accordingly, systematic differences between cohorts may, in principle, reflect either time-related or cohort-related effects or both. In order to construe such differences as a manifestation of (only or mainly) time-related influences, it is essential to be able to rule out 'cohort effects' as an explanation or to show that such an explanation is unlikely. Before discussing this possibility it is necessary to consider briefly the concept of cohort effects.

COHORT EFFECTS

In a general sense, *cohort effects* are systematic differences, over and above possible, age-related differences, between cohorts measured or observed at the same point in time. Such differences may be a consequence of qualitatively different conditions or experiences, before the actual study, for different cohorts (or a relatively large proportion of their members). They may also reflect the way or the degree to which certain conditions ('historical events') have influenced members of different cohorts.

To exemplify, three cohorts of subjects born in 1910, 1930 and 1950, and interviewed in 1970, would have had qualitatively very different experiences of the Great Depression; for a majority of the members of the youngest cohort this period would be seen only as a historical epoch or a set of events with little emotional significance. For the older cohorts, the years of depression would probably have had a considerable impact but in quite distinct ways since the Depression struck them at very different ages.

Although it is reasonable to postulate that certain conditions or historical events have some generalized effects on members of different cohorts (or a relatively large proportion of their members), which is implied in the concept of cohort effects, it should also be emphasized that members *within a particular cohort* are likely to have been exposed to the events in different ways and to different degrees. The degree and nature of exposure to distinctive events will depend on a number of factors including the person's position in the social hierarchy, and chance. For instance, the effects of the depression years would certainly be quite different for an unemployed industrial worker than for a well-educated person of the same age with a secure position in the state bureaucracy. This has been called the Differential-Effects Problem in the literature on cohort analysis; see Rosow (1978).

If we return to our own empirical study, it is natural to state as a basic assumption that there are no, or only negligible, cohort effects. As mentioned, the modal ages of subjects in successive cohorts were separated by only one year and there are no grounds for expecting that members of different cohorts were exposed (before 1983) to distinctly different conditions that would affect their probability of being involved in bully/victim problems. The majority of the members in the various cohorts had been students in the same schools for several years and there had occurred no systematic changes in the local school system to which all participating schools belonged. It is also difficult to conceive of particular events in the society at large or marked parental changes in child-rearing practices or attitudes that would have resulted in non-negligible cohort effects (over and above possible age differences). Further support for the assumption about the lack of cohort effects comes from the observation that the cross-sectional age trends at Time 1 (before intervention) in this study (Figure 6.8) agree fairly well with the relevant age curves derived from a nationwide survey of more than 80 000 students from all over Norway (Olweus, 1986, 1991).

It should also be noted that what might appear as cohort effects could be the consequence of *sampling or selection bias*. Such apparent, or *non-genuine, cohort effects* could result from inadvertent changes in the recruitment of subjects to the various cohorts so that the cohorts in fact represented populations with different compositional characteristics. Such sampling bias could certainly complicate interpretation of the time-lagged comparisons. In the present study, however, the basic sampling units (classes) were distributed on the cohorts by an essentially random procedure, so there is little reason to suspect 'cohort effects' because of sampling bias. (Non-genuine cohort effects of this kind do not seem to have received much attention in the literature on cohort analysis.)

In addition, the present design using adjacent cohorts provides partial protection against non-genuine cohort effects that might jeopardize the time-lagged comparisons. We here refer to the fact that two of the cohorts serve as a base line group in one set of comparisons and as a treatment group in another. This is the case with Cohort 5 at Time 1, the data for which are used as a base line in comparison with the Cohort 4 data collected at Time 2 (after 8 months of intervention; see Figure 6.1). In addition, the Cohort 5 data obtained at Time 2 serve to evaluate the possible effects of 8 months of intervention when they are compared with the data for Cohort 6 at Time 1. The same situation applies to Cohort 6 in comparisons with Cohorts 5 and 7, respectively.

The advantage of this aspect of the design is that a possible bias in the sampling of the cohorts would operate in opposite directions in the two sets of comparisons, thus making it difficult to obtain consistent 'intervention effects' across cohorts as a consequence of such non-genuine cohort effects. This feature of the design would provide the same kind of protection against faulty conclusions in case the base line data for one or both of these cohorts were unusually high or low simply as a function of chance (*non-genuine cohort effects due to sampling variability*).

Summarizing the foregoing discussion, we can conclude that in the present study possible differences in time-lagged contrasts between age-equivalent groups cannot easily be explained by (genuine) cohort effects. In addition, the design provides good protection against faulty interpretation of the results as a consequence of non-genuine cohort effects associated with sampling bias and sampling variability. Accordingly, presence of systematic differences in time-lagged comparisons very likely reflect time-related changes. This is not to say that such differences necessarily are effects of the anti-bullying intervention program. A conclusion on this point can be reached only after consideration of hypotheses about alternative time-related changes such as effects of repeated measurement and attitude change. These issues will be explored briefly after a presentation of some aspects of the procedure and main results.

OUTCOME VARIABLES

The main variables on which possible effects of the intervention could be expected to show up are of course related to different aspects of bully/victim problems. In the present context mainly data for the key individual items reflecting these problems will be reported. In later publications, analyses of more reliable composites of items will be presented.

The three key items were worded as follows.

1. How often have you been bullied in school? (Being exposed to direct bullying or victimization, with relatively open attacks on the victim.)
2. How often have you taken part in bullying other students in school? (Bullying or victimizing other students.)
3. How often does it happen that other students don't want to spend recess with you and you end up being alone? (Being exposed to indirect bullying or victimization by means of social isolation, exclusion from the group.)

To avoid idiosyncratic interpretations the students were provided with a detailed but simple 'definition' of bullying before answering question 1. And in both the written and the oral instructions, it was repeatedly emphasized that their answers should refer to the situation 'this spring', i.e., the period 'from Christmas until now'. All three questions had the same seven response alternatives, ranging from 'it hasn't happened this spring' (scored 0) over 'now and then' (scored 2) and 'about once a week' (scored 3) to 'several times a day' (scored 6).

Other items referred to being bullied or bullying others respectively on the way to and from school. Several items also concerned the individual's attitude toward victims of bullying (e.g., 'How do you usually feel when you see a student being bullied in school?') and bullying students (e.g., 'What do you think of students who bully others?').

With regard to the validity of self-reports on variables related to bully/victim problems, it may be mentioned that in my early Swedish studies (Olweus, 1978) composites of 3–5 self-report items on being bullied or bullying and attacking others respectively correlated in the range 0.40–0.65 (Olweus, in press, unpublished) with reliable peer ratings on related dimensions (Olweus, 1977). Similarly, Perry, Kusel & Perry (1988) have reported a correlation of 0.42 between a self-report scale of three victimization items and a reliable measure of peer nominations of victimization in elementary schoolchildren.

In the present study we also obtained a kind of peer rating in that each student (in Cohorts 5–7) had to estimate the number of students in his or her class who were bullied or who bullied others during the reference period. These data were aggregated for each class and the resulting class means were correlated with the means derived from the students' own reports of being victimized or victimizing others. The two sets of class means were quite substantially correlated, the average correlations being 0.61 for the victimization dimension and 0.58 for the bullying variable (Time 1). Corresponding coefficients for estimated average *proportion* of students in the class being bullied or bullying others (which measure corrects for differing number of students in the classes) were even somewhat higher, 0.62 and 0.68 respectively. There was thus considerable agreement across classes between class estimates derived from self-reports and from this form of peer ratings. *The results presented above certainly attest to the validity of the self-report data employed.*

Since a link has been established between bullying behavior and antisocial/criminal activities (Olweus, 1978, 1986, 1991) it was hypothesized that the intervention program against bullying *might* also lead to a reduction in antisocial behavior. To measure different aspects of antisocial behavior in relatively young people, preadolescents and adolescents, a new self-report instrument was developed (Olweus & Endresen, in preparation; Olweus, 1989). This inventory shows many similarities with the instruments recently developed by Elliott & Ageton

(1980) and by Hindelang, Hirschi & Weis (1981) but our inventory contained fewer items on serious crimes and more items related to school problems.

Psychometric analyses of the inventory have given quite encouraging results indicating that the scales have satisfactory or good reliability, stability, and validity as well as theoretical relevance (Olweus, 1989).

Finally, it was thought important to assess possible effects on student satisfaction with school life, in particular during recess time. (In Norwegian comprehensive schools, students usually have a break of approximately ten minutes every 45 minutes. In addition, they have a lunch break of 20–30 minutes in the middle of the day.) Since most of the bullying takes place at school (during recess and on the way to and from classes, and not on the way to and from school, see Olweus, 1986, 1991) the following question was considered relevant: 'How do you like recess time?'

STATISTICAL ANALYSES

Since classes rather than students were the basic sampling units (with students nested within classes), it was considered important to choose a data analytic strategy that reflected the basic hierarchical features of the design (see, e.g., Kirk, 1982). Accordingly, data were analyzed with ANOVA (analysis of variance) with students nested within classes nested within schools nested within cohorts (in these particular analyses, nested within times/occasions). Sex of the subjects was crossed with times, schools (within times), and classes (within schools).[1] This means that variation due to schools nested within cohorts, rather than individuals within classes and schools, is the appropriate error term for testing the effects of the intervention program (Time 1 vs Time 2, Time 1 vs Time 3). Since several of the cohorts figured in two comparisons, the analyses had to be conducted separately for each combination of cohorts.

For several of the variables (or derivatives of them such as percentages), less refined (and in some respects, less informative) analyses with *t* tests and *chi-square* were also carried out. The findings from these analyses were in general agreement with those obtained in the ANOVAs.

MAIN RESULTS

The results for some of the variables discussed above are presented separately for boys and girls in Figures 6.2–6.7. Since the design of the study is relatively complex, a few words about how to read the figures are in order.

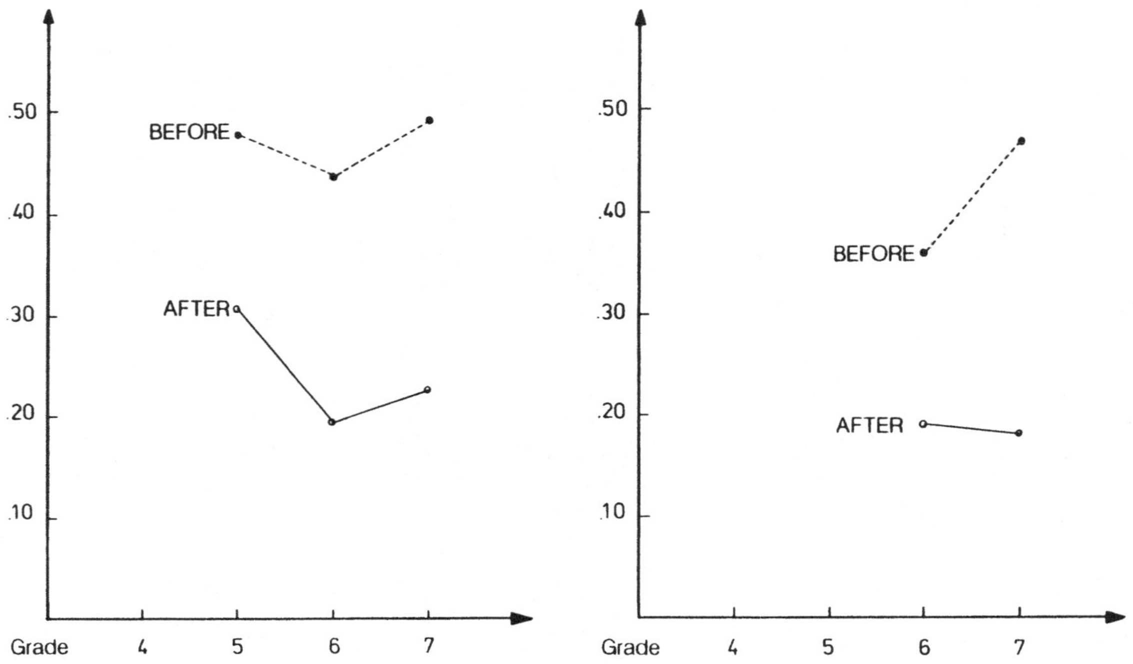

Figure 6.2. Effects of intervention program on 'Being exposed to direct bullying' for boys. The left graph shows effects after 8 months of intervention, and the right graph displays results after 20 months of intervention. Upper curves (labelled Before) show base line data (Time 1), and lower curves (labelled After) display data collected at Time 2 in the left graph and at Time 3 in the right graph.

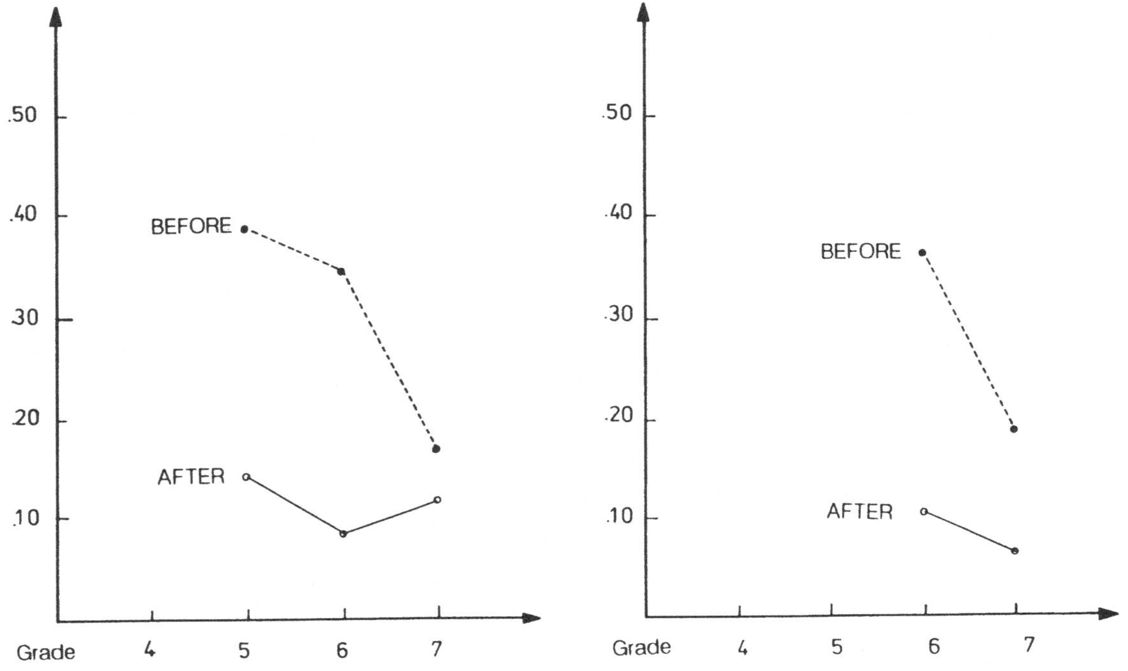

Figure 6.3. Effects of intervention program on ‘Being exposed to direct bullying’ for girls. See Figure 6.2 for explanation of the figure.

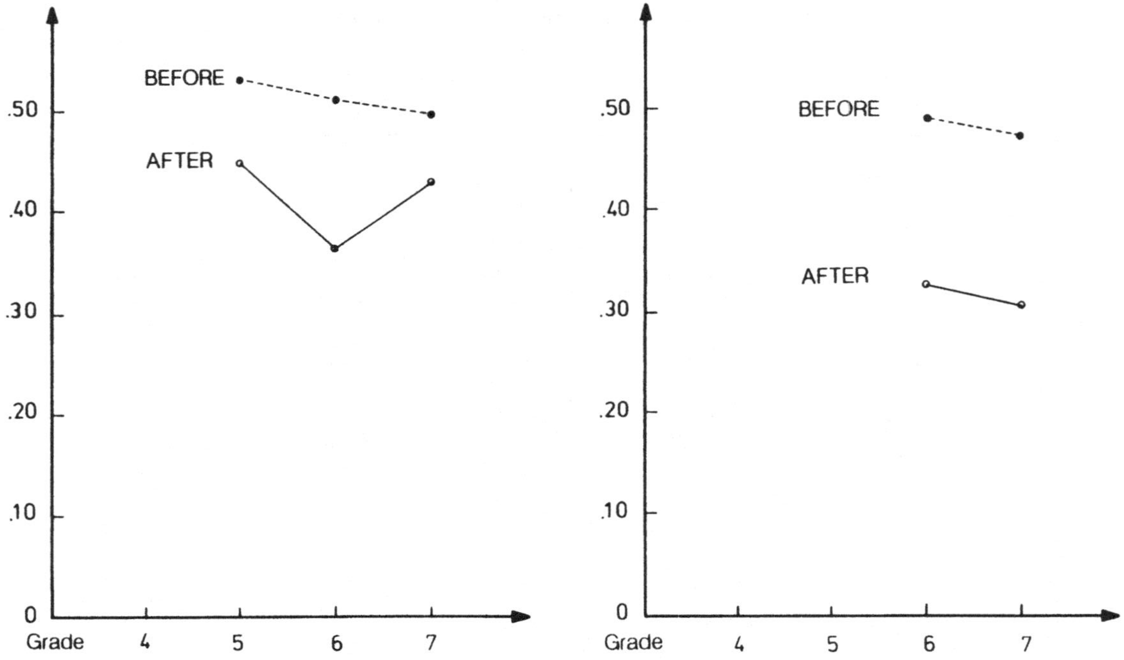

Figure 6.4. Effects of intervention program on 'Bullying other students' for boys. See Figure 6.2 for explanation of the figure.

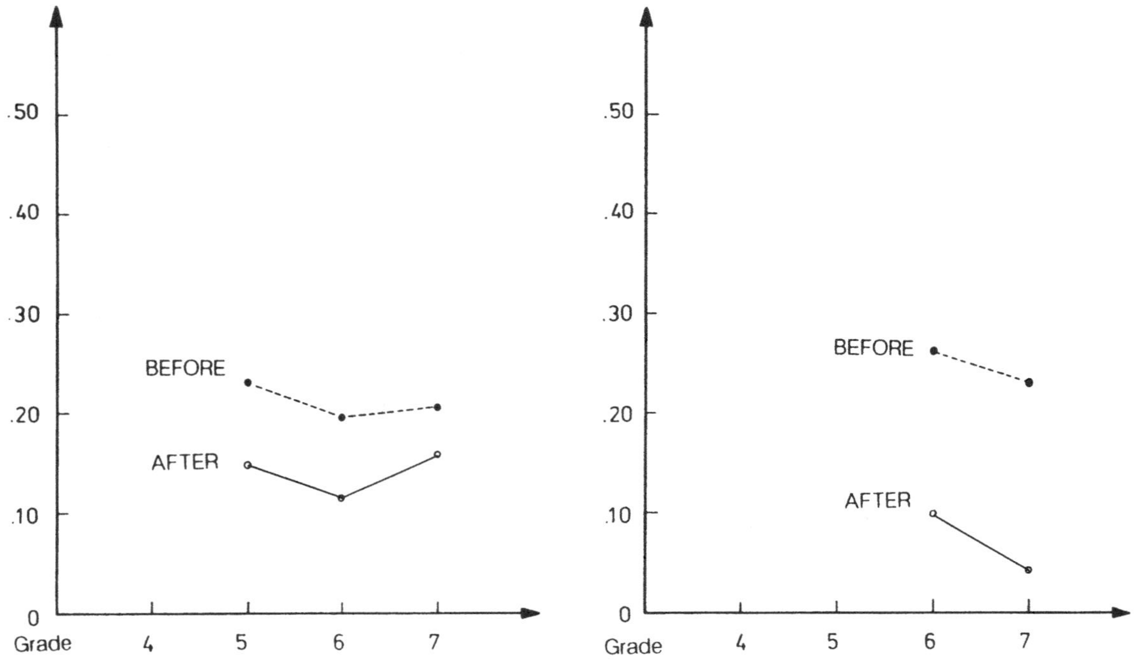

Figure 6.5. Effects of intervention program on 'Bullying other students' for girls. See Figure 6.2 for explanation of the figure.

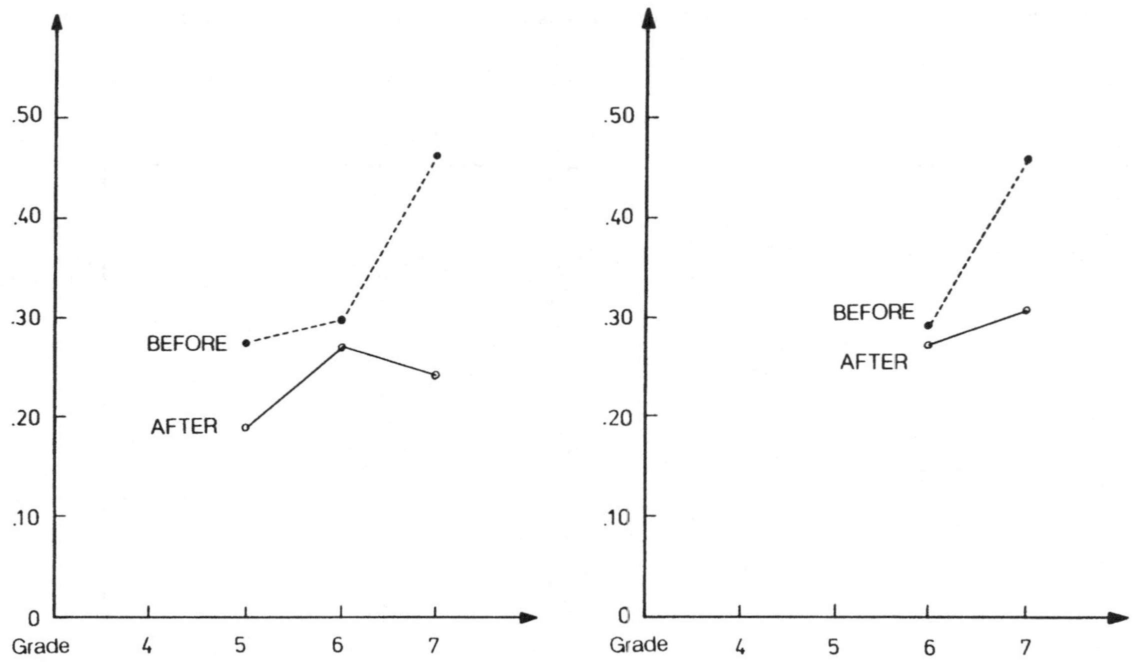

Figure 6.6. Effects of intervention program on 'Total scale of antisocial behavior' (TAS) for boys. See Figure 6.2 for explanation of the figure.

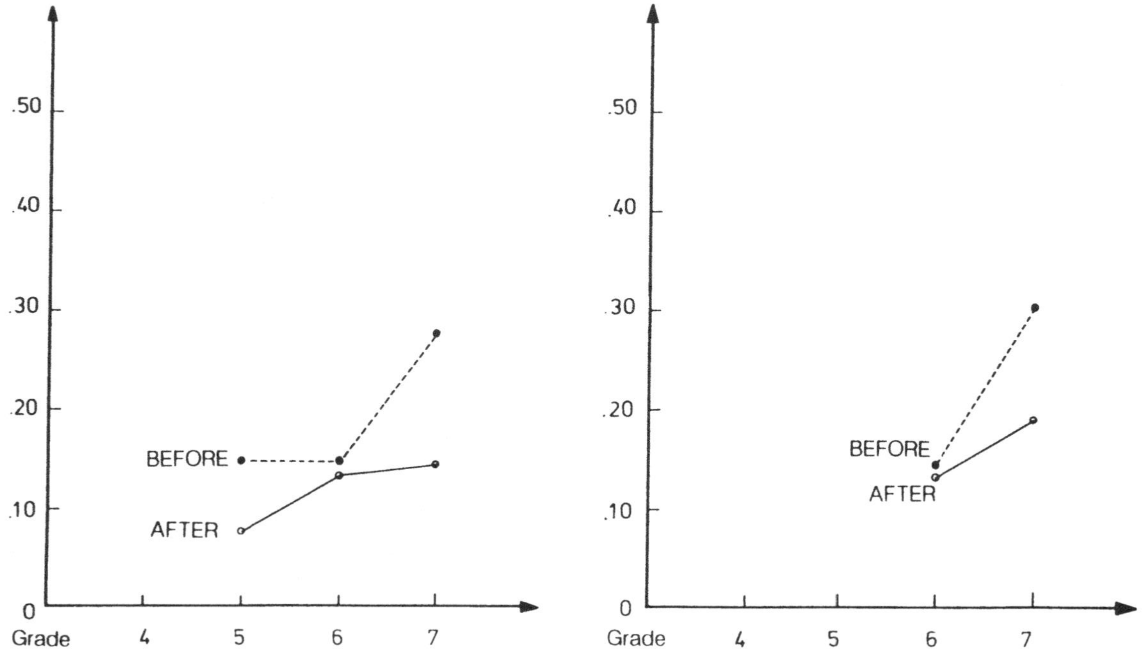

Figure 6.7. Effects of intervention program on 'Total scale of antisocial behavior' (TAS) for girls. See Figure 6.2 for explanation of the figure.

The left graph shows the effects after 8 months of intervention, and the right graph displays the results after 20 months. The upper curves (labelled Before) show the base line data (Time 1) for the relevant cohorts (Cohorts 5, 6, and 7 in the left graph and Cohorts 6 and 7 in the right). The lower curves (labelled After) display data collected at Time 2 (after 8 months of intervention) in the left graph and at Time 3 (after 20 months of intervention) in the right graph for the age-equivalent cohorts (Cohorts 4, 5, and 6 at Time 2, and Cohorts 4 and 5 at Time 3).

It should be noted that in some of the figures there are minor differences in base line data (Before) for Cohorts 6 and 7 when presented in the left and right graphs respectively. This is a consequence of the restriction of the analyses to subjects who had valid data at both time points (below); accordingly, it is not exactly the same subjects who entered the two sets of analyses.

The scales on the vertical axis are in some sense arbitrary simply reflecting the system used in scoring the variables.

The *main findings* of the analyses can be summarized as follows.

- There were marked reductions in the levels of bully/victim problems for the periods studied, 8 and 20 months of intervention respectively (Figures 6.2–6.5). By and large, reductions were obtained for both boys and girls and across all cohorts. For the longer time period the effects persisted in the case of 'Being exposed to direct bullying' and 'Being exposed to indirect bullying' and were strengthened for the variable 'Bullying others'.
- Similar reductions were obtained for the aggregated 'peer rating' variables 'Number of students being bullied in the class' and 'Number of students in the class bullying others'. There was thus consensual agreement in the classes that bully/victim problems had decreased during the periods studied.
- In terms of percentages of students reporting being bullied or bullying others 'now and then' or more frequently, the reductions amounted to approximately 50% or more in most comparisons (Time 1 – Time 3 for 'Bullying others'.)
- There was no displacement of bullying from the school to the way to and from school. There were reductions or no changes on the items measuring bully/victim problems on the way to and from school.
- There was also a reduction in general antisocial behavior (Figures 6.6 and 6.7) such as vandalism, theft, and truancy. (For the grade 6 comparisons the effects were marginal for both time periods.)
- At the same time, there was an increase in student satisfaction with school life as reflected in 'liking recess time'.

- There were weak and inconsistent changes for the questions concerning attitudes to different aspects of bully/victim problems.

In the majority of comparisons for which reductions were reported above, the differences between base line and intervention groups were highly significant or significant (in spite of the fact that many of them were based on single items).

QUALITY OF DATA AND POSSIBLE ALTERNATIVE INTERPRETATIONS

It is beyond the scope of this chapter to discuss in detail the quality of the data collected and the possibility of alternative interpretations of the findings. An extensive discussion of these matters can be found elsewhere (Olweus, 1991). Here I limit myself to summarizing the conclusions in the following 'point statements'.

- Self-reports, which were implicated in most of the analyses conducted so far, are in fact the best data source for the purposes of this study.
- It is very difficult to explain the results obtained as a consequence of (a) underreporting by the students; (b) gradual changes in the students' attitudes to bully/victim problems; (c) repeated measurement; and (d) concomitant changes in other factors. All in all, it is *concluded that the reductions in bully/victim and associated problems described above are likely to be mainly a consequence of the intervention program and not of some other 'irrelevant' factor.*

A TIME BY COHORT ANALYSIS

In addition to the time-lagged comparisons, it may be informative also to consider briefly the results from a time by cohort ANOVA with repeated measurements on the time factor (see Figure 6.1). The hierarchical nature of the data with nesting of students, classes and schools within higher-order units was of course retained in these analyses. The nesting also entered the 'within' part of the analyses involving repeated measurements, thus making the design quite complex. For the present chapter, the time by cohort ANOVA will be restricted to two time points (Time 1 and Time 2) and to one variable, a composite (mean) of the two variables covering exposure to direct and indirect bulllying, respectively (above). An overview of the results can be gained from Figure 6.8. For ease of reading, the figure is drawn as an age by cohort rather than as a time by cohort plot.

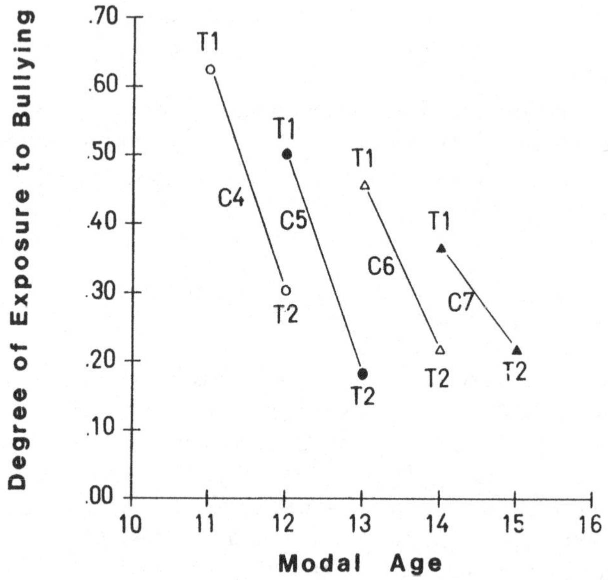

Figure 6.8. Age by cohort (C) plot. Comparison of Time 1 (*T*1) and Time 2 (*T*2) on 'Being exposed to direct and indirect bullying' for boys plus girls.

We can imagine a line connecting all the T(ime)1-points which would show the expected age curve for the relevant ages. The data actually obtained for these ages, after 8 months of intervention, are indicated by the T2 points. The differences between T1 and T2 for a particular age thus represents the kind of effects tested in the time-lagged comparisons reported above. The figure seems to suggest that the effects obtained at age 14 (Cohort 7 vs Cohort 6) are somewhat weaker than at ages 12 and 13.

The most striking finding from the time by cohort ANOVA was a very highly significant main effect of time ($F = 243.88$; d.f. $= 1/51$; $p = 0.000$). There was also a significant, though much weaker, main effect associated with the cohort classification ($F = 6.32$; d.f. $= 3/51$; $p = 0.001$). It should be noted that the latter result can in principle reflect both cohort effects (in the sense discussed above) and age variation between cohorts: the four levels of cohort (C4–C7) covered a span of modal age differences amounting to three years (11.5 vs 14.5). In this study, however, both genuine and non-genuine cohort effects were very unlikely, as previously pointed out, and consequently the significant main effect linked to the cohort classification can be best understood as an effect of the average age differences between cohorts.

Main effects associated with the time factor can reflect time-related changes but also age effects: the average age of the four cohorts was 12.5

years at Time 1 and 13.5 years at Time 2. Despite the much smaller age variation implicated in the main time effects (one year, from 12.5 to 13.5) compared with the main effect due to cohort (three years, from 11.5 to 14.5), the effects associated with the time factor were much larger. This finding strongly supports the general conclusion, based on the time-lagged contrasts, that there were very marked effects in the data due to time-related changes, over and above age-related differences (cf. Nesselroade & Baltes, 1974).

THE DOSAGE–RESPONSE RELATIONSHIP

In the previous analyses, both the longitudinal and cross-sectional aspects of the design were utilized. However, the longitudinal analyses can be carried further through an examination of the relationship between the *degree of change* from Time 1 to Time 2 and components of the intervention program. The research question can be formulated in the following way: *Did those units that showed greater reductions in bully/victim problems from Time* 1 *to Time* 2 *implement more of the intervention program* (*or particular components of the program*) *than those units that evidenced smaller changes*? This question is a version of the *dosage–response relationship* which states that, at least up to a certain limit, it is natural to expect greater effects of a treatment or an intervention strategy the larger its 'dosage' is. Even though the preceding analyses in my view constitute very strong evidence for the effects of the intervention program, findings of a positive dosage–response relationship would certainly further strengthen such a conclusion.

Information on the intervention program and its implementation in the various classes and schools at Time 2 (8 months after initiation of the program) was obtained from the main (class) teachers through a questionnaire. Three presumably important aspects of the intervention program concerned whether there were class rules against bullying in the class, whether there had been (more-or-less) regular class meetings about bully/victim problems, and whether the class had set up roleplays about bully/victim problems in the course of the academic year. The main responses from teachers to these three items were combined into a composite which reflected to some extent the degree of implementation of the intervention program in each particular class. All of these program components work primarily at the class level and, accordingly, the natural unit for an analysis of change is the class in this case. For other aspects of the program the school might be the most appropriate unit of analyses.

Valid data were obtained for 89 classes but, for nine of them, the composition of the class had undergone major changes in the transition from elementary to junior high school which prevented meaningful comparisons from Time 1 to Time 2 at the class level. Consequently, the following analyses will be based on 80 classes. The variable for the measurement of change in bully/victim problems was the same as that used in the time by cohort ANOVA, a composite of exposure to direct and indirect bullying.

RESIDUAL CHANGE SCORES OR SIMPLE DIFFERENCE SCORES?

Before embarking on the correlational analysis, a decision must be made about how to measure degree of change from $T1$ to $T2$ (at the class level in the present case; the conclusions drawn are likely to apply equally well to changes at the individual level).

In a situation with only two waves of data available, it has been common practice in the social sciences to measure change by means of a *residual 'gain' score*, that is, the deviation or residual from the 'expected' value of the dependent variable at Time 2 ($Y2$) derived from the regression of $Y2$ on $Y1$ (value of the dependent variable at Time 1), or some attenuation-corrected estimate of the 'true residual change' (Rogosa, Brandt & Zimowsky, 1982). It should be noted that techniques for the study of longitudinal change such as path analysis and LISREL typically implicate a kind of residual change score.

There are a number of problems, however – both psychometric, statistical, and conceptual – associated with the use of residual change scores, as convincingly argued by Rogosa and his associates (Rogosa *et al.*, 1982). According to these authors, the issue of measuring change should rather be considered in a 'growth curve' framework, in which *individual* (*or class*) *time paths* are the proper focus of analysis and the basic source of information on change is the regression of the dependent variable on time (and not of $Y2$ on $Y1$). This approach clears up a number of misconceptions in the analysis-of-change literature including several incorrect views of the simple difference score. One of the main conclusions of these authors is in fact 'when only two waves of data are available, the difference score is a natural and useful measure of individual change' (Rogosa *et al.*, 1982: 744).

It is interesting to note that most authors discussing the problem of change in situations with more than two waves of data seem to agree that one should use a growth curve approach. Extrapolating from that perspective, it is the difference score (with regression of the dependent variable on time) that is the obvious choice when there are data from only two time points: the natural 'downward' extension of the growth curve approach is the difference score (with slope $b = (Y2 - Y1)/(T2 - T1)$), and not the residual gain score (with regression of $Y2$ on $Y1$). It is surprising that this argument in favor of the difference score has figured so infrequently in the lively and often bewildering debate on the measurement of change.

At the same time, it should be emphasized that data from two time points and the difference score are less than optimal for the study of change and that data should preferably be collected for three or more time points. Parenthetically, it may be mentioned that several of the variables included in the present study were measured at three time points or more. For the present purposes, however, we have restricted our analyses of change to two waves of measurement.

Following the basic recommendation of the Rogosa *et al.* paper, degree of change was measured in the present study as the difference between the class average of bully/victim problems (degree of exposure to bullying) at Time 1 and the corresponding value at Time 2 ($Y1 - Y2$), the difference being weighted by number of students in the class. This measure was then correlated with the variable on degree of implementation of the intervention program, as previously discussed. The correlation between these two variables amounted to a substantial 0.51 ($n = 80$), thereby confirming the assumed relationship between 'dosage' and 'response': those classes that showed larger reductions in bully/victim problems had implemented the three components of the program to a greater extent than those with smaller changes. As pointed out, this kind of finding provides corroborating evidence for the effects of the intervention program. At the same time, it should be underscored that this is only a preliminary analysis which will be followed up by more comprehensive and detailed examinations. In particular, the program consists of several other components which will have to be included in a more complete analyses.

A presentation of the intervention program[2] is outside the scope of this chapter; the interested reader will find a practically oriented description of it in Olweus (1986, in preparation) and a more theoretical discussion of its conceptual background and principles in Olweus (1991).

THE HIERARCHICAL NATURE OF THE DATA

In the present study, the sampling units were intact classes drawn from a collection of schools. However, on a large number of variables, including those discussed in this chapter, data were obtained from each individual student, and for these variables the student was the 'observational unit'. The project thus comprises data at different levels with students nested within classes which were nested within schools nested within conditions. The hierarchical structure of the data must be taken into account in the statistical analyses (see, e.g., Kirk, 1982; Winer, 1971).

A common error in analyzing data of this kind is to ignore the nesting or clustering and generally treat the data as if they constituted a simple random sample of individuals (rather than a sample of clusters of individuals; see Kish, 1965). In consequence, an inappropriate error term will be used in testing the effects of interest, for example the effects of time of measurement (the intervention program) in the time-lagged contrasts design (above). More specifically, in this particular case the error term would involve variation between individuals within time points (conditions) rather than variation among schools within time points.

Use of variation between lower-level units as the error term rather than variation among the relevant higher-level units commonly results in an inflated alpha level with too many significant *F* tests. The positive bias in the *F* test is due to the fact that the variance (and the standard error) of a cluster sample is typically larger than that of a simple random sample of the same *n*. The ratio of these two variances has been termed the 'design effect' (Kish, 1965; 162) and, the greater the design effect, the greater the bias in the *F* test.

The usually larger variance of the cluster sample (e.g., the variance of the class means or schools means) is a consequence of the homogeneity of individuals within clusters: students within a class tend to 'resemble' each other, that is, be more similar on the dependent variable than students selected at random. The degree of homogeneity or similarity among individuals within a cluster can be expressed as the *intraclass correlation, rho* (Kish, 1965). The greater the homogeneity within clusters, the greater the between-clusters variance and the design effect. The extreme case is when all individuals within clusters have the same value and clusters are completely separated. This results in a *rho* of 1.0.

The reasoning above is based on a model in which the time-related changes (the effects of the intervention program) are seen as a fixed effect while schools, classes and students are considered random variables (Kirk, 1982; Winer, 1971): We want to generalize the results to schools, classes and students 'like those included in the project'. However, if schools and classes are defined as fixed factors, the between-students (nested within classes, schools and conditions) variation will serve as the error term for all *F* tests. In most situations, this is not a very useful strategy since it severely restricts generalizability of the findings to the particular schools and classes included in the research.

The reason why many researchers may want to disregard the nested structure of their data is probably that an error term involving higher-level units (such as classes or schools) rather than lower-level units (such as individuals) has fewer, often much fewer, degrees of freedom and thus results in a less powerful test of the effects of interest.

The lower sensitivity of the statistical tests is of course no excuse for using an incorrect error term.

It should be noted, however, that for situations in which higher-level random effects (due to, e.g., schools or classes) are tested against the appropriate between-individuals error term and found not to be significant (usually at a somewhat larger alpha level than usual), these sources of variation and their respective degrees of freedom may be pooled to form a combined error term (Glass & Stanley, 1970; Kirk, 1982). The result is often similar to using the between-individuals variation as the error term. The pooling strategy is defensible, however, *only after* effects due to higher level random effects have been tested and found nonsignificant.

The basic message of this section can be summarized as follows: *If the data at hand have a hierarchical structure,* as is often the case in psychological and educational research, *this must be taken into account in the statistical analyses.*

SUMMARIZING DISCUSSION

The chapter opened by asking the question: How can we document possible effects of an anti-bullying program in school when an experimental set-up is not feasible?

The approach taken here was to use a cohort-longitudinal (or selection cohorts) design with adjacent cohorts. Since there were developmental ('maturational') changes in the dependent variables of interest, the main focus of analysis was on time-lagged contrasts between age-equivalent cohorts. These analyses were supported by a time-by-cohort ANOVA and by correlational analyses (at the class level) documenting a positive 'dosage–response' relationship, that is, a clear association between extent of reduction in bully/victim problems between Time 1 and Time 2 and degree of implementation of important components of the intervention program. Additional analyses (not reported in detail in this chapter) involving a separate sample have been conducted to control for possible effects of repeated measurement. Several other alternative interpretations of the findings have been discussed and found to be very unlikely (see Olweus, 1991). For an adequate statistical analysis of the data, the importance of taking into account the hierarchical nature of the data, with lower-level units nested or clustered within higher-level units, was strongly emphasized. It was generally concluded that the documented marked reductions in bully/victim problems over time were likely to be mainly a consequence of the intervention program and not of some other 'irrelevant' factor.

All in all, a cohort-longitudinal design with adjacent cohorts must be considered a fairly strong design for the study of planned change (such as introduction of an anti-bullying program), when an experimental set-up is not practically feasible or ethically defensible (cf. Reichardt, 1979). However, interpretation of the results is greatly facilitated if reasonable assumptions about the nature of some effects in the design can be made. When using adjacent cohorts it is often natural to postulate on conceptual grounds that there are no, or only negligible, cohort effects. The reasonableness of such an assumption can also be checked to some extent by looking at the pattern of findings. Graphs of age by cohort (and time), time by cohort (and age) and cohort by time (and age) can be very helpful in such an examination.

As with other designs, including experimental ones, the validity of the conclusions drawn are strengthened if alternative interpretations can be ruled out through supplementary analyses, or if links can be established between putative causal factors and degree of change as in the 'dosage–response' relationship. Accordingly, it is important to try to incorporate such possibilities already at the planning stage.

An attractive feature of the cohort-longitudinal design is generally the possibility of examining a particular hypothesis or issue (see Alsaker & Olweus, 1991) in several different comparisons and with both cross-sectional and longitudinal data. The opportunity to compare and evaluate cross-sectional and longitudinal analyses and, more generally, to replicate results from one analysis in one or more additional analyses within the same study, are likely to lead to more robust and dependable findings. The inclusion of several different age groups or cohorts also considerably extends the basis for generalizing the results.

Despite the considerable advantages associated with a cohort-longitudinal design with adjacent cohorts it seems to have been used by only a handful of researchers in developmental or educational psychology, such as Nesselroade & Baltes (1974) and Dusek & Flaherty (1981). For the study of planned change, we have come across only one study in the research literature, that by Ball & Bogatz (1970), and this study was limited to two 'cohorts'. We believe that more frequent use of this design, in particular with more than two cohorts, would be of considerable advantage for the field.

ACKNOWLEDGEMENTS

The research reported was supported in various periods by grants to Dan Olweus from the William T. Grant Foundation, the Norwegian Ministry of Education, the Norwegian Council for Social Research, and the Swedish Delegation for Social Research (DSF). Several of the ideas presented were developed while Olweus was a Fellow at the Center for Advanced Study in the Behavioral Sciences, Stanford, USA. He is indebted to the University of Bergen, the Spencer Foundation, the Norwegian Council for Social Research, and the Center for Advanced Study in the Behavioral Sciences for financial support of the year at the Center.

NOTES

1. We would like to express our gratitude to professor Hans Magne Eikeland whose deep insights into the logic of analysis of variance were of great help in deriving the expected mean squares and in selecting the appropriate error terms in the complex ANOVAs.
2. The 'program-package' related to the intervention program against bully/victim problems consists of a questionnaire for the measurement of bully/victim problems, a copy of a small book *Bullying in school – what we know and what we can do* (Olweus, in preparation) aimed at teachers and parents, a video about bullying, and a parent folder. (Additional materials are being developed.) These materials are copyrighted which implies certain restrictions on their use. For more information, please write to Dan Olweus, University of Bergen, Oysteinsgate 3, N-5007 Bergen, Norway.

REFERENCES

Adam, J. (1978). Sequential strategies and the separation of age, cohort, and time-of-measurement contributions to development data. *Psychological Bulletin, 85,* 1309–1316.

Alsaker, F. D. & Olweus, D. (1991). *Global self-evaluation and perceived stability of self in early adolescence: A cohort-longitudinal study.*

Ball, S. & Bogatz, G. A. (1970). *The first year of Sesamestreet: An evaluation.* Princeton, N.J.: Educational Testing Service.

Baltes, P. B. (1968). Longitudinal and cross-sectional sequences in the study of age and generation effects. *Human Development, 11,* 145–171.

Baltes, P. B., Cornelius, S. W. & Nesselroade, J. R. (1979). Cohort effects in developmental psychology. In J. R. Nesselroade & P. B. Baltes (eds.), *Longitudinal research in the study of behavior and development.* New York: Academic Press.

Cook, T. D. & Campbell, D. T. (1979). *Quasi-experimentation.* Chicago: Rand McNally.

Dusek, J. B. & Flaherty, J. F. (1981). The development of the self-concept during the adolescent years. *Monograph of the Society for Research in Child Development, 46.*

Elliott, D. S. & Ageton, S. S. (1980). Reconciling race and class differences in self-reported and official estimates of delinquency. *American Sociological Review, 45,* 95–110.

Glass, G. V. & Stanley, J. C. (1970). *Statistical methods in education and psychology.* Englewood Cliffs, N.J.: Prentice-Hall.

Glenn, N. D. (1976). Cohort analysts' futile quest: Statistical attempts to separate age, period, and cohort effects. *American Sociological Review, 41,* 900–904.

Hindelang, M. J., Hirschi, T. & Weis, J. G. (1981). *Measuring delinquency.* Beverly Hills, CA: Sage.

Kish, L. (1965). *Survey sampling.* New York: Wiley.

Kirk, R. E. (1982). *Experimental design: Procedures for the behavioral sciences* (2nd edn). Belmont, CA: Brooks/Cole.

Nesselroade, J. R. & Baltes, P. B. (1974). Adolescent personality development and historical change: 1970–1972. *Monographs of the Society for Research in Child Development, 39* (1, Serial No. 154).

Nesselroade, J. R. & Baltes, P. B. (1984). Sequential strategies and the role of cohort effects in behavioral development: Adolescent personality (1970–72) as a sample case. In S. A. Mednick, M. Harway & K. M. Finello (eds.), *Handbook of longitudinal research* (Vol. 1, pp. 55–87). New York: Praeger.

Olweus, D. (1973). *Hackkycklingar och översittare: Forskning om skolmobbning.* Stockholm: Almqvist & Wiksell.

Olweus, D. (1977). Aggression and peer acceptance in adolescent boys: Two short-term longitudinal studies of ratings. *Child Development, 48,* 1301–1313.

Olweus, D. (1978). *Aggression in the schools: Bullies and whipping boys.* Washington D.C.: Hemisphere (Wiley).

Olweus, D. (1986). *Mobbning – vad vi vet och vad vi kan göra.* (Translated: *Bullying in school – what we know and what we can do*). Stockholm: Liber.

Olweus, D. (1989). Prevalence and incidence in the study of antisocial behavior: Definitions and measurement. In M. Klein (ed.), *Self-report methodology in criminological research* (pp. 187–201). Dordrecht: Kluwer.

Olweus, D. (1991). Bully/victim problems among school-children: Basic facts and effects of a school based intervention program. In D. Pepler & K. H. Rubin (eds.), *The development and treatment of childhood aggression* (pp. 411–448). Hillsdale, N.J.: Erlbaum.

Olweus, D. (in press). Victimization by peers: Antecedents and long-term outcomes. In K. H. Rubin & J. B. Asendorf (eds.), *Social withdrawal, inhibition, and shyness in childhood.*

Olweus, D. (in preparation). *Bullying in school – what we know and what we can do.* Book manuscript.

Olweus, D. & Endresen, J. (in preparation). *Assessment of antisocial behavior in preadolescence and adolescence.* Manuscript.

Olweus, D. & Roland, E. (1983). *Mobbing – bakgrunn og tiltak.* Oslo, Norway: Kirke-og undervisningsdepartementet.

Perry, D. G., Kusel, S. J. & Perry, L. C. (1988). Victims of peer aggression. *Developmental Psychology, 24,* 807–814.

Reichardt, C. (1979). The statistical analysis of data from nonequivalent groups designs. In T. D. Cook & D. T. Campbell, (eds.), *Quasi-experimentation.* Chicago: Rand McNally.

Rogosa, D., Brandt, D. & Zimowsky, M. (1982). A growth curve approach to the measurement of change. *Psychological Bulletin, 92,* 726–748.

Rosow, J. (1978). What is a cohort and why? *Human Development 21,* 65–75.

Ryder, N. B. (1965). The cohort as a concept in the study of social change. *American Sociological Review, 30,* 843–861.

Winer, B. J. (1971). *Statistical principles in experimental design* (2nd edn). New York: McGraw-Hill.

7 Statistical and conceptual models of 'turning points' in developmental processes

ANDREW PICKLES AND MICHAEL RUTTER

INTRODUCTION

During recent years there has been a growing interest in what have been termed transitions or 'turning points' in a person's development or life course (see, e.g., Elder, Caspi & Burton, 1988; Hareven, 1978; Maughan & Champion, in press; Rutter, 1989). The focus is on two main types of everyday events or happenings that bring about a potential for long-term psychological change. First, there are those in which the potential stems from an opening up or closing down of opportunities. Going to university and dropping out of school respectively provide obvious examples. Secondly, there are those that involve a radical lasting change in life circumstances. Such changes may come about as a result of key additions or subtractions from a person's nexus of intimate family relationships (as with marriage or divorce), or from alterations in life pattern (as from the transition to parenthood or being made redundant in midlife), or from a major social change stemming from a geographical move (as with immigration to a different country or a move from a metropolis to a rural village). The general concept is easy to understand and the operational definition of potential turning points is also straightforward, with the proviso that it is necessary to consider whether the events actually changed opportunities or life circumstances in the individual case. Thus, marriage may, but need not, involve a major change in social network, pattern of relationships or way of life.

Before considering the concept in more detail, it should be noted that, as we are using it here, three main classes of events are excluded. First, we are not considering rare dramatic 'internal' psychological experiences such as are exemplified by religious conversions. Many years ago William James (1902) portrayed the reality of their occurrence but they fall outside the realm of more ordinary turning points that we seek to study. The same applies to rare dramatic 'external' experiences such as those brought about by earthquake or shipwreck or being taken hostage (Garmezy & Rutter, 1985). Thirdly, we exclude universal age-defined transitions such as the hypothesized 'mid-life crisis' postulated by Levinson *et al.* (1976).

There is no doubt, of course, that there are everyday events or happenings that so alter subsequent life experiences that they carry the potential for bringing about psychological change. Nevertheless, it remains an empirical question whether major changes in life experiences in fact make a significant impact on psychological functioning. There is evidence that they do. This has been shown, for example, in relation to bereavement (Raphael, 1984) and unemployment (Warr, 1987). However, most of the findings apply to relatively short-term psychological effects and it remains to ask whether there are also lasting consequences. Again, there is evidence that in some circumstances there may be (Rutter & Madge, 1976; Rutter, 1987*a*). Moreover, there are also some well-documented examples of instances in which apparently 'positive' experiences have seemed to alter the consequences of earlier 'negative' ones, so that it may be supposed that a risk trajectory has been diverted onto a more adaptive path (Rutter, 1989). Thus, Furstenberg, Brooks-Gunn & Morgan (1987) showed that, among teenage mothers, those that went on to complete high school after the birth of the child were several times more likely to be economically secure in their mid-30s than those who dropped out of school following the pregnancy.

It might be thought that the analytic task of testing for the psychological effects of life transitions involving potential turning points should, therefore, be relatively straightforward. Longitudinal data will be needed to test for the postulated change over time in psychological functioning. However, the pattern of findings indicate that in most cases it would be misleading to conceptualize what happens as a once-and-for-all change that stems from some event that arises out of the blue. Rather, the findings suggest a dynamic model involving interlinked chain effects both before and after the turning point (Elder, in press; Rutter, 1987*a*, 1987*b*, 1989). For example, Hofferth (1987) has outlined the multiple steps in the decision tree leading to becoming a teenage mother: becoming sexually active at an early age, not using contraceptive methods (or doing so ineffectively), persisting with the pregnancy rather than having a termination, and keeping the child rather than giving it up for adoption or foster care. Moreover, the long-term consequences may be greatly influenced by later decisions: such as whether to continue with schooling. The example makes clear the need to consider most turning points as part of a process over time and not as a dramatic lasting change that takes place at any one time. There is a need, therefore, to study linkages over time that involve the several points at which alternatives present themselves. At each point some individuals choose one way; others choose another, and it is necessary to examine both the consequences of their choices and the mechanisms resulting in one choice rather than the other.

The scope for change, not only in actual behavior but for redefining roles and concepts of self, are clearly greater at some points in the developmental path than others. Thus, as the examples illustrate, there is a strong association between the occurrence of turning points with the transition to young adulthood (reviewed in Maughan & Champion, in press), a period during which many decisions and acts of lasting consequence may occur. The supposed interdependence of many of the events that occur around this time, such as leaving school, starting work, getting married and so on, provides great opportunity for chains of experiences that redirect or confirm earlier trajectories.

It is evident that any investigation of these postulated interdependencies or chain effects is likely to be complex, but in principle at least, these may be dealt with by the application of standard path analytic procedures. These are relatively straightforward where a natural ordering may be assumed in the event or choice sequence (Hogan, 1978; Neugarten, Moore & Lowe, 1965), a circumstance that we later exploit. However, the complexities do not derive just from the chain effects as such. First, apparent interdependency through third variables are always possible. Winship (1986) illustrated how heterogeneity in the form of individual differences in time-tables or a shared dependency of events upon an omitted variable, could lead to spurious interdependency among events, a generalization of the well-known problem of spurious duration dependency in event histories (see for example Pickles, Davies & Crouchley, 1982). In Winship's example of the interdependence of the age at leaving school and the age at marriage, a third unobserved variable, 'maturity', could, for certain types of model, explain any pattern of observed interdependence. Although important, this problem of distinguishing true from spurious interdependency, an example of potential non-identifiability, is mathematically difficult and tedious and can often depend critically on the details of each study and analysis. For example, the risk of non-identifiability may be substantially eased where continuous explanatory variables are present (Elbers & Ridder, 1982).

Second, it cannot be assumed that the transitions impinge similarly on everyone. Rather, the content or meaning of the transitions must be personalized in ways that go beyond their mere occurrence to take account of qualities of the transition, the timing of the transition and characteristics of the subjects. For example, Knight, Osborn & West (1977) showed that marriage as such made little if any difference to male delinquent careers. On the other hand, the characteristics of the spouse did make a difference; marriage to a non-delinquent woman was followed by a substantial fall-off in criminal activities whereas marriage to a delinquent woman had the reverse effect (this differential effect being significant even after partialling out the effect of prior characteristics). Similarly, moving house in itself made little difference but if the move was away from London this was followed by a reduction in delinquent acts (West, 1982).

The timing of the occurrence of turning points may be of importance. Thus, for example, teenage marriages are much more likely than those in the 20s or 30s to be followed by divorce (Thornes & Collard, 1979), and may thus be associated with rather different patterns of long-term change. In addition, the meaning of events may be altered by their timing; thus, maternal employment has no overall effects on children's development (Gottfried & Gottfried, 1988) but if the mother first takes a job outside the house at the time of divorce this does have an adverse effect on some children – presumably because it implies loss of the mother as well as the father (Hetherington, Cox & Cox, 1982). Also, challenging events may have an effect when they coincide in time with other potentially stressful events but not when they occur in isolation – as seems to be the case with the move to high school (Simmons & Blyth, 1987).

The turning point potential may also apply only to subgroups of individuals who have the specified transition experiences. Thus, Elder (1986) showed that military service had beneficial effects for disadvantaged youths which did not apply to those from a more privileged background. This seemed to be because in the disadvantaged subgroup the Army provided the opportunity of further education that might not otherwise have been experienced and also made early marriages less probable.

Not surprisingly, pursuing such questions typically requires detailed empirical investigation of potentially complex processes involving a sequence of events and experiences. Throughout such an investigation there are the risks of missing systematic effects for a well-defined subgroup within the sea of random fluctuations of a larger group or of missing individually insignificant subgroup effects that are systematic across subgroups. In addition, there is the conflicting risk of the over-exploitation of chance outcomes and of isolating subgroups without theoretical or practical importance. These problems of finding the right balance between the risks of making type I and II errors are, of course, commonplace but they appear to be particularly acute in this kind of investigation. There are several general statistical procedures for attempting to formalize this balance (see, e.g., Gabriel, 1966; Aitkin, 1979), but perhaps more important is the undertaking of sensitive, efficient and theoretically informed data analysis followed by an emphasis upon the need for replication.

Third, the happening that brought about the transition or turning point may be connected only indirectly with the process leading to psychological change. For example, Magnusson, Stattin & Allen (1986) showed that unusually early puberty in girls was associated with an increased tendency to drop out of school and not go onto tertiary education. Further analysis, however, showed that the mechanism did not derive from the physiological changes of puberty as such but rather from joining a peer group of much older teenagers. The effects were not seen in those early maturing girls who remained part of a same age peer group.

In complementary fashion, it may be necessary to consider the extent to which psychological changes extend beyond the domain directly affected by the transition. For example, if young people leave school before taking public examinations it necessarily follows that they will lack the scholastic credentials and the required 'passport' for tertiary education. However, a more interesting question is whether or not this makes a difference to their later earnings or to the sort of person they marry or to the likelihood that they will experience depression.

Fourthly, in many cases the turning point cannot be reduced to an altered sum or balance of 'good' and 'bad' experiences. In some instances, stressful experiences can involve benefits if the person copes successfully with the challenges involved. This seemed to be the case, for instance, in Elder's (1974) study of older children who had to take on additional responsibilities during the Great Economic Depression. Conversely, apparently 'good' experiences may have negative effects, for example as seems to apply to the changes consequent upon the birth of a younger sibling (Dunn & Kendrick, 1982) or the entry into the home of a step-parent (Hetherington, 1988): effects stemming from feelings of jealousy or rivalry.

In this chapter we will illustrate several methods for the investigation of turning points, including cross-tabulation, discrete structural equation, latent class and event history models. The major emphasis is upon methods that can be applied to processes in which the responses are discrete or are defined categorically. As Brown, Harris & Lemyre (Chapter 4 of this volume) argue, such categorically defined variables may bear a closer theoretical relationship to the quantities of interest in psychiatry than apparently similar, though potentially more efficient, continuous equivalents. Thus, several more standard procedures suitable for the analysis of turning points in continuous response variables (e.g. profile analysis forms of MANOVA (multiple analysis of variance: see Kenward, 1987) and LISREL (linear structural relation: Joreskog & Sorbum, 1984)) have not been pursued here. It must also be emphasized that the work presented here is exploratory. Both the empirical issues and the methods to address them are complex and we have no doubt that further work with these methods, or with more standard alternatives, will offer greater clarification. Our objective in this paper is very much one of learning from this exploration rather than presenting pedagogic examples.

Instead of presenting an abstract explanation of these methods that is then followed by an application, we have decided to present the example and the methods used in analysis in tandem in order to illustrate how the choice and definition of the method and problem grows out of the apparent needs indicated by previous results.

THE EXAMPLE DATA: THE TRANSITION TO EARLY ADULT LIFE FOR YOUNG PEOPLE IN CARE

The longitudinal data analyzed in this chapter are taken from a study of the effects of institutional rearing on psychosocial functioning in early adulthood. 81 women and 91 men raised in children's homes (out of 93 and 123 originally selected) were compared with a quasi-random sample of 41 women and 42 men reared in the inner city and of broadly similar socioeconomic background (out of 51 and 58 originally selected). The comparison group were taken from the classroom controls for a study of the children of psychiatric patients. Contemporaneous teacher ratings of emotional and behavioral disturbance in childhood were available together with delinquency records. The subjects were also interviewed in their early to mid-20s on their life histories and their current functioning using standardized methods. Further details of the study and measurements are given in Quinton & Rutter (1988), Rutter, Quinton & Hill (1990) and Zoccolillo, Pickles, Rutter & Quinton (in preparation). Although the sample size was not large in relation to the needs of many of the more complex multivariate methods, their richness had already been demonstrated and cross-tabulation methods had identified an important turning point for the sample of women (Quinton & Rutter, 1988). We now summarize those findings but using both men and women and somewhat different measures. The pattern of results, while generally very consistent with previous findings, shows some important differences.

CROSS-TABULATION ANALYSES OF TURNING POINTS

The main initial focus of the statistical analyses was the adult outcome for young people who had spent most of their growing years in institutions owing to breakdown in their parenting. Was this outcome, as measured by the presence of adult criminality, poor social functioning with peers or poor work record, different from that for young people from a similar socially disadvantaged background who were reared by their parents in the family home in the usual way? (see Quinton & Rutter, 1988; Quinton, Rutter & Liddle, 1984; Rutter &

Quinton, 1984; Rutter, Quinton & Hill, 1990). Direct case-control comparisons were clear-cut in showing that the institution-reared group fared worse in all respects. However, there was marked heterogeneity, with some of the institution-reared individuals functioning well in early adult life. The next step was to search for possible explanations for these differences in outcome; accordingly, cross-tabulations were undertaken comparing cases and controls on variables thought likely to be influential on the basis of previous research. In each comparison, the possible differentiating variables were related to outcome within each subgroup and the cases and controls were then combined to see if the variable accounted for the case-control difference in outcome. Various factors were found to be relevant (see references cited above) but the presence of marital support at the time of follow-up stood out as providing a particularly powerful effect (see Figure 7.1a). This seemed to constitute what we would now term a potential 'turning point', one that we have now examined in detail. Before concluding that the presence of marital support truly had an effect on psychosocial

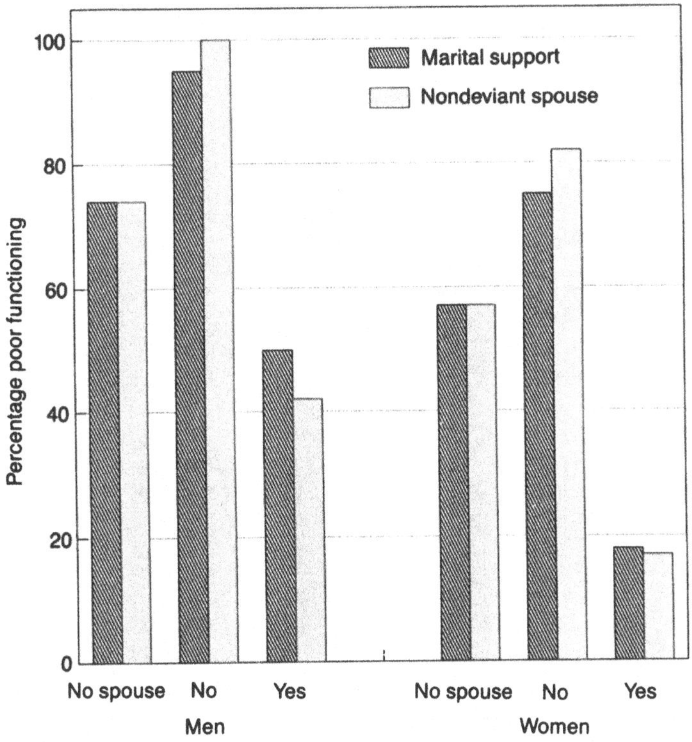

Figure 7.1. Adult social functioning by sex and (a) marital support, (b) nondeviant spouse (ex-care sample only).

functioning it was necessary first to explore the possibility that the finding was an artefact deriving from prior differences in the characteristics of the subjects with and without a harmonious marital relationship with a nondeviant spouse: the operational definition of marital support.

Figure 7.1b shows that the effect remains where marital support is defined as the presence of a nondeviant spouse, in order to exclude the subjects' own contribution to the supportive relationship. Previous research suggested that behavioral disturbance in childhood was likely to predict poor psychosocial functioning in adult life. The findings (here based on Rutter B-score of conduct disorder or mixed conduct/emotional, delinquency record and retrospective interview: see Zoccolillo, Pickles, Rutter & Quinton (in preparation) for further detail on this measure) showed that it did, though the effect was substantially stronger in males. It seemed possible also that those who were behaviorally deviant when young might be more likely to make poor marital choices and hence land up without a nondeviant spouse. The

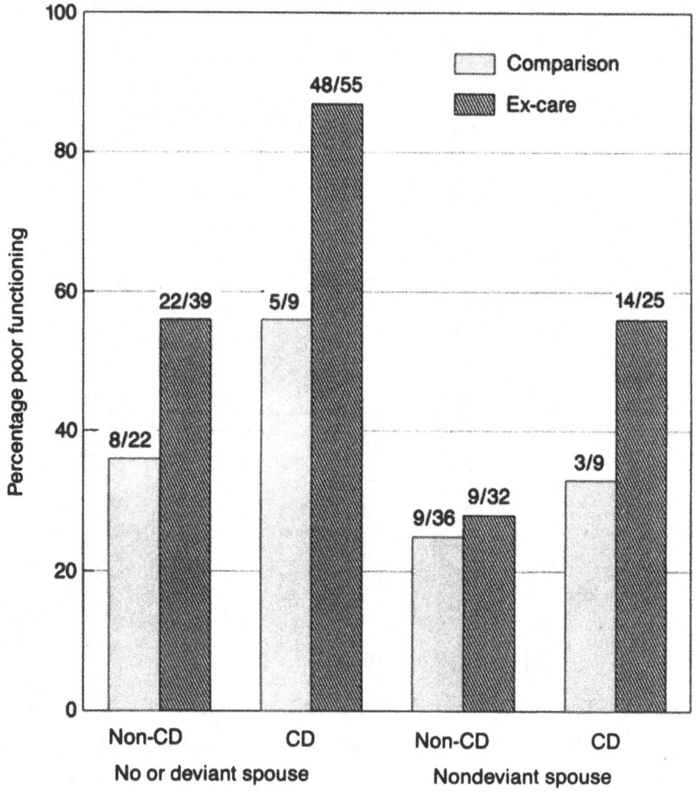

Figure 7.2. Adult social functioning by group, childhood conduct disorder and nondeviant spouse.

Table 7.1. *Adult social functioning by childhood rearing (GP), conduct disorder (CD) and nondeviant spouse (NDS): Logit model backward selection sequence*[a] *(N = 227)*

Model	Scaled deviance	Chi-square	p
Full 3-way interaction	260.82		
−GP · CD · NS		0.01	0.7
All 2-way interactions	260.83		
−GP · CD		1.47	0.2
−GP · NDS		1.17	0.3
−CD · NDS		0.51	0.5
All main effects	264.48		
−GP		5.46	0.02
−CD		15.16	<0.001
−NDS		14.61	<0.001

[a] In all cases tests are made against the model for which a scaled deviance has been given.

apparent effect of nondeviant spouse in adult life might be merely a continuity in poor psychosocial functioning and not a turning point at all. This appeared to be the case for the women (at least for the ex-care women, the comparison women showing too little conduct disorder to examine this effectively), among whom those with conduct disorder, although no more or less likely to lack a current spouse ($p = 0.5$), had spouses more likely to be deviant ($p < 0.001$). Conduct disorder in men showed no relationship to gaining a spouse or their deviance ($p = 0.6$ and 0.2, respectively).

The overall effect is expressed graphically in Figure 7.2 and in the form of linear logistic analyses in Table 7.1. It is clear that an effect of childhood deviance on adult psychosocial functioning was present and that a significant main effect for group remained, though weakened in size and smaller than that for nondeviant spouse. These results suggested that much of the long-term risk associated with an institutional upbringing stemmed from an increased likelihood of making an unhappy marriage to a deviant man.

The findings seemed largely to rule out an artefactual effect of marital support and hence to support the hypothesis of a turning point effect associated with the quality of marriage. But the analysis left open the question of why some subjects landed up with a nondeviant spouse whereas others did not. Further analyses indicated the importance of a characteristic of 'planning', meaning that the individuals showed forethought at decision making about their life choices. The variable

Table 7.2. *Adult social functioning for ex-care subjects by marital support (NDS) and planning for work and marriage (PL): Logit model backward selection sequence*[a] *(N = 151)*

Model	Scaled deviance	Chi-square	p
Full 2-way interaction	182.20		
NDS · PL		0.69	0.4
Main effects	182.89		
NDS		12.50	<0.001
PL		0.80	0.4

[a] In all cases tests are made against the model for which a scaled deviance has been given.

used was a combined measure for planning marriage and/or work. The findings showed that 'planners' were more than three times as likely to choose nondeviant spouses (63% vs 16%). Moreover, this was not merely a reflection of a lack of behavioral deviance. Planning by itself appeared to have little direct effect on psychosocial outcome in adult life but the more important effect appeared to be through its effect upon the likelihood of having a nondeviant spouse. That is, if non-planners 'struck lucky' in their marital choice, they were almost as likely as planners to have a good outcome. In short, from this and other related analyses, it seemed that 'planning' constituted a crucial mediating link in the chain but, in itself, it did not have much direct effect on outcome. The linear logistic analysis findings are summarized in Table 7.2.

It should be added that the frequency of planning also helped explain why nondeviant spouses were so much less frequent in the institution-reared group. Whereas nearly half (47%) of that group were non-planners, this was so for only a fifth (21%) of controls. The next question was why this was the case; how did the planning tendency develop? It was hypothesized that various aspects of an institutional upbringing (both the lack of close family ties and the fact that there are few opportunities for the young people in institutions to take decisions for themselves) might make it less likely that planning would become habitual. If so, however, why did planning develop in some institution-reared individuals? It was postulated that positive school experiences might serve to counteract the institutional effect. The findings suggested they did. Within the institutional group, those with positive school experiences were more likely to have planned either work or marriage (66% vs 47%). This effect was not found in the control group (80% vs 78%) (other considerations suggested that this was because they had

Table 7.3. *Planning for work and marriage by childhood rearing (GP), conduct disorder (CD) and positive school experience (SE): Logit model backward selection sequence*[a] *(N = 227)*

Model	Scaled deviance	Chi-square	p
Full 3-way interaction	273.66		
GP · CD · SE		2.50	0.1
All 2-way interactions	276.21		
GP · CD		0.01	0.9
GP · SE		0.60	0.4
CD · SE		4.60	0.03
Main effects + CD · SE interaction	276.85		
GP		14.29	<0.001

[a] In all cases tests are made against the model for which a scaled deviance has been given.

sources of self esteem in the family, so that additional sources at school made little difference). Again, it was necessary to check that positive school experiences were not just a reflection of behavioral non-deviance; previous analyses showed that they were not. The data are put together in the form of a linear logistic analysis in Table 7.3 and confirm those earlier findings.

In summary, then, these cross-tabulations, brought together through linear logistic analyses, showed significant effects for two postulated 'turning points' – positive school experiences and marital support – and indicated that a 'planning' tendency constituted a key mediator across these two links in the chain of development. Other analyses pointed to other elements in the chain; these included a discordant/harmonious family environment on leaving the institution, a teenage pregnancy, and poor material circumstances (see Quinton & Rutter, 1988). However, the style of analysis is sufficiently exemplified without the need to consider these further. We would argue that this 'piece-meal' approach to analysis will usually be required as a first stage in any exploration of possible 'turning points' in development. It is essential in order to sort out likely contenders for mechanisms and to see how they might operate in different subgroups. Imaginative consideration of alternative explanations is essential if artefactual interpretations are to be avoided and linear logistic analyses are required in order to examine combinations of variables. This approach can take one quite a long way in testing hypotheses on each separate link in the chain. Moreover, it has the important advantage of examining effects on the frequency of occurrence of dependent variables, as well as on their quality.

However, there are several limitations to this piece-meal cross-tabulation approach when the steps are put together in the form of a hypothesized chain of interlinked connections. First, the links over time are put together conceptually rather than statistically. The analyses do not correspond to the estimation of a 'structural model' and therefore do not allow any formal discernment of causal paths or the breakdown of effects into 'direct' and 'indirect' mechanisms. Secondly, the analyses at each point in the chain have been treated as if they were independent, when in fact they may have been influenced by the same (or related) 'error' variables that are intercorrelated over time. Thirdly, the impact of measurement error has not been considered. Lastly, issues of timing and detailed sequencing of events are not directly addressed.

A SYSTEM OF SIMULTANEOUS EQUATIONS OR STRUCTURAL MODEL

In general, log-linear and logit models, the standard procedures for analyzing multivariate categorical data, are not consistent with any structural model of the process and are not amenable to path analytic interpretation. However, if the process can be assumed to possess a natural ordering then an analysis can be performed as a set of recursive relationships and a structural model can be estimated using these simple methods (Goodman, 1973; Maddala, 1983, Section 5.5). Such recursive relationships might seem appropriate here, with the measures being interrelated according to the following triangular system of simultaneous equations

$$\begin{aligned}
\text{conduct} &= f_1\,(\text{sex, care}, e_1)\\
\text{school} &= f_2\,(\text{sex, care, conduct}, e_2)\\
\text{planning} &= f_3\,(\text{sex, care, conduct, school}, e_3)\\
\text{spouse} &= f_4\,(\text{sex, care, conduct, school, planning}, e_4)\\
\text{adult outcome} &= f_5\,(\text{sex, care, conduct, school, planning,}\\
&\qquad \text{spouse}, e_5)
\end{aligned}$$

where $e_1, \ldots, e_5$ are error terms. The impact of all prior measures can occur directly upon any later measure and can occur indirectly through any of the intermediate measures. Similar triangular systems have been explored in the analysis of continuous measures of ability and schooling on subsequent economic success (see, e.g., Chamberlain & Griliches, 1975) and Hsiao (1986, Section 5.4). For discrete outcomes Winship & Mare (1983) and Maddala (1983) provide a succinct discussion of identification and estimation issues for two equation systems.

A major attraction of a recursive system is that, if the error terms e_1 to e_5 are independent, then each of the equations (that might correspond to, say, separate logit models) could be separately estimated. There are however several complications to consider. The first concerns how the dependent variables arise, whether as discrete categorical responses or as values of a latent variable above or below a threshold. The second concerns the mechanism by which they act as independent variables on later outcomes, whether as a 'structural shift' associated with the category or a covariation with the value of an underlying latent variable. As an example, the influence of a deviant spouse on social functioning may be as a 'handicap' with an effect of a certain fixed magnitude, or it may be an indicator of a continuous feature in the choice of spouse (reflecting both the spouse and the ability of the subject to choose) with a corresponding effect of varying magnitude. Indeed simultaneous and separate effects from both the category and the underlying continuous feature are possible. Those models that allow for effects via the latent variable rather than just the category of response involve correlations among the errors (i.e., e_1 to e_5 above) and are therefore substantially more difficult to estimate. However, it seems that the forms with latent explanatory variables fit at least as well as the categorical forms. This is discussed with examples in Winship & Mare (1983).

Table 7.4 presents results from the independent estimation of each equation, with the effects of preceding measures occurring through their categorical outcome. The fitted equations included all main effects together with significant two-factor interaction effects. Similar links as before are indicated along this causal chain with positive school experiences having an effect on planning (for those with conduct disorder), planning on gaining a nondeviant spouse, and nondeviant spouse on adult outcome, though direct effects of intermediate variables are also seen, as is evidence of assortative mating among the conduct-disordered girls. The cumulative effects may be decomposed into direct and indirect in the manner of Winship & Mare (1983, equation 43) and summarized in Appendix 1, where it is also explained how nonlinearity in the equations results in the magnitude of the effects depending upon subgroup. Thus, for example, the direct effect of a positive school experience on adult dysfunction is smaller for ex-care girls with conduct disorder, compared with those without (−0.18 and −0.21), as too are the total indirect effects (−0.05 and −0.08). For the conduct-disordered girls those indirect effects are made up of the two-step effects via nondeviant spouse (−0.03) and via planning (−0.02), and the three-step effect via planning and thence nondeviant spouse (−0.00).

The indirect effects, in particular the last, are much smaller than expected from the impression left by the cross-tabulation results. The discrete outcome path calculus accounts for the probabilistic nature of

Table 7.4. *Parameter estimates from recursive models of adult social functioning (N = 227)*

Constant	Coefficient	Standard error
Child conduct disorder		
Constant	−0.272	
Sex	−2.646	(0.796)
Care	0.721	(0.406)
Sex × Care	1.980	(0.862)
School experience		
Constant	0.114	
Sex	−0.488	(0.303)
Care	−0.073	(0.312)
Child × CD	−1.375	(0.331)
Planning		
Constant	0.432	
Sex	−0.368	(0.349)
Care	−1.892	(0.456)
Child CD	−1.069	(0.401)
Sch. exp.	0.014	(0.485)
Care × Sch. exp.	1.067	(0.665)
Marital support		
Constant	−0.589	
Sex	0.241	(0.389)
Care	−0.306	(0.327)
Child CD	0.319	(0.418)
Sch. exp.	0.570	(0.314)
Planning	1.239	(0.352)
Sex × Child CD	−1.709	(0.682)
Adult outcome		
Constant	−0.853	
Sex	−0.942	(0.332)
Care	0.890	(0.358)
Child CD	1.138	(0.378)
Sch. exp.	−0.893	(0.336)
Planning	0.485	(0.444)
Support	−1.142	(0.329)
Child CD × Planning	−1.728	(0.786)

the links at each stage, a process that may tend to attenuate the indirect effects rather more than we intuitively do ourselves when examining each link separately, particularly where intermediate outcomes in the chain have a probability of occurrence far from 0.5. In this instance, the strong effect of school experience on planning for those with conduct disorder is being attenuated by the low probability of a nondeviant spouse, a result of assortative mating. This is important contextual information, but this attenuation also reflects the focus of interest of the path analysis method, namely the decomposition of the total sample variance of the final outcome measure. Effects occurring to only a small subgroup of the sample, even effects of substantial magnitude and scientific importance, will often represent only a small proportion of this total variance. A restriction of interest to those variables showing substantial *total* effects in terms of path analysis of the whole sample can wrongly eliminate important turning points from the field of study.

A LATENT CLASS TRANSITION OR MARKOV MODEL

The previous linear logistic models of social functioning (SF) that included childhood conduct disorder (CD) as an explanatory variable can be thought of as forms of Markov transition models and these are typically represented by matrices of transition probabilities between states, of the following form:

		Outcome state (SF)	
		Poor	Good
Initial state (CD)	Poor	$1-p$	p
	Good	q	$1-q$

Linear logistic models in which covariates (in addition to CD) were included but not interacted with CD (the initial state) correspond to Markov transition models in which the effects (on the logit scale) of covariates on the transition from poor to good is assumed to be equal but opposite to their effect on the transition from good to poor. Logit models with covariates introduced interacting with CD correspond to more general models with transition probabilities p and q that are influenced quite independently. However, in both cases, the logit estimation assumes that the categories defining state membership are determined without error and their results can be misleading where error is present.

The use of the three childhood CD and three adult outcome measures to determine membership of an underlying behavioral state at each occasion was explored through the use of a latent class Markov model.

Latent variable models consist of two components; the measurement model that describes how the observed variables are related to the latent variables, and the structural model that describes the relationship between the latent variables (and any others measured without error). The measurement model defining the relationship of the latent class to each of the binary indicator measures $\{Y_{ij}\}$ was specified by logit equations of the form

$$\Pr[Y_{ij} = 1 \mid XC_i = 0] = \text{logit}(a_j)$$

$$\Pr[Y_{ij} = 1 \mid XC_i = 1] = \text{logit}(a_j + b_j)$$

where XC_i is the latent class membership of child i, with values 0 (poor) or 1 (good) and the parameters $\{a_j, b_j\}$ allow for false positives and negatives among the CD indicators. Similar equations were specified for each of the adult measures. The structural model first required the specification of the prior probability or 'prevalence' of the latent state

$$\Pr[XC_i = 1] = c.$$

By denoting the latent class membership in adulthood by XA_i, the latent Markov model was specified by the transition probabilities between the latent states

$$\Pr[XA_i = 1 \mid XC_i = 0] = p$$

and

$$\Pr[XA_i = 1 \mid XC_i = 1] = 1 - q,$$

where p and q are the probabilities of making a transition from poor to good and good to poor respectively. Further extensions of the model allowed the prior probability c, and transition rates p and q to depend upon sex, childhood rearing and gaining a nondeviant spouse. A full appreciation of the workings of this model in practice was gained only after some effort. Results from the model depended upon a careful specification of the measurement models, or in more practical terms upon how the childhood and adult indicators were combined to define the states of interest. If measures were assumed equivalent, by imposing equality constraints within the $\{a_j\}$ and $\{b_j\}$, then measurement error was at risk of being identified as discontinuity, elevating estimates of transition probabilities. With no restrictions on the measurement equations evidence of real discontinuity in latent disorder was easily absorbed into measurement error resulting in tests of the structural model having little power. Some preliminary investigation suggested that no restrictions on the $\{a_j\}$ could be justified. These parameters were concerned with the prevalence of the indicators among individuals without the latent disorder, a disorder that has been implicitly defined

Table 7.5. *Measurement characteristics and prevalence estimates from a latent class model of continuity in disorder*

	False positive	False negative
B-Score (CD or mixed)	3.2%	58.5%
Delinquency <age 15	1.8%	71.9%
Retrospective interview	10.2%	29.3%
Adult crime (Boys)	6.8%	42.2%
(Girls)	2.9%	64.2%
Social	14.4%	54.9%
Work	12.1%	27.8%
Prevalence of CD		
Ex-care boys	64.6%	
Ex-care girls	38.8%	
Control boys	26.3%	
Control girls	2.3%	
Log-likelihood	−648.715	

as having effects that are pervasive across the relevant set of measures. However, some of the *b* coefficients, which measure the difference in indicator prevalence between those with and without the latent disorder, could be equated (those of the childhood indicators and the adult indicators crime and work). The remaining adult indicator, concerned with social relationships, appeared to be a rather poor discriminator of those with or without pervasive problems. In addition, the crime indicator seemed to occur less frequently among women than among men, for both those with and without disorder.

These comments are reflected in the parameter estimates of Table 7.5 obtained from a model where the transition probabilities representing discontinuity between childhood and adulthood were restricted to zero. In practice, the actual frequencies of false positives and false negatives depend not only on the characteristics of the indicators but also upon the prevalence of disorder. Thus, among the comparison girls where conduct disorder was rare, more of the errors of classification were false positives, compared with the ex-care boys, where rather more false negatives occurred. As a result, although for most groups the estimated rates of disorder (as represented by the latent state) were higher than rates identified using the observed indicators, they were lower where the prevalence of disorder was low. The latent class model therefore provided a clearer separation of groups with high and low levels of disorder than could be done using combinations of observed indicators.

Table 7.6. *Tests of discontinuity between childhood and adulthood*

	Chi-square	d.f.	*p*
Childhood non-disorder to adult disorder			
Simple homogeneous non-zero transition rate	0.00	1	1
Transition rate dependent on care status	0.00	2	1
Transition rate dependent on sex	1.13	2	0.6
Transition rate dependent on care × sex	1.36	4	0.9
Childhood disorder to adult non-disorder			
Simple homogeneous non-zero transition rate	2.60	1	0.1
Transition rate dependent on care status	6.39	2	0.04
Transition rate dependent on sex	2.60	2	0.3
Transition rate dependent on care × sex	8.01	4	0.09

Table 7.6 presents the results of allowing for discontinuity. The results suggest that there was no significant adult onset of pervasive poor functioning in this sample. However, there was significant discontinuity out of the childhood disorder state, and this varied with the care status of the child, the estimated transition rates being 0.21 for ex-care boys, 0.27 for ex-care girls, 0.57 for comparison boys and 1.00 for the comparison girls (a virtually non-existent group).

Table 7.7 presents a cross-tabulation of posterior probabilities. A posterior probability is the probability with which an individual can be assigned to a particular latent state, or history of latent states in a longitudinal context such as this, given their observed indicators and covariate values and the parameter estimates of the model. Summed across the sample, or a cross-classification of the sample, these give some indication of the sample process as seen by the latent Markov analysis and allow a direct comparison with a cross-tabulation using the original indicators or some simple combination of them. The specific combinations of childhood indicators chosen (positive if one of the three childhood indicators is positive – even where missing data) and of adult indicators (positive if two of three indicators positive) were selected to give similar prevalences to those identified by the latent Markov analysis. Indeed, it has been these combinations that have been used everywhere else in this chapter, not only to provide consistency across analyses, but because the latent Markov approach was able to provide explicit clues as to the prevalences and corresponding thresholds most appropriate to use. This was a noteworthy strength of this approach. Comparisons of the two cross-tabulations clearly illustrated the increased continuity arising from our attempt to reduce the impact of measurement errors.

Table 7.7. *A comparison of continuity between childhood and adult disorder as measured by observed and latent classifications*

		Boys		Girls	
		Observed disorder[a] (Sample frequencies)			
		Adult		Adult	
		No	Yes	No	Yes
Childhood CD	No	42	9	76	2
	Yes	29	34	18	17
		Latent classification (Estimated frequencies derived from posterior probabilities)			
		Adult		Adult	
		No	Yes	No	Yes
Childhood CD	No	47.9	0	80.1	0
	Yes	10.6	55.6	5.2	27.8

[a] Conduct disordered if 1 or more in 3 childhood indicators positive. Adult dysfunction if 2 or more in 3 indicators positive.

Table 7.8. *Assortative mating, discontinuity and the marital support of a nondeviant spouse*

Assortative Mating	Marital support & discon-tinuity	Marital support on outcome indicators	Chi-square	d.f.	*p*
No	No	No			
Yes	Yes	Yes	30.90	6	<0.001
No	Yes	Yes	11.02	2	0.004
Yes	No	Yes	3.18	2	0.2
Yes	Yes	No	4.22	2	0.12
Yes	No	No	13.67	4	0.008

An examination of how the discontinuity that remained was associated with marital support is presented in Table 7.8. The null model allowed the transition rate out of conduct disorder to vary only with care status. The full model allowed for three additional effects. Firstly, the prevalence of the latent childhood state could vary with deviance of spouse, reflecting assortative mating. Secondly, the transition rate out of childhood disorder could vary with the presence or absence of a nondeviant spouse. Thirdly, the occurrence of positive adult indicators could vary as the result of the supportive effect of the spouse regardless of the childhood state of the subject. All three effects could differ between the sexes. An overall test showed highly significant effects to be present. The sequence of tests isolated significant assortative mating and significant effects for either or both of the nondeviant spouse effects. In this model these last two effects were highly colinear and essentially could not be distinguished. With the three effects included, the difference in the transition rate out of disorder did not differ significantly by care status (2.58, 1 d.f., $p = 0.1$).

In the above analysis, a deviant spouse and no spouse were pooled to form a single category of a lack of marital support. Although there was some evidence that no spouse appeared intermediate in effect, there was no significant difference between the transition rates with a deviant spouse or with no spouse for either men or women (1.84, 2 d.f., $p = 0.4$).

EVENT-HISTORY MODEL FOR THE PROCESS OF GAINING A SUPPORTIVE RELATIONSHIP

These foregoing results suggested that a closer look at the process of spouse selection might prove valuable. In addition, there was a need to consider alternative methods which might prove more appropriate to sequences of events that possessed no natural ordering (see Rindfuss, Swicegood & Rosenfeld, 1987) and which began to address issues concerned with timing. Between leaving care and the follow-up interview the women may well have been through several cohabiting relationships and even before such relationships will also have been at risk of teenage childbearing. Does the value of a planning disposition lie in being able to avoid entering into unsupportive relationships or single parenthood or does it lie in the ability and decisiveness necessary to get out of such potential 'traps' (Harris, Brown & Bifulco, 1987)? The process of moving into, out of and between various relationships and levels of support/burden might be investigated using multistate event-history models.

Such a model could estimate the impact of covariates, such as planning, on the transition rates or intensities between recurrent states (potentially revisitable) in much the same way that survival models do for transitions in the non-recurrent state of death. Unfortunately, the information on the intervening relationships, being based on retrospective questioning, is not as complete as that for the current spouse. Although some progress is possible, the estimation of formal multistate models using incomplete information is difficult in situations of realistic complexity (Cox & Miller, 1965, Ch. 5; DeStavola, 1985, Ch. 3). We

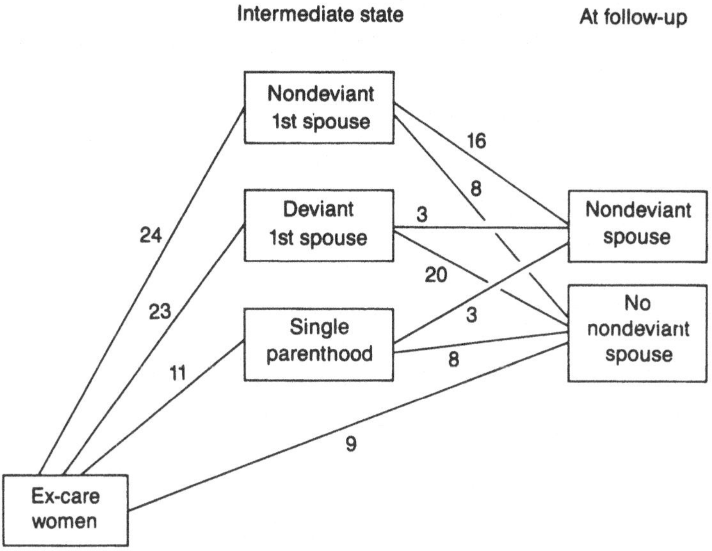

Figure 7.3. Paths to marital support (numbers refer to sample frequencies).

therefore compromised on the structure of the model that was investigated, to that shown in Figure 7.3.

The first part of the model focused upon their earliest experiences in this arena and consisted of a competing risk model where the women were at risk of three transitions; cohabitation with a nondeviant spouse, cohabitation with a deviant spouse, and single parenthood prior to any cohabitation. Behaviour subsequent to this was then modeled by a less formal model that simply examined the probability of being in a supportive relationship given these first outcomes, the exact path between the two being left unspecified.

Throughout the model, but in particular in the first part, it might also have been valuable to have distinguished the further states of living at home and living independently, the possible value of a harmonious parental home in screening peers and potential spouses having already been noted. However, the data proved too sparse to allow this.

In the analysis that follows the relative shapes of the three hazards have not been assumed but have been estimated from the data as Weibull hazards with different shape and scale parameters. A non-parametric specification of them is possible using partial likelihood (Cox, 1972; see also Clayton, 1988, for a review and problems in multistate models) but in preliminary analyses using partial likelihood the results differed little from those reported here. Aalen *et al.* (1988) described simple models that offer some intuitive justification for the use of the Weibull hazard function in biology and the social sciences.

Table 7.9. *Weibull model for the effects of conduct disorder, planning disposition and harmonious family home on the competing risks of nondeviant spouse, deviant spouse and single parenthood (N = 67)*

Hazard to	Coefficient	Standard error	Relative risk	Confidence interval (95%)
Nondeviant spouse				
Constant	−1.742			
Weibull	2.165	0.341		
Conduct	−0.194	0.562	0.82	0.28–2.48
Planning	0.357	0.437	1.43	0.61–3.37
Deviant spouse				
Constant	−1.437			
Weibull	1.783	0.300		
Conduct	0.409	0.443	1.51	0.63–3.59
Planning	−1.258	0.724	0.28	0.07–1.18
Single parenthood				
Constant	−2.456			
Weibull	2.369	0.526		
Conduct	0.490	0.636	1.63	0.47–5.68
Planning	−1.279	1.028	0.28	0.04–2.09

The choice of a parametric hazard simplified further exploration of models that allowed for correlations across the various risk processes due to unobserved heterogeneity. In the analysis this was treated as a normally distributed component of variance. Alternative approaches to omitted variables for event-history data, such as the stable law models of Hougaard (1987) or non-parametric maximum likelihood (Heckman & Singer, 1984; Pickles & Davies, 1985) appeared less tractable. As was the case in the recursive logistic model, the various parts of the model that ignored heterogeneity could be separately estimated.

Table 7.9 gives the parameter estimates from data on the 67 ex-care women for whom data were available for the first part of the model. Relatively few of the effects of covariates were significant, but in terms of the magnitudes of the estimated effects planning appeared important. Plots of the estimated hazard functions between the ages of 13 and 22 are shown in Figure 7.4 for both non-planners and planners. Very clearly shown are the substantially lower hazards for planners to the poor intermediate states of deviant first spouse and single parenthood, in contrast to their very similar hazard function to a nondeviant first spouse. The effects of conduct disorder also failed to achieve sig-

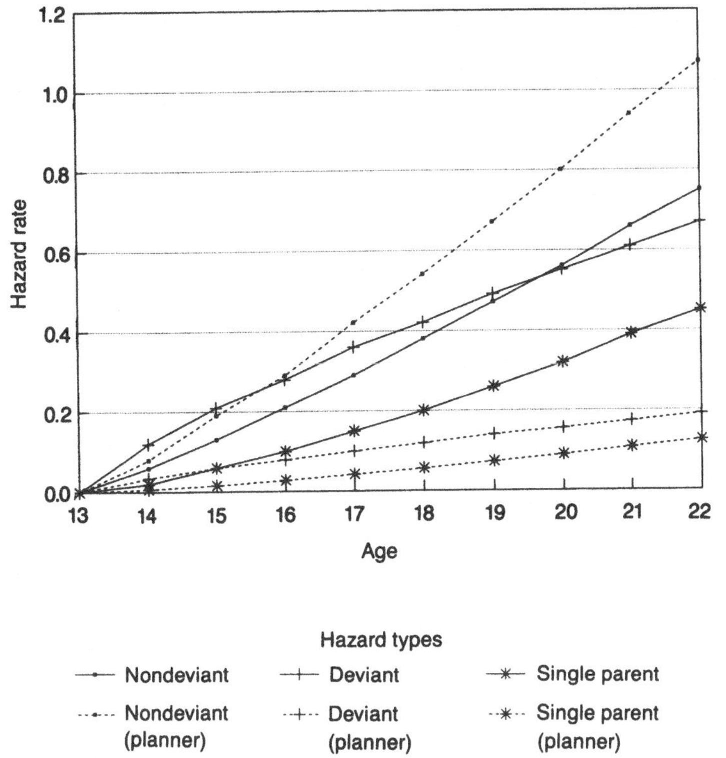

Figure 7.4. Hazard functions to nondeviant spouse, deviant spouse and to single parenthood.

nificance, but were of the expected sign, with a reduced hazard to a nondeviant first spouse but increased for those to a deviant first spouse and single parenthood.

Figure 7.4 also shows how the hazards to each of the intermediate states vary independently with age. Of particular note is that the hazard function to deviant spouse was, for these women, higher at the younger ages than the hazard to a nondeviant spouse, but was lower when they were older. This is shown more clearly in the plot of the risk ratio in Figure 7.5. Although for these data this difference in hazard function shapes (and thus non-constant risk ratio) was not statistically significant, it is interesting to pursue its possible consequences.

What this curve suggests is that cohabitations in the younger ages are more at risk of being with a deviant spouse than at older ages. As a consequence a characteristic, attribute or constraint that lowers the risks of any cohabitation in these younger ages will also reduce the eventual probability that the first cohabitation will be with a deviant spouse and

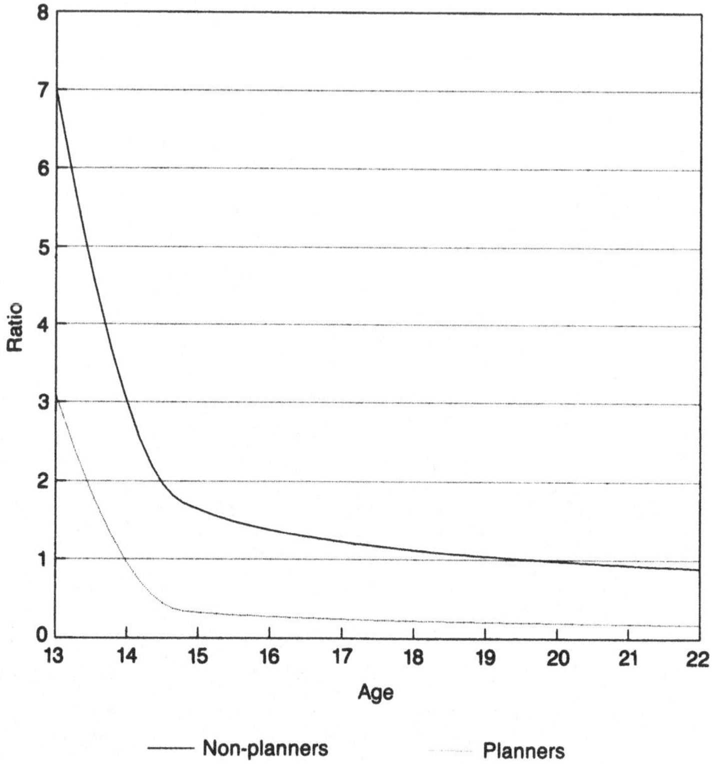

Figure 7.5. The ratio of hazards to deviant and nondeviant spouse.

increase that with a nondeviant spouse. Thus the law, a 'protective' home or a characteristic such as trepidation that simply delays cohabitation can, in an environment of age/time dependent risks, positively (or negatively) alter the nature of final outcomes. A competing risk framework allows emphasis to be given to these questions of timing and illustrates possible conceptual links with other work on the risks associated with early maturity.

The second part of the model, a logit model of the probability of being with a nondeviant spouse at the time of follow-up, included both the intermediate states of deviant first spouse and single parenthood (nondeviant spouse being the reference group) and the explanatory variables conduct disorder and planning. The results are shown in Table 7.10.

In comparison with an intermediate state with a nondeviant first spouse, those of single parenthood and particularly deviant first spouse

Table 7.10. *From first spouse or single parenthood to nondeviant spouse at follow-up (N = 58)*

	Constant	Coefficient	Standard error
Constant	0.0853		
Deviant			
1st spouse		−2.398	0.904
Single parent		−1.175	0.915
Conduct		−0.659	0.895
Planning		3.257	1.195
Scaled deviance		29.47	d.f. 53

appear to reduce substantially the probability of a supportive relationship at follow-up. Given the intermediate state, the effect of conduct disorder was of the expected sign but was neither large nor significant. By contrast, that for a planning disposition was substantial and significant. Interactions between the intermediate state dummy variables and covariates provide a crude test of the paths along which the covariates have their effect. The data were too sparse for the fitting of many interaction terms and so a more parameter-efficient approach was sought. The main focus of interest lay in whether the covariates, in particular planning, had a general effect or whether their effect was specifically associated with those experiencing a poor intermediate state. Redefining the covariate to limit its effect to just these states gave only a slightly worse fitting model but with a substantially increased parameter estimate. This appeared to confirm the value of a planning disposition for 'getting out' from potential long-term problems.

Although we had already encountered problems associated with the sparseness of data, some exploration of the possible impact of omitted variables was undertaken. In this instance, the inclusion of the variance component also began to deal with the problem of potential sample selection that occurs between the two halves of the model. The addition of a normally distributed variance component (see Brillinger & Preisler (1986) for a more detailed outline of the genetal approach) to each of the three hazards and to the logit choice component of the previous model required a further four parameters and gave a reduction of 25.03 in the overall scaled deviance. There was little change in the estimates for the covariates from those of Tables 7.9 and 7.10, with the effects of planning remaining important.

DISCUSSION

Unquestionably, the analysis of turning points can become extremely complex. The prospect of attempting to identify the important chain of effects for the relevant subgroup in the presence of measurement error, omitted variables, time-dependencies and so on, can be overwhelming. However, the experience recounted in this chapter suggests that progress can be made, at least for those circumstances where an ordering of events is possible, by the use of relatively simple cross-tabulation/logit methods, guided by a clear conception of the kinds of mechanisms and effects expected and of the alternatives to be checked.

The additional knowledge gleaned from the application of the more complex multivariate methods was considerable, but the nature of that new knowledge was often quite unexpected. Our initial implicit question was whether the original analyses would 'hold up' under these alternative and less familiar methods of data analysis. The more interesting points that emerged related to discovering the empirical implications of the different conceptualizations of the process that were embodied in each of the methods.

Structural models provide a valuable tool for formalizing the decomposition of direct and indirect effects over several links in the chain and, where the appropriate data are available, would allow more thorough checking of omitted variable explanations. Nevertheless, the standard programs for the estimation of such models lack an easy treatment of what is an essential ingredient of the turning point argument, namely that the effects vary across subjects. Critical is the opportunity to explore interacting effects, so easily done within logit models, or – and more generally – to allow for random coefficients (as in so-called multilevel models; see Goldstein (1987)). The latter are particularly suitable where the covariates to explain differing response are unmeasured or at least as yet unidentified. The application in this chapter illustrated clearly how the decomposition of effects in a discrete data model is dependent upon the prevalence of initial, intermediate and outcome events in the chain. Major individual effects can be substantially attenuated as the result of the small proportion of the population to whom the effect applies. Moreover, the prevalences, and thus the attenuation, vary across sub-groups, implying that several different decompositions of direct and indirect effects may need to be examined. The example showed that unless the effect sizes at each step in the chain are very substantial, progressive attenuation is likely to occur at each link in a chain. This should caution us against stringing together large numbers of events in a chain purely on the basis of each being significant and then expecting this path to explain a large proportion of the population variance. However, neither does this mean that the chain should be ignored, for the size of the final effect can still be very substantial for some individuals.

The insights from the latent Markov model emerged only after an initial period of familiarization. The dangers in the casual use of multiple measures as indicators of a meaningful latent variable became clear. Considerable attention must be given to the specification of the measurement models and consideration given to the power of the statistical tests that are likely to be achieved. Additional calculation beyond the simple computation of the parameter estimates was required, in particular the cross-tabulation of posterior probabilities, to grasp properly the characteristics of the latent process being identified. However, under appropriate conditions the estimated structural relationships, when swept of measurement error, can be substantially sharpened and the measurement models can provide great insight into the performance and characteristics of the indicators.

Cross-tabulation methods are particularly cumbersome where the chain of events does not allow a fixed ordering to be imposed upon them, or where the timing of events rather than just their order becomes of importance. Competing risk survival methods, in the form of multistate event-history models, would appear to offer advantages, at least in terms of the conceptual framework that they bring. As yet their application to processes beyond even moderate complexity (not to say realism) often requires a sophistication of mathematics and programming beyond those usually available. Moreover, several problems, in particular the initial conditions problem (Heckman, 1981; Pickles, 1987), remain to be solved or restrict the scope for generalization (Chesher & Lancaster, 1983). In spite of these problems our results suggest that even very simplified versions can yield a greater understanding of the process, bringing to the fore questions of timing that should be central to any analysis of developmental processes.

It should not be forgotten that the nature of the expected methods of analysis influences the nature of the study design and the data that are collected. The data used in this chapter were collected and initially processed largely with cross-tabulalation in mind. Thus repeat measures and the detailed dating of life-histories were not given major emphasis. Although, in this case, we doubt whether their availability would substantially alter the eventual story to be told, the presence of such measures would have made the more complete application of those other methods used in this chapter both more straightforward and more powerful.

Regardless of the technique, the complexity of the 'individualized' mechanisms that are postulated makes replication more than usually necessary because of the possibility of capitalizing on chance associations. In the case of the hypotheses that we have considered here, replication is available (albeit with somewhat different samples and outcome variables) with all the key variables – including positive school experiences (Rutter *et al.*, 1979), planning (Clausen, 1986), premarital pregnancy (Harris *et al.*, 1987), and marital support (Brown & Harris, 1978; Parker & Hadzi-Pavlovic, 1984). That is reassuring so far as it does, although clearly there is the further need to replicate the dynamic chain process involving turning points that has been postulated here.

APPENDIX 1

Direct and indirect effects for categorical data

In the case of the models estimated here (type III in the classification of Winship & Mare (1983)) the discrete endogeneous variables have a direct effect. Since the relationships between variables are nonlinear the effects, and associated paths, must be evaluated at specified levels of all the covariates and, following usual practice, mean values have been used here.

For a two-equation system,

$$Z = a_0 + a_1 X + a_3 \cdot d_Y + e_Z \quad \text{and} \quad Y = b_0 + b_1 X + e_Y,$$

where $\mathrm{cov}(e_Y, e_Z) = 0$ and where Y and Z are observed discretely; then the effects of the variable X on the variable Z can be decomposed into direct effects and those indirect through Y as follows:

$$dp(d_Z = 1) = a_1 \cdot f(a_0 + a_1 X + a_3 d_Y)$$

(total effect) (direct effect)

$$+ a_3 \cdot f(a_0 + a_1 X + a_3 d_Y) b_1 \cdot f(b_0 + b_1 X)$$

(indirect effect)

The a's and b's are regression coefficients of one type or another (e.g. probit, logistic, etc.) and the e's are error terms assumed to have distributions of the corresponding form. The intermediate variable Y influences the final outcome Z only through the discrete binary variable d_Y, related to Y by means of a threshold. For a probit model f is given by $\exp[-(t ** 2/2)]/sqrt(2 * pi)$ and for a logit model by $\{\exp(t)/[1 + \exp(t)]\}\{1/[1 + \exp(t)]\}$.

As an example, the direct effects of positive school experience on adult outcome that are given in the text for ex-care girls with and without conduct disorder are calculated from $-0.893 \times \exp(0.995)/[1 + \exp(0.995)] ** 2 = -0.18$ for those with CD and $-0.893 \times \exp(-0.532)/[1 + \exp(-0.532)] ** 2 = -0.21$ for those without CD, where -1.002 is the estimated coefficient for positive school experience given in Table 7.4 and 0.995 and -0.532 are the rates, on the logistic scale, of poor adult outcome among ex-care girls with and without CD.

The extension over several equations is obvious.

APPENDIX 2

Weibull competing risk model

Individuals, subscripted i, were from age 13 assumed to be exposed simultaneously to several risks, subscripted j. The hazard for individual i from risk j was of a Weibull form given by

$$h_{ij}(t) = c_j t^{c_j - 1} \exp[b_{j0} + b_{j1}x_{i1} + b_{j2}x_{i2} + \ldots + b_{jp}x_{ip})$$

where c_j is a parameter that determines the pattern of time variation in the risk and the parameters b_{j1} to b_{jp} and corresponding explanatory covariates determine the relative risks among individuals. Density functions for the age at the first event are then constructed in the standard fashion as the product of the event-specific hazard and the survivor function from all risks.

As a member of the proportional hazards family with log link function, exponentiation of the estimated coefficients for the risk factors gives the estimated relative risks. The Weibull parameter estimates how the instantaneous risk varies with age, a value of 1 representing a constant risk with larger and smaller values representing increasing and decreasing risks respectively.

In the treatment of omitted heterogeneity, the constants b_{j0} rather than being assumed fixed constants were taken to have been normally distributed random variables. A mean a_{j0} and standard deviation a_{j1} were estimated for these exactly correlated random variables by means of marginal maximum likelihood, their distribution being represented by means of 10 point Gaussian quadrature at locations d_k. This gives expressions of the form

$$a_{jik} = a_{j0} + a_{j1} \cdot d_k$$

for the 'constant' for individual i on the jth risk and kth quadrature point.

The procedure assumes the random component to be independently and identically distributed over individuals. Thus it is implicitly assumed that the omitted covariate has constant variance across individuals and that it is uncorrelated with included covariates. In addition, all covariates are assumed exogeneous (see Crouchley & Pickles (1989) for further discussion of marginal maximum likelihood in a renewal model).

ACKNOWLEDGEMENTS

We are grateful to David Quinton for providing the data, and to both him and Barbara Maughan for valuable discussion.

REFERENCES

Aalen, O. (1988). Heterogeneity in survival analysis. *Statistics in Medicine 7*, 1121–1137.

Aalen, O., Borgan, O., Keiding, N. & Thormann, J. (1988). Interaction between life-history events. Nonparametric analysis for prospective and retrospective data in the presence of censoring. *Scandinavian Journal of Statistics, 7*, 161–171.

Aitkin, M. (1979). A simultaneous test procedure for contingency table models. *Applied Statistics, 28,* 233–42.

Brillinger, D. R. & Preisler, H. K. (1986). Two examples of quantal data analysis: (a) multivariate point processes, (b) pure death process in an experimental design. *Proceedings of the 13th International Biometric Conference,* Seattle.

Brown, G. & Harris, T. (1978). *The social origins of depression.* London: Tavistock Publications.

Chamberlain, G. & Griliches, Z. (1975). Unobservables with a variance components structure: ability, schooling and the economic success of brothers. *International Economic Review, 16,* 422–450.

Chesher, A. & Lancaster, T. (1983), The estimation of models of labour market behaviour. *Review of Economic Studies, 50,* 609–624.

Clausen, J. A. (1986). Early adult choices and the life course. *Zeitschrift für Sozialisations Forschung und Erzielungsozioligie, 6,* 313–320.

Clayton, D. (1988). The analysis of event history data: a review of progress and outstanding problems. *Statistics in Medicine, 7,* 819–841.

Cox, D. R. (1972). Regression models and life tables. *Journal of the Royal Statistical Society, 34B,* 187–220.

Cox, D. R. & Miller, H. D. (1965). *The theory of stochastic processes.* London: Methuen.

Crouchley, R. & Pickles, A. R. (1989). An empirical comparison of conditional and marginal likelihood methods in a longitudinal study. *In* C. Clogg (ed.), *Sociological methodology 1989* (pp. 161–183). New York: Jossey–Bass.

Davies, R. B. & Pickles, A. R. (1985). Longitudinal vs cross-sectional methods for behavioural research: a first round knock-out. *Environment and Planning, A 17,* 1315–1329.

DeStavola, B. L. (1985). Multi-state Markov Processes with Incomplete Information. Unpublished PhD Thesis, Imperial College, London.

Dunn, J. & Kendrick, C. (1982). *Siblings: Love, envy and understanding.* London: Grant McIntyre.

Elbers, C. & Ridder, G. (1982). True and spurious duration dependence: the identifiability of the proportional hazards model. *Review of Economic Studies, 49,* 403–409.

Elder, G. H. (1974). *Children of the Great Depression.* Chicago University Press.

Elder, G. H. (1986). Military times and turning points in men's lives. *Development Psychology, 22,* 233–245.

Elder, G. H. (in press). Family transitions, cycles and social change. In P. Cowan & M. Hetherington (eds.), *Family transitions.*

Elder, G. H., Caspi, A. & Burton, L. (1988). Adolescent transitions in developmental perspective: Sociological and historical insights on adolescence. In M. R. Gunner (ed.), *Minnesota Symposia on Child Psychology.* Hillsdale, NJ: Erlbaum.

Furstenberg, F. F., Brooks-Gunn, J. & Morgan, P. J. (1987). *Adolescent mothers in later life.* Cambridge University Press.

Garmezy, N. & Rutter, M. (1985). Acute reactions to stress. In M. Rutter and L. Hersov (eds.), *Child and adolescent psychiatry: Modern approaches.* (2nd edition) (pp. 152–176). Oxford: Blackwell Scientific.

Gabriel, K. R. (1966). Simultaneous test procedures for multiple comparisons on categorical data. *Journal of the American Statistical Association, 61,* 1081–1096.

Goldstein, H. (1987). *Multilevel models in educational and social research.* London: Griffin.

Goodman, L. A. (1973). Causal analysis of panel study data and other kinds of survey data. *American Journal of Sociology, 78,* 1135–1191.

Gottfried, A. E. & Gottfried, A. W. (eds.) (1988). *Maternal employment and children's development: Longitudinal research.* New York: Plenum Press.

Hareven, T. K. (ed.) (1978). *Transitions: the family and life course in historical perspective.* New York: Academic Press.

Harris, T., Brown, G. W. & Bifulco, A. (1987). Loss of parents in childhood and psychiatric disorder: the role of social class position and pre-marital pregnancy. *Psychological Medicine, 17,* 163–183.

Heckman, J. J. (1981). The incidental parameter problem and the problem of initial conditions in estimating a discrete time discrete data stochastic process. In C. F. Manski & D. McFadden (eds.), *Structural analysis of discrete data with econometric applications* (pp. 179–195). Cambridge, Mass.: MIT Press.

Heckman, J. J. & Singer, B. (1984). A method for minimizing the impact of distributional assumptions in econometric models of duration. *Econometrica, 52,* 271–320.

Hetherington, E. M. (1988). Parents, children and siblings: six years after divorce. In R. A. Hinde & J. Stevenson-Hinde (eds.), *Relationships within families: Mutual influences* (pp. 311–331). Oxford: Clarendon Press.

Hetherington, E. M., Cox, M. & Cox, R. (1982). Effects of divorce on parents and children. In M. E. Lamb (ed.), *Nontraditional families: Parenting and child development* (pp. 233–288). Hillsdale, NJ: Erlbaum.

Hinde, J. (1982). Compound Poisson regression models. In R. Gilchrist (ed.), *GLIM82* (pp. 109–121). Berlin: Springer-Verlag.

Hofferth, S. L. (1987). Teenage pregnancy and its resolution. In S. Hofferth & C. Hayes (eds.), *Risking the future: Adolescent sexuality, pregnancy and childbearing,* vol. 2. Washington, D.C.: National Academy Press.

Hogan, D. P. (1978). The variable order of events in the life-course. *American Sociological Review, 43,* 573–586.

Hougaard, P. (1987). Modelling multivariate survival. *Scandinavian Journal of Statistics, 14,* 291–304.

Hsiao, C. (1986). *Analysis of panel data.* New York: Wiley.

James, W. (1902). *The varieties of religious experience.* London: Longman.

Jőreskog, K. G. & Sőrbum, D. (1984). *LISREL VI: Analysis of linear structural relationships by maximum likelihood, instrumental variables, and least squares methods* (3rd edition). Mooresville, IN: Scientific Software.

Kenward, M. G. (1987). A method for comparing profiles of repeated measurements. *Applied Statistics, 36,* 296–308.

Knight, B. J., Osborn, S. G. & West, D. J. (1977). Early marriage and criminal tendency in males. *British Journal of Criminology, 17,* 348–360.

Levinson, D., Darrow, D. N., Klein, E. B., Levinson, M. H. & McKee, D. (1976). *The seasons of a man's life.* New York: Alfred Knopf.

Maddala, G. S. (1983). *Limited-dependent and qualitative variables in econometrics.* Cambridge University Press.

Mare, R. D. & Winship, C. (1985). School enrolment, military enlistment and the transition to work: implications for the age pattern of employment. In J. J. Heckman & B. Singer (eds.), *Longitudinal analysis of Labour Market Data* (pp. 364–400). Cambridge University Press.

Magnusson, D., Stattin, H. & Allen, V. L. (1986). Differential maturation among girls and its relations to social adjustment: a longitudinal perspective. In P. B. Baltes, D. L. Featherman & R. M. Lerner (eds.), *Life-span development and behaviour* (vol. 7, pp. 136–172). Hillsdale NJ: Erlbaum.

Maughan, B., & Champion, L. (in press). Risk and protective factors in the transition to young adulthood. In P. B. Baltes & M. M. Baltes (eds.), *Successful ageing: Research and theory.* Cambridge University Press.

NAG (1983). *Fortran library manual.* Oxford: Numerical Algorithms Group.

Neugarten, B. L., Moore, J. W. & Lowe, J. C. (1965). Age norms, age constraints and adult socialization. *American Journal of Sociology, 70,* 710–717.

Parker, G. & Hadzi-Pavlovic, D. (1984). Modification of levels of depression in mother-bereaved women by parental and marital relationships. *Psychological Medicine, 14,* 125–136.

Pickles, A. R. (1987). The problem of initial conditions in longitudinal analysis. In R. Crouchley (ed.), *Longitudinal data analysis* (pp. 129–149). Aldershot: Avebury.

Pickles, A. R. & Davies, R. B. (1985). The analysis of housing careers. *Journal of Regional Science, 25,* 85–101.

Pickles, A. R., Davies, R. B. & Crouchley, R. (1982). Heterogeneity, non-stationarity and duration-of-stay effects in residential mobility. *Environment and Planning, A14,* 615–622.

Quinton, D. & Rutter, M. (1988). *Parental breakdown: The making and breaking of inter-generational links.* Aldershot: Avebury.

Quinton, D., Rutter, M. & Liddle, C. (1984). Institutional rearing, parenting difficulties and marital support. *Psychological Medicine, 14,* 107–124.

Raphael, B. (1984). *The anatomy of bereavement.* London: Hutchinson.

Rindfuss, R. R., Swicegood, C. G. & Rosenfeld, R. A. (1987). Disorder in the life-course: how common and does it matter? *American Sociological Review, 52,* 785–801.

Rutter, M. (1987*a*). Continuities and discontinuities from infancy. In J. D. Osofsky (ed.), *Handbook of infant development* (2nd edition) (pp. 1256–1296). New York: Wiley.

Rutter, M. (1987*b*). Psychosocial resilience and protective mechanisms. *American Journal of Orthopsychiatry, 57,* 316–33.

Rutter, M. (1989). Pathways from childhood to adult life. Jack Tizard Memorial Lecture. *Journal of Child Psychology and Psychiatry, 30,* 23–51.

Rutter, M. & Madge, N. (1976). *Cycles of disadvantage.* London: Heinemann Education.

Rutter, M. & Quinton, D. (1984). Long-term follow-up of women of institutionalized in childhood: factors promoting good functioning in adult life. *British Journal of Developmental Psychology, 18,* 225–234.

Rutter, M., Maughan, B., Mortimore, P., Ouston, J. & Smith, A. S. (1979). *Fifteen thousand hours: secondary schools and their effects on children.* London: Open Books.

Rutter, M., Quinton, D. & Hill, J. (1990). Adult outcome of institution reared children: Males and females compared. L. Robins & M. Rutter (eds.) *Straight and devious pathways from childhood to adult life* (pp. 135–157). New York: Cambridge University Press.
Simmons, R. G. & Blyth, D. A. (1987). *Moving into adolescence: The impact of pubertal change and school context.* Hawthorne, NY: Aldine de Gruyton.
Thornes, B. & Collard, J. (1979). *Who divorces?* London: Routledge and Kegan Paul.
Warr, P. (1987). *Work, unemployment and mental health.* Oxford: Clarendon Press.
West, D. J. (1982). *Delinquency: Its roots, careers and prospects.* London: Heinemann.
Winship, C. (1986). Age dependence, heterogeneity and the interdependence of life-cycle transitions. In N. Tuma (ed.), *Sociological methodology 1986* (pp. 249–264). New York: Jossey-Bass.
Winship, C. & Mare, R. D. (1983). Structural equations and path analysis for discrete data. *American Journal of Sociology, 89,* 54–110.
Zoccolillo, M., Pickles, A., Rutter, M. & Quinton, D. (in preparation). The outcome of conduct disorder: Implications for defining adult personality disorder.

8 Qualitative analyses of individual differences in intraindividual change: examples from cognitive development

EBERHARD SCHRÖDER, WOLFGANG EDELSTEIN, AND SIEGFRIED HOPPE-GRAFF

INTRODUCTION

The aim of the present chapter is twofold: on the one hand, qualitative analyses of individual developmental trajectories in cognition are presented; on the other hand, conceptual, methodological and statistical implications of the qualitative analysis of individual differences in intraindividual change are discussed. In contrast to the variable-oriented approaches most often applied in the analysis of individual development, a person- or individual-oriented approach will be used (Magnusson, 1985; Schröder, 1989). Person- or individual-oriented approaches are applied in clinical case studies, medical research and biostatistics, where the individual's patterns of characteristics, attributes or trajectories over time are the unit of analysis. This approach thus focuses mainly on configurations or constellations of attributes. In developmental research the individual-oriented approach is infrequent in spite of the fact that the empirical evaluation of important theories about development depends on the analysis of individual paths of development. Thus, for example, Piaget's theory of cognitive development postulates different stages or levels in cognitive development and that certain levels of cognitive functioning always precede, and are a necessary condition for, the emergence of subsequent levels of development (invariable developmental sequence). Empirically, questions concerning *décalages* in development and developmental sequences can be adequately evaluated only on the basis of the individual developmental patterns, since aggregate developmental curves for groups do not show how the individual develops over time (Bakan, 1967). Therefore, in this chapter we will use an analytical and methodological approach that is designed for the analysis of sequential data, in particular for the study of intraindividual change and intraindividual differences in development. Further, we will focus on interindividual differences as generated by *internal* constraints on development and analyze whether the acquisition of cognitive operations within the individual forms an invariable developmental sequence or whether uniformity in developmental trajectories does not obtain.

The analysis of individual development will be exemplified by the domain of cognitive development, especially the development of conservation of area at ages 7 and 8, and the development of syllogistic reasoning at ages 9, 12 and 15. The data of the present research derive from a longitudinal study conducted in Iceland (Edelstein, Keller & Schröder, 1990). Subjects were 121 children from an urban community who were tested at ages 7, 8, 9, 12, and 15. As we shall focus on methodological issues, in particular the modeling of assumptions about individual development in cognition and the statistical examination of these models, specific theoretical issues such as the hypothesis for the order-theoretical models presented in this chapter will not be discussed extensively.

CONCEPTUAL AND METHODOLOGICAL IMPLICATIONS IN THE ANALYSIS OF DEVELOPMENTAL SEQUENCES

The constructs of developmental sequence and stage are central to the theory of cognitive development as they represent intraindividual change in the acquisition of cognitive abilities and operations. In developmental theory the concept of sequence refers to the ordered acquisition of distinct developmental steps or stages. Two types of developmental sequences are distinguished (see also Campbell & Richie, 1983): prerequisite structures, and precursor sequences. A prerequisite structure is a necessary condition for the emergence of a later ability. Precursor sequences merely reflect the empirical order in the acquisition of different tasks within one developmental dimension. This implies that some tasks are easier to solve than others, because specific performance conditions (difficulty of tasks or mode of presentation) result in differences when solving the tasks. The postulation of prerequisite or precursor sequences, however, in turn requires structural analysis of the relations between tasks or operations. Conceptual arguments are needed to validate the interrelationship examined (see Harré & Madden, 1975; Toulmin, 1981). Therefore, the concept of developmental sequence commands explanatory status only if theoretical and conceptual arguments support the postulated order of acquisition. Such arguments are, therefore, required for meaningful empirical analyses of developmental sequences.

A review of the empirical research shows that assumptions about sequentiality in the emergence of cognitive operations are mostly based on the analysis of group sequentiality in one-group designs or across-groups sequentiality in cross-sectional designs. Few studies examine intraindividual change, in spite of the fact that sequence hypotheses focus explicitly on individual development. To emphasize this argument, hypotheses dealing with intraindividual change will be represented within the methodological framework offered by Buss (1979). Three analytical dimensions are relevant in the analysis of individual development; the person (individual), the variable (developmental tasks), and the measurement occasion. According to Buss, intraindividual change and intraindividual differences in development can only be analyzed with respect to the following two types of data aggregations:

> case 1: interindividual differences in intraindividual differences, where individuals are compared in terms of sampling across variables at one occasion;
> case 5: interindividual differences in intraindividual change, where individuals are compared in terms of sampling across occasions with regard to one variable.

Figure 8.1 shows the two analytical perspectives within a two-dimensional data-matrix (where the third dimension 'individuals' is not represented).

When analyzing individual differences in intraindividual differences and intraindividual change, the two data aggregation strategies mentioned above correspond to the following analytical perspectives. First: the synchronous perspective represents the analysis of developmental sequences within one measurement point, that is, *configurations* of variables within the subject (synchronous profiles). In the case of synchronous analysis the sequence of acquisition is not observed but inferred since the individuals have only been tested once. Second: the diachronous perspective represents the examination of the observed developmental changes, that is temporal *constellations* across measurement occasions (diachronous profiles). The second analytical perspective necessitates longitudinal designs, because it focuses on the analysis of change across different measurement occasions.

Three different procedures have been used for the statistical evaluation of sequence hypotheses (see Spiro, 1984[1]). These strategies are as follows.

1. Difference-testing procedures: differences in one or more developmental variables in different age groups are taken as evidence of intraindividual change in development. The inference from the developmental function of a population or a sample to intraindividual changes within the subjects is valid only if the developmental function of the group is congruent with those of the individuals. This implicit assumption is unlikely, as interindividual differences that are not

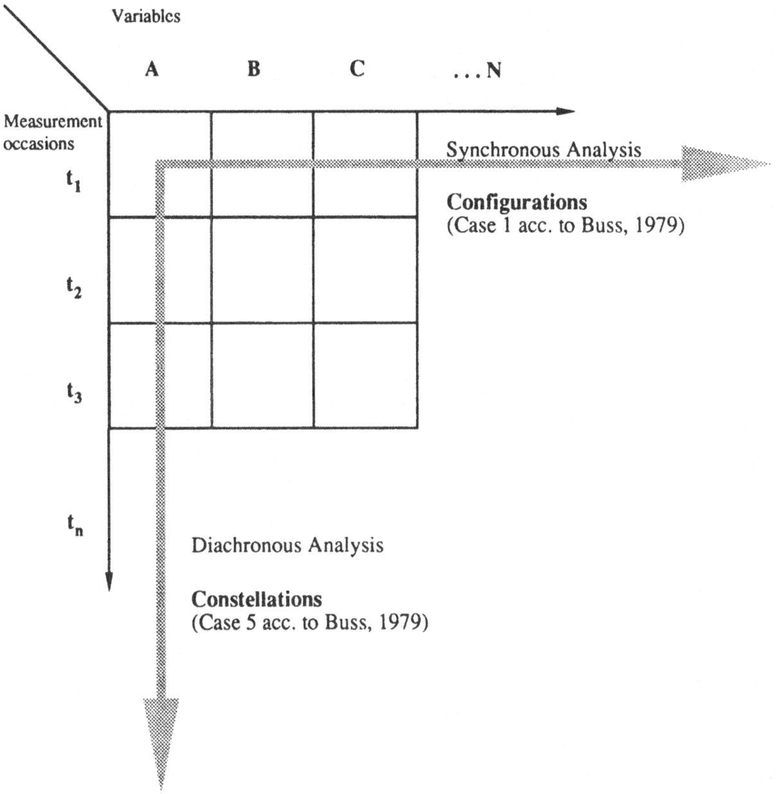

Figure 8.1. Methodological framework for the analysis of development sequences.

revealed in the global developmental function of the sample will usually exist between the individual developmental courses (Bakan, 1967). Therefore, developmental paths of individuals cannot be predicted or approximated by the developmental function of the group.

2. Correlational procedures: according to Winer (1980) correlational testing procedures are appropriate to the analysis of developmental sequences as they focus on the functional or formal (structural) relations between developmental variables. Correlations are taken to represent the degree of consistency between variables or the degree of stability of an attribute over time. However, sequential relationships between variables (in the sense of implicative relationships) cannot be justified using correlational analysis. It has been shown in different studies that, when order-theoretical statistical procedures were successfully employed to ascertain hierarchical relations between variables, statistically significant covariations between those variables could not be

found (Edelstein, Keller & Wahlen, 1984; Henning, 1981; Hudson, 1978; Rudinger, 1978; Schröder, 1989).

3. Unidimensional Guttman scaling: this procedure appears to be adequate for the analysis of developmental sequences because it takes into account the individual patterns or configurations. Each individual can be definitively classified on the developmental scale. Unfortunately, Guttman scaling is restricted to transitive (linear) relationships and does not permit investigation of cumulative or synchrony relationships. Further, it is not readily applicable to the longitudinal analysis of developmental sequences.

As these procedures are inadequate for the analysis of intraindividual change, new empirical and methodological strategies have been developed which are more appropriate to the analysis of developmental sequences (Bart & Airasian, 1974; Bart & Krus, 1973; Dayton & Macready, 1976; Hildebrand, Laing & Rosenthal, 1977; Rudinger, Chaselon, Zimmermann & Henning, 1985; von Eye, 1985, von Eye & Brandtstädter, 1988). These procedures, which in part derive from the field of biostatistics, latent attribute scaling or order theory, can be systematically characterized by reference to the distinction between variable- and person- (individual-)oriented approaches (Bergman & Magnusson, 1983; Magnusson, 1985). As mentioned earlier, within the individual-oriented approach assumptions about individual development can be formulated and expressed in terms of configuration- or constellation-hypotheses based on intraindividual differences or intra-individual change according to the methodological framework formulated by Buss (1979). In this case the variables will be aggregated to form specific configurations of attributes or constellations of time occasions which represent appropriate individual courses of development in either a synchronous or a diachronous perspective.

Within the individual-oriented approach the formal or functional relations between variables or time occasions, as postulated and validated by structural or task analysis, can be formulated in terms of *statement calculus*. Formulations in terms of statement calculus make it possible to specify whether occurring patterns are admissible or inadmissible according to the sequence hypothesis. For example, if attribute A is the precursor of B (A and B coded in dichotomous form) the combination of non-A and B is inadmissible because of the implicative relationship of A and B. The other three combinations (A B, A non-B, and non-A non-B) are admissible, as they do not contradict the sequence hypothesis. In Figure 8.2 the first contingency table represents an implicative relation between two developmental variables A and B. Logical implication, however, only matches the ordered series of variables on the synchronous level; it adequately describes the ordered set of relationships between variables at one time of measure-

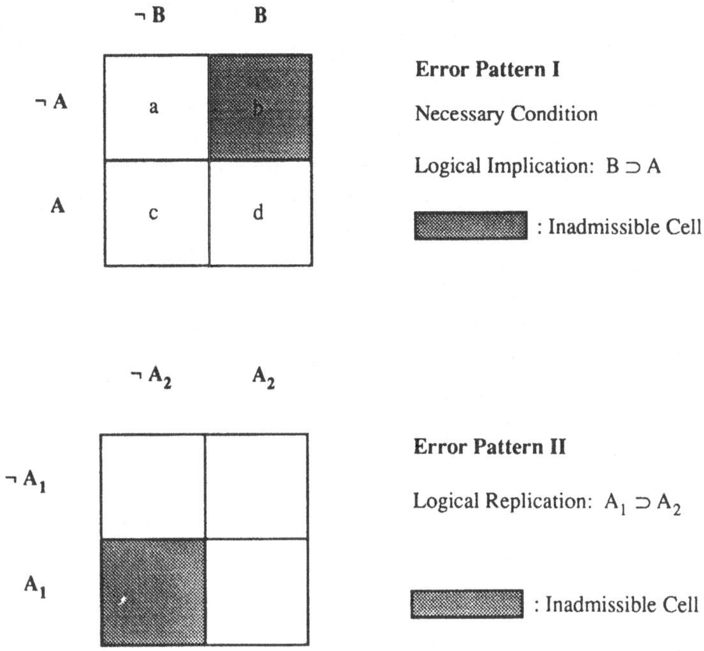

Figure 8.2. Error patterns of logical implication and replication.

ment (configurations). In contrast, the diachronous level of analysis focuses on the emergence of concepts across times of measurement. In this case an additional assumption has to be examined and included in the developmental model. It concerns the maintenance of an acquired ability. Assuming progressive consolidation and integration of cognitive structures, it is postulated that different tasks emerge during development (cumulativity); that is, once an ability is acquired, it must be retained across development. This relation can be formulated as a sufficient condition corresponding to the logical proposition type of replication. Considering the case of two measurement occasions (t_1 and t_2), replication implies that an ability existing at the first time of measurement (A_1) must be present on the follow-up measurement occasion (A_2). For instance, the occurrence of ability A on the first measurement occasion represents a sufficient condition for the occurrence of the same ability at the following time of measurement. Note that this is not the case in most instances of psychological assessment of a trait. The second contingency table in Figure 8.2 represents the replicative relation (cumulativity) between two measurement occasions A_1 and A_2. The error (inadmissible) cells are shaded. These examples of bivariate relations can easily be extended to multivariate relationships.

ORDER-THEORETICAL STATISTICAL PROCEDURES

For the statistical evaluation of the order-theoretical analyses to be reported below, two different procedures were used. One of these is Dayton & Macready's (1976) probabilistic validation procedure, a procedure known as 'scalability model' (Henning & Rudinger, 1985). The other is prediction analysis according to Hildebrand, Laing & Rosenthal (1977). For reasons to be detailed below, the unconditional prediction analysis (von Eye & Brandtstädter, 1988) was applied. Both procedures are adequate for the testing of developmental hypotheses and have been applied in the context of order-theoretical analyses, as they permit the reconstruction of a postulated developmental model from observed developmental data.

Dayton and Macready's method of analysis is a two-step procedure (see also Rudinger *et al.*, 1985): The first step is used for the estimation of the so-called 'recruitment probabilities'. In order to classify the observed patterns according to the admissible patterns postulated by theory (true-score patterns) the conditional probability is calculated for each configuration by means of the maximum-likelihood method. Because inadmissible patterns may occur empirically, parameters for 'false' classifications are needed. The number of misclassifications is expressed by the guessing and forgetting probability parameters (positive error α_i and negative error β_i). On the basis of the estimation of the model the predicted frequencies for each possible pattern and the probability of each true-score pattern θ_i are calculated.

In a second step the predicted and the observed frequencies of the patterns are compared by means of chi-square statistics in order to test the fit of the two distributions. If both distributions belong to the same population, it can be assumed that the theoretical model represents the distribution of the observed patterns. Unfortunately, chi-square statistics are adequate only if the frequency of an expected cell is equal to or greater than 1. If the sample size is relatively small and the model examined is quite complex, then the expected frequencies of some patterns may be less than 1 and the prerequisites of chi-square statistics are not fulfilled.

The prediction analysis of Hildebrand *et al.* (1977) serves to analyze the prediction from specific states or categories of an independent variable to specific states or categories of a dependent variable. A measure for the proportional reduction in error (PRE) is computed which tests whether the order-theoretical hypothesis is true. The PRE-measure evaluates only those patterns or cells that are inadmissible under the hypothesis. Unconditional prediction analysis (UPA: von Eye & Brandtstädter, 1988; a computer program is described in von Eye &

Krampen, 1987) makes use of the same algorithm as Hildebrand *et al.*'s prediction analysis but it is assumed that all variables, not only the predictor and the criterion variables, are independent of each other. Thus, developmental hypotheses that do not assume conditional relationships between predictor and criterion variables can also be tested. As an inferential procedure the binomial test is used. This statistical test is relatively robust with regard to the distribution of the frequencies.

SUBJECTS, METHOD, DESIGN, AND INSTRUMENTS

The data for the present research are taken from a longitudinal study conducted in Iceland. This study was designed to analyze individual developmental trajectories in the domains of cognition, sociomoral cognition, personality and ego resources as a function of different life worlds and social conditions in a society exposed to processes of rapid modernization since the end of the Second World War (Edelstein, Keller & Schröder, 1990). Subjects were 121 urban children who were tested at the ages 7, 8, 9, 12, 15, and 17. Table 8.1 presents the longitudinal measurement design of the study. As there is not enough space to show analyses of various design variables (gender, social class, general ability) here, the stratification of the sample will not be described (for details see Edelstein, Keller & Schröder, 1990).

To measure the development of cognition, a variety of instruments were administered depending on the age and the developmental status of the subjects (for details see Schröder, 1989). The order-theoretical analysis of individual development will be exemplified by the concept of conservation of area at ages 7 and 8 and the domain of syllogistic reasoning at ages 9, 12 and 15. These empirical examples were not chosen for their theoretical impact, but in order to demonstrate the order-theoretical approach in the analysis of developmental sequences.

Conservation of area was measured in the following manner (Goldschmid & Bentler, 1968): The subjects were presented two same-sized cardboard squares. They were told that each cardboard field represented a meadow for grazing cows. A farmer is building barns on the meadows. On each meadow the same number of barns have been built, but the location of the barns is different in each field. In the first field a systematic arrangement of the barns was presented to the subject, while in the second field the barns were placed unsystematically. In the first task two barns were placed on each field, in the second task six barns, and in the third twelve barns. A cow is grazing on each of the fields. After the presentation of the materials the subject was asked if the cows in the two fields have the same amount of grass to eat or if one of the cows has more grass. Every response (*judgment*) was probed for the

Table 8.1. *Measurement design of the longitudinal study*

Urban sample	*N*	Measurement	Grade	Age
1976/1977	121	1	1	7
1977/1978	59	2	2	8
1978/1979	113	3	3	9
1981/1982	109	4	6	12
1984/1985	105	5	9	15
1986	61	6	11	17

subjects' justification (*explanation*). Judgment and explanation were protocolled. Subjects whose explanations involved equivalence of both settings (identity) were classified as conservers. Subjects who referred to differences in the location of the barns when explaining differences in the amount of grass available to the cows were scored as non-conservers.

Conservation of area 1: conservation of equivalent areas of grass, while two barns are located differently on each field.

Conservation of area 2: conservation of equivalent areas of grass, while six barns are located differently on each field.

Conservation of area 3: conservation of equivalent areas of grass, while twelve barns are located differently on each field.

Syllogistic deductions with verbal material are based on the propositional logic of formal operations, more specifically on the binary operation of logical implication (see Table 8.2; Haars & Mason, 1986; Overton, 1990; Staudenmeyer, 1976). Three syllogistic tasks were presented to the subjects at age 9, and again at ages 12 and 15. The statements contained different propositions and were applied to different contexts. The first proposition refers to an experimental context available to all school children ('When there is a fire drill at school, the school bell rings'). The second syllogistic proposition is based on a counterintuitive statement beyond concrete experience ('During the summer it snows constantly in Iceland'). The third proposition involves abstractly symbolized content ('If I travel to A, I pass B'). The three syllogistic statements thus involve different reference contexts.

For each syllogistic task four basic forms of syllogistic arguments were presented: affirmation of antecedent, denial of antecedent, affirmation of consequent, and denial of consequent. If all four syllogistic forms were answered correctly, the subject used conditional deductions (an unequivocal truth value is assigned to the affirmation of

Table 8.2. *Basic forms of a syllogistic proposition*

	Premise:
$P \subset Q$	If there is a fire drill at school (antecedent symbolized as P), the school bell rings (consequent symbolized as Q).
	Affirmation of antecedent or modus ponens:
$P \supset Q$	
P	There is a fire drill at school.
Q	Does the school bell ring?
	Correct answer: yes
	Denial of antecedent:
$P \supset Q$	
$\neg P$	There is no fire drill at school.
Q	Does the school bell ring?
	Correct answer: maybe
	Affirmation of consequent:
$P \supset Q$	
Q	The school bell rings.
P	Is there a fire drill at school?
	Correct answer: maybe
	Denial of consequent or modus tollens:
$P \supset Q$	
$\neg Q$	The school bell does not ring.
P	Is there a fire drill at school?
	Correct answer: no

$\supset$ logical implication, $\neg$ negation

antecedent and to the denial of consequent and an equivocal truth value is assigned to denial of antecedent and to affirmation of consequent). This form of conditional deduction corresponds to the logical proposition of implication, emerging in cognitive development at the stage of formal operations (Inhelder & Piaget, 1958).

EMPIRICAL EXAMPLES: ANALYSES OF INDIVIDUAL TRAJECTORIES IN COGNITIVE DEVELOPMENT

In the following section the two examples of order-theoretical analysis in the field of cognitive development will be reported.

Developmental model: conservation of area

Task-analysis and developmental hypothesis. In the conservation of area task, children were asked whether the quantity of grass is

Figure 8.3a. Synchronous model: conservation of area.

Conservation of area 1 → Conservation of area 2 → Conservation of area 3

→ is precursor (necessary condition)

the same in both fields or whether one of the fields contains more grass. Note that the two fields differ only with respect to the location of the barns. Although the three tasks of conservation of area are homological in structure, the number of schemas represented and variables included (barns) increase (from 2 barns to 6 and in the third task to 12). It was hypothesized that the difficulty of the tasks should increase with their complexity. Therefore *décalages* in the acquisition of the three tasks can be expected. Hypotheses about performance *décalages* in cognition have been examined empirically in the tradition of neo-Piagetian research (see Chapman, 1987). In these researches it is assumed that the increase of complexity is determined by the attentional capacity of the subject. If this is true, an increase in complexity will lead to *décalages* in the acquisition of the tasks.

Formulation of the developmental model. According to the *décalage* hypothesis conservation of area 1 should be acquired earlier than conservation of area 2 and 3 and conservation of area 2 should be acquired earlier than conservation of area 3 (hypothesis of transitivity in acquisition; see Figure 8.3*a*).

The acquisition sequence in the synchronous model is formulated as an implicative relation. This was postulated independent of the developmental status or age of the child. Therefore the same sequence was assumed for the second measurement occasion (see Figure 8.3*b*).

In addition it was assumed that the synchronous relationships are also valid for the diachronous perspective. Therefore it was postulated that the concept of conservation of area develops cumulatively. This means

Figure 8.3b. Synchronous model for two measurement occasions: conservation of area.

Conservation of area 1 → Conservation of area 2 → Conservation of area 3

Conservation of area 1 → Conservation of area 2 → Conservation of area 3

→ is precursor (necessary condition)

Figure 8.3c. Sequential model for two measurement occasions: conservation of area.

Conservation of area 1 → Conservation of area 2 → Conservation of area 3

↓ ↓ ↓

Conservation of area 1 → Conservation of area 2 → Conservation of area 3

→ is precursor (necessary condition)

↓ cumulative development

that a task solved adequately at the first time of measurement is retained at the next measurement occasion. According to propositional logic this diachronous relationship can be formulated as logical replication (see Figure 8.3*c*).

Statistical examination of the model and results. The transformation of the developmental model into a binary coded representation is shown in Table 8.3. The developmental patterns differ with respect to the course and the rate of development: stagnation, progression, regression in development, and invariant developmental courses. There are 64 possible patterns of individual development, but only admissible patterns are listed in the table.

Table 8.4 presents the results of the two statistical procedures described earlier. In columns 3 to 5 we present the results of the structural analysis according to Dayton & Macready (1976) and in column 6 those of the unconditional prediction analysis according to von Eye & Brandtstädter (1988). In the first column all 64 possible patterns of development are listed. Patterns that are admissible in the model are in bold. In the second column the observed frequencies are listed. The next parameter, listed in column 3, represents the probability of pattern *i*. These probabilities as well as the next two parameters are analyzed by Dayton & Macready's procedure. In column 4 the frequencies predicted according to the specified model are tabulated. Chi-square statistics are tabulated in the fifth column. Summary statistics according to Dayton & Macready's procedure are listed at the foot of the table, where measures for the alpha- and beta-error as well as the summary chi-square statistics are given. The last column in the table represents the predicted frequencies examined by the unconditional prediction analysis. This procedure is based on the assumption of total independence among all six variables.

Table 8.3. *Admissible patterns in the sequential model: conservation of area*

	COA17	COA27	COA37	COA18	COA28	COA38
Stagnation	0	0	0	0	0	0
Progression	0	0	0	1	0	0
Stagnation	1	0	0	1	0	0
Progression	0	0	0	1	1	0
Progression	1	0	0	1	1	0
Stagnation	1	1	0	1	1	0
Progression	0	0	0	1	1	1
Progression	1	0	0	1	1	1
Progression	1	1	0	1	1	1
Stagnation	1	1	1	1	1	1

COA17,8: Conservation of area 1 at age 7 (8) years
COA27,8: Conservation of area 2 at age 7 (8) years
COA37,8: Conservation of area 3 at age 7 (8) years

The frequencies predicted by the procedure of Dayton & Macready appear to fit the observed frequencies well. While only one observed developmental trajectory is inadmissible according to the postulated model, no relevant discrepancies between observed and expected frequencies were found. The model was reconstructed under the constraint that only about 1% of the developmental trajectories were to be reclassified as positive errors and none as negative errors (see the alpha- and beta-errors at the foot of the table). Both parameters are quite low. The statistical test of the fit between observed and predicted data yields acceptable results. The hypothesis that the predicted and the observed data derive from the same distribution (fit), was accepted statistically, as the observed chi-square is smaller than the critical value ($\chi^2 = 14.72$, 53 d.f.)

However, the statistical results are indeed problematic. On the one hand, the chi-square statistic should be interpreted with the proviso that the expected frequency of each cell is greater than 1 (otherwise problems of over-fit must be expected, see Rudinger *et al.*, 1985). On the other hand, no subject should have inadmissible patterns. For this reason a statistical procedure (UPA) was applied to the data that does not lead to problems of chi-square statistics in cases where cell frequency is below 1.

In column 6 of Table 8.4 the frequencies predicted by unconditional prediction analysis are listed. The frequencies were computed under the assumption that all variables are independent of each other. As shown at the bottom of the table, the fit between the observed data and the postulated developmental model is statistically acceptable. According to

Table 8.4. *Results of order-theoretical analyses, developmental model: conservation of area* ($N = 59$)

Pattern	Observed frequency (N)	Theta	Predicted frequency (DM5)	Chi-square	Predicted frequency (UPA)
000000	**3**	**0.0448**	**2.8051**	**0.0135**	**0.0130**
000001	0		0.0379	0.0379	0.0323
000010	0		0.0379	0.0379	0.0641
000011	0		0.0006	0.0006	0.1585
000100	**4**	**0.0852**	**4.7384**	**0.1151**	**0.2444**
000101	0		0.0641	0.0641	0.6040
000110	**0**	**0.0000**	**0.0641**	**0.0641**	**1.1979**
000111	**9**	**0.1546**	**8.7619**	**0.0065**	**2.9596**
001000	0		0.0379	0.0379	0.0083
001001	0		0.0005	0.0005	0.0206
001010	0		0.0005	0.0005	0.0410
001011	0		0.0000	0.0000	0.1012
001100	0		0.0641	0.0641	0.1561
001101	0		0.0009	0.0009	0.3859
001110	0		0.0009	0.0009	0.7653
001111	0		0.1185	0.1185	1.8909
010000	0		0.0379	0.0379	0.0126
010001	0		0.0005	0.0005	0.0312
010010	0		0.0005	0.0005	0.0620
010011	0		0.0000	0.0000	0.1532
010100	1		0.0641	13.6531	0.2363
010101	0		0.0009	0.0009	0.5838
010110	0		0.0009	0.0009	1.1580
010111	0		0.1185	0.1185	2.8610
011000	0		0.0005	0.0005	0.0080
011001	0		0.0000	0.0000	0.0199
011010	0		0.0000	0.0000	0.0396
011011	0		0.0000	0.0000	0.0979
011100	0		0.0009	0.0009	0.1509
011101	0		0.0000	0.0000	0.3730
011110	0		0.0000	0.0000	0.7398
011111	0		0.0017	0.0017	1.8278
100000	0		0.0380	0.0380	0.0323
100001	0		0.0005	0.0005	0.0799
100010	0		0.0005	0.0005	0.1585
100011	0		0.0000	0.0000	0.3917

Table 8.4. (*Cont.*)

Pattern	Observed frequency (*N*)	Theta	Predicted frequency (DM5)	Chi-square	Predicted frequency (UPA)
100100	**3**	**0.0503**	**2.8815**	**0.0049**	**0.6040**
100101	0		0.0390	0.0390	1.4922
100110	**3**	**0.0515**	**2.9601**	**0.0005**	**2.9596**
100111	**7**	**0.1174**	**6.9065**	**0.0013**	**7.3121**
101000	0		0.0005	0.0005	0.0206
101001	0		0.0000	0.0000	0.0510
101010	0		0.0000	0.0000	0.1012
101011	0		0.0000	0.0000	0.2502
101100	0		0.0390	0.0390	0.3859
101101	0		0.0005	0.0005	0.9534
101110	0		0.0400	0.0400	1.8909
101111	0		0.0935	0.0935	4.6716
110000	0		0.0005	0.0005	0.0312
110001	0		0.0000	0.0000	0.0772
110010	0		0.0000	0.0000	0.1532
110011	0		0.0000	0.0000	0.3786
110100	0		0.0390	0.0390	0.5838
110101	0		0.0005	0.0005	1.4425
110110	**3**	**0.0508**	**2.9599**	**0.0005**	**2.8610**
110111	**3**	**0.0492**	**3.0000**	**0.0000**	**7.0684**
111000	0		0.0000	0.0000	0.0199
111001	0		0.0000	0.0000	0.0493
111010	0		0.0000	0.0000	0.0979
111011	0		0.0001	0.0001	0.2419
111100	0		0.0005	0.0005	0.3730
111101	0		0.0001	0.0001	0.9216
111110	0		0.0401	0.0401	1.8278
111111	**23**	**0.3891**	**22.9995**	**0.0000**	**4.5159**
Σ	59			14.7184	

$\chi^2 = 14.7184$ (53 d.f.)
$\alpha_i = 0.013$
$\beta_i < 0.001$

PRE = 0.967
$z = 7.6752$
$p(z) < 0.0001$
Precision = 0.5163 (measure of specificity of hypothesis)

Pattern: configuration of items COA17, COA27, COA37, COA18, COA28, and COA38 (see notes below Table 8.3)
θ_i: probability of pattern *i*
α_i: positive error (guessing probability)
β_i: negative error (forgetting probability)

the postulated order-theoretical model, a proportional reduction in error approaching 100% was reached (PRE = 0.97). In spite of the goodness of fit using the UPA procedure, this procedure has a disadvantage for developmental research. It concerns the procedure for predicting frequencies. In unconditional prediction analysis the prediction of frequencies is based on the assumption of total independence between the variables. In contrast, Dayton & Macready's procedure predicts frequencies on the basis of conditional probabilities according to the postulated developmental or theoretical model.

DEVELOPMENTAL MODEL: SYLLOGISTIC REASONING

Task analysis and developmental hypothesis. Syllogistic reasoning was measured by presenting four basic forms of a conditional proposition to the subjects. Subjects were requested to keep the syllogistic premise in mind and to judge the four conditional statements. Subjects were scored as formal reasoners when all four basic propositions were answered correctly. In order to construct a developmental model for three measurement occasions which did not exceed the total amount of six variables (otherwise the model would be too constrained), only two out of three syllogisms could be included in the model. In order to maintain the contrast between concrete and abstract modalities, the experimental and the abstract syllogism were included in the model, while the counterintuitive syllogism was dropped. Although the experiential and the abstract syllogism require the same inferential logic, the contextualization of the propositions differ. While the experiential syllogism refers to experiences that are well known to every child, the abstract syllogism is symbolic and decontextualized. It was assumed that the experiential syllogism is acquired earlier than the abstract syllogism as experiential contextualization facilitates deductive reasoning.

Formulation of the developmental model. According to the *décalage* hypothesis formulated above, the experiential syllogism should be acquired earlier than the abstract syllogism (hypothesis of transitivity in acquisition; see Figure 8.4*a*). The acquisition sequence in the

Figure 8.4a. Synchronous model: syllogistic reasoning.

Experiential syllogism → Abstract syllogism

→ is precursor

Figure 8.4b. Synchronous model for three measurement occasions: syllogistic reasoning.

Experiential syllogism → Abstract syllogism

Experiential syllogism → Abstract syllogism

Experiential syllogism → Abstract syllogism

→ is precursor

synchronous model was postulated independent of the developmental status or age of the adolescent. Therefore the same sequence was assumed to be valid for the second and third measurement occasions (see Figure 8.4*b*).

Further it was assumed that the synchronous relationships are also valid for the diachronous perspective. Therefore it was postulated that syllogistic reasoning develops cumulatively. A syllogistic proposition that has been deduced adequately at the first time of measurement must be deduced in the same way at the following measurement occasions (see Figure 8.4*c*).

Statistical examination of the model and results. The transformation of the developmental model into binary coded representation is shown in Table 8.5. The developmental patterns differ with respect to

Figure 8.4c. Sequential model for three measurement occasions: syllogistic reasoning.

Experiential syllogism → Abstract syllogism

↓ ↓

Experiential syllogism → Abstract syllogism

↓ ↓

Experiential syllogism → Abstract syllogism

→ is precursor

↓ cumulative development

Table 8.5. *Admissible patterns in the sequential model: syllogistic reasoning*

	SyE9	SyA9	SyE12	SyA12	SyE15	SyA15
Stagnation	0	0	0	0	0	0
Progression	0	0	0	0	1	0
Progression	0	0	1	0	1	0
Stagnation	1	0	1	0	1	0
Progression	0	0	0	0	1	1
Progression	0	0	1	0	1	1
Progression	1	0	1	0	1	1
Progression	0	0	1	1	1	1
Progression	1	0	1	1	1	1
Stagnation	1	1	1	1	1	1

SyE9,12,15: Experiential syllogism at age 9 (12 or 15) years
SyA9,12,15: Abstract syllogism at age 9 (12 or 15) years

the course and the rate of development: stagnation, progression, regression in development, and invariant developmental courses. There are 64 possible patterns of individual development but only admissible patterns are listed in the table.

In Table 8.6 again the results of two statistical procedures, Dayton & Macready's and UPA, are presented. The description of the table corresponds to the description given in the previous empirical example. The frequencies predicted by the Dayton & Macready's procedure do not fit well with the observed frequencies. About 36% of the observed developmental patterns are not admissible according to the sequential model. Thus, large discrepancies were found between the predicted and observed frequencies. An adequate reconstruction of the data according to the postulated model was not possible, as the model was reconstructed under the constraint that about 7% of the developmental trajectories were reclassified as positive errors and 21% as negative errors (see the alpha- and beta-errors at the bottom of the table). Concerning the statistical test of the fit between observed and predicted data, the results were in agreement with the findings. The hypothesis that the theoretical patterns and the observed data derive from the same distribution (fit) was rejected, as the observed chi-square was much larger than the critical value ($\chi^2 = 123.89$, 53 d.f.).

The frequencies predicted by unconditional prediction analysis are listed in the last column. These frequencies were computed under the assumption that all variables are independent of each other. The fit between the observed data and the postulated developmental model was statistically significant. According to the postulated order-theoretical

Table 8.6. *Results of order theoretical analyses, developmental model: syllogistic reasoning (N = 101)*

Pattern	Observed frequency (*N*)	Theta	Predicted frequency (DM5)	Chi-square	Predicted frequency (UPA)
000000	**37**	**0.5467**	**36.5464**	**0.0056**	**16.2803**
000001	2		4.8383	1.6650	8.2616
000010	**7**	**0.0256**	**6.9401**	**0.0005**	**11.5893**
000011	**8**	**0.1525**	**7.9633**	**0.0002**	**5.8811**
000100	4		2.9261	0.3941	6.2444
000101	1		0.7897	0.0560	3.1688
000110	1		0.9515	0.0025	4.4452
000111	5		2.1435	3.8068	2.2557
001000	5		3.6784	0.4748	5.3553
001001	0		0.9333	0.9333	2.7176
001010	**2**	**0.0588**	**3.7101**	**0.7882**	**3.8122**
001011	**1**	**0.0000**	**2.6697**	**1.0443**	**1.9345**
001100	2		0.7005	2.4108	2.0541
001101	1		1.6025	0.2265	1.0423
001110	1		1.8162	0.3668	1.4622
001111	**3**	**0.1723**	**5.8183**	**1.3652**	**0.7420**
010000	0		2.8126	2.8126	1.2123
010001	0		0.3733	0.3733	0.6152
010010	0		0.5350	0.5350	0.8630
010011	0		0.6164	0.6164	0.4379
010100	0		0.2262	0.2262	0.4650
010101	0		0.0644	0.0644	0.2359
010110	0		0.0768	0.0768	0.3310
010111	1		0.1782	3.7909	0.1679
011000	0		0.2840	0.2840	0.3988
011001	0		0.0754	0.0754	0.2023
011010	1		0.2891	1.7481	0.2838
011011	0		0.2187	0.2187	0.1440
011100	0		0.0575	0.0575	0.1529
011101	0		0.1365	0.1365	0.0776
011110	0		0.1530	0.1530	0.1088
011111	1		0.4962	0.5114	0.0552
100000	5		2.8364	1.6503	3.5306
100001	0		0.4607	0.4607	1.7916
100010	1		0.6225	0.2289	2.5133
100011	1		0.9371	0.0042	1.2754
100100	0		0.2280	0.2280	1.3542
100101	1		0.0711	12.1343	0.6872
100110	0		0.0836	0.0836	0.9640
100111	2		0.2028	15.9225	0.4892
101000	1		0.3715	1.0633	1.1614
101001	0		0.3961	0.3961	0.5893

Table 8.6. (*cont.*)

Pattern	Observed frequency (N)	Theta	Predicted frequency (DM5)	Chi-square	Predicted frequency (UPA)
101010	**0**	**0.0000**	**0.6098**	**0.6098**	**0.8267**
101011	**2**	**0.0361**	**1.3945**	**0.2629**	**0.4195**
101100	0		0.0642	0.0642	0.4454
101101	0		0.1612	0.1612	0.2260
101110	0		0.1777	0.1777	0.3171
101111	**1**	**0.0000**	**0.5867**	**0.2911**	**0.1609**
110000	0		0.2193	0.2193	0.2629
110001	0		0.0391	0.0391	0.1334
110010	0		0.0515	0.0515	0.1871
110011	0		0.0853	0.0853	0.0949
110100	0		0.0212	0.0212	0.1008
110101	0		0.0187	0.0187	0.0511
110110	0		0.0197	0.0197	0.0717
110111	0		0.0641	0.0641	0.0364
111000	0		0.0322	0.0322	0.0864
111001	0		0.0437	0.0437	0.0438
111010	0		0.0601	0.0601	0.0615
111011	0		0.1558	0.1558	0.0312
111100	0		0.0182	0.0182	0.0331
111101	0		0.0609	0.0609	0.0168
111110	0		0.0622	0.0622	0.0236
111111	**4**	**0.0076**	**0.2230**	**63.9846**	**0.0119**
Σ	101			123.8961	

$\chi^2 = 123.8961$ (53 d.f.)
$\alpha_i = 0.0714$
$\beta_i = 0.2142$

PRE = 0.3933
$z = 4.7179$
$p(z) < 0.001$
Precision = 0.5875
(measure of specificity of hypothesis)

Pattern: configuration of items SyE9, SyA9, SyE12, SyA12, SyE15, and SyA15 (see notes below Table 8.5)
θ_i: probability of pattern i
α_i: positive error (guessing probability)
β_i: negative error (forgetting probability)

model the proportional reduction in error achieved was nearly 40% (PRE = 0.39).

When comparing the results of the two statistical procedures, it is surprising that unconditional prediction analysis achieved a satisfactory fit in spite of the fact that about 36% of the developmental trajectories are not admissible according to the postulated developmental model. These contradictory results in the case of syllogistic reasoning are due to the fact that the two statistical procedures are based on different basic assumptions. While UPA is based on the assumption of independence between variables, Dayton & Macready's procedure predicts frequencies on the basis of conditional probabilities according to the developmental model. Thus, the model of syllogistic reasoning is a critical case in evaluating both statistical procedures.

CONCLUSIONS

In order to analyze developmental sequences an order-theoretical approach was attempted. Order-theoretical analysis can be characterized as an individual-oriented approach to the analysis of individual development, since the main focus of the analysis lies on the configurations of attributes or the constellations of an attribute over time. The analysis of configurations of attributes relates to the synchronous perspective and the analysis of constellations of an attribute over time to the diachronous perspective. Within this framework, hypotheses about developmental sequences can be formulated in terms of statement calculus. With regard to the synchronous perspective an implicative relationship between the variables was assumed. With regard to the diachronous perspective cumulative development was postulated. On the basis of these two basic hypotheses, admissible and inadmissible patterns of development were distinguished.

The two statistical procedures investigated were specially designed for the analysis of sequential data. However, the two statistical procedures differ with respect to the basic assumptions. While in Dayton & Macready's procedure frequencies were predicted on the basis of recruitment probabilities, in the UPA procedure the distribution of frequencies of the inadmissible patterns is tested against a distribution model of total independence. With respect to the specificity of the order-theoretical hypothesis, the UPA model is based on weaker statistical assumptions, because the PRE measure only reflects the difference between observed inadmissible patterns and the predicted patterns under the assumption of independence. In contrast, in Dayton & Macready's procedure, developmental patterns were predicted according to the sequential model assumed by theory (conditional probabilities).

In the first empirical example, where only one inadmissible pattern was found, both statistical procedures appear to reconstruct the postulated structure in the observed data quite well. While Dayton & Macready's procedure predicted the frequencies very accurately compared with the empirical distribution and without relevant misclassifications, the prediction of the UPA procedure was less precise. In the second empirical example, where about 36% of the observed paths of development were inadmissible, Dayton & Macready's procedure reconstructed the observed data under the restriction of frequent misclassifications. The UPA procedure, however, led to acceptable results, in spite of the fact that more than a third of the developmental trajectories are inadmissible according to the theoretical model of development. When the results of the two developmental models are compared with the basic assumptions in the statistical procedures, the statistical model underlying Dayton & Macready's procedure appears more adequate for testing sequential hypotheses than the model underlying the UPA procedure. However, with respect to the inferential test Dayton & Macready's procedure was less robust than the UPA procedure because in both developmental models summary chi-square statistics were calculated on the basis of cells with predicted frequencies less than 1 per cell.

With respect to the different domains of cognition that were analyzed in the two empirical examples, order-theoretical analysis appears to fit the data gathered in experimental settings better than verbal reasoning data. While in an experimental setting the influence of various performance factors can be controlled, so that different influences remain unconfounded, verbal reasoning refers to semantic categories and experiences the effects of which interfere with the operational structure of the task. Therefore, verbal reasoning depends on a variety of performance conditions which interact with each other. In other words, in the case of syllogistic reasoning we expect an interaction between operational and representational schemes. Thus, in the domain of verbal reasoning, individual differences occur in the order of acquisition: subjects use different rather than invariable paths of development. In contrast, in the domain of experimentally controlled tasks, such as the conservation tasks, no individual differences were found in the order of acquisition (invariability in intraindividual change). Nevertheless, large differences between individuals were observed with respect to their level of maximal development.

The methodological construct of individual differences is located on two different levels in the analysis of developmental change. In the present study, with its focus on the order-theoretical approach, *internal* constraints on development were analyzed, highlighting individual differences in micro-developmental processes. This is the question of interindividual variability in intraindividual change. The study of *external* constraints in development is a different step in the analysis of individual differences in development. Under this perspective, differences between individual developmental trajectories would be traced to external conditions such as opportunities or constraints in the social life-worlds or in the developmental ecologies of the subjects that affect different subjects in different ways.

NOTES

1. Spiro, A. (1984, June). Methods for the analysis of categorial data on developmental sequences. Paper presented at the 14th Annual Symposium of the Jean Piaget Society, Philadelphia, USA.

REFERENCES

Bakan, D. (1967). *On method: Toward a reconstruction of psychological investigation.* San Francisco: Jossey-Bass.

Bart, W. M. & Airasian, P. W. (1974). Determination of the ordering among seven Piagetian tasks by an ordering-theoretic method. *Journal of Educational Psychology, 66*(2), 277–284.

Bart, W. M. & Krus, D. J. (1973). An ordering-theoretic method to determine hierarchies among items. *Educational and Psychological Measurement, 33,* 291–300.

Bergman, L. R. & Magnusson, D. (1983). The development of patterns of maladjustment: Report of the Project 'Individual Development and Environment'. Psychological Department, 50, University of Stockholm, Stockholm.

Buss, A. R. (1979). Toward a unified framework for psychometric concepts in multivariate developmental situations. In J. R. Nesselroade & P. B. Baltes (eds.), *Longitudinal research in the study of behavior and development: Design and analysis* (pp. 41–59). New York: Academic Press.

Campbell, R. L. & Richie, D. M. (1983). Problems in the theory of developmental sequences. *Human Development, 26,* 156–172.

Chapman, M. (1987). Piaget, attentional capacity, and the functional implications of formal structure. In H. W. Reese (ed.), *Advances in child development and behavior* (Vol. 20, pp. 289–334). Orlando, FL: Academic Press.

Dayton, C. M. & Macready, G. B. (1976). A probabilistic model for validation of behavioral hierarchies. *Psychometrika, 41*(2), 189–204.

Edelstein, W., Keller, M. & Schröder, E. (in press). Child development and social structure: Individual differences in development. In P. B. Baltes, D. L. Featherman & R. M. Lerner (eds.), *Life-span development and behavior* (Vol. 10). Hillsdale, NJ: Lawrence Erlbaum.

Edelstein, W., Keller, M. & Wahlen, K. (1984). Structure and content in social cognition: Conceptual and empirical analyses. *Child Development, 55,* 1514–1526.

Goldschmid, M. L. & Bentler, P. M. (1968). *Manual: Concept assessment kit – conservation.* San Diego, CA: Educational & Industrial Testing Service.

Haars, V. J. E. & Mason, E. J. (1986). Children's understanding of class inclusion and their ability to reason with implication. *International Journal of Behavioral Development, 9,* 45–63.

Harré, R. & Madden, E. H. (1975). *Causal powers.* Oxford: Basil Blackwell.

Henning, H. J. (1981). Suche und Validierung kognitiver Struktur, Entwicklungssequenzen und Lern-/Verhaltenshierarchien mit Hilfe probabilistischer Modelle (Search for and validation of cognitive structures, developmental sequences and learning or behavioral hierarchies by means of probabilistic models). *Zeitschrift für Psychologie, 189,* 437–461.

Henning, H. J. & Rudinger, G. (1985). Analysis of qualitative data in developmental psychology. In J. R. Nesselroade & A. von Eye (eds.), *Individual development and social change: Explanatory analysis* (pp. 295–341). New York: Academic Press.

Hildebrand, D. K., Laing, J. D. & Rosenthal, M. (1977). *Prediction analysis of cross-classifications.* New York: Wiley.

Hudson, L. M. (1978). On the coherence of role-taking abilities: An alternative to correlational analysis. *Child Development, 49,* 223–227.

Inhelder, B. & Piaget, P. (1958). *The growth of logical thinking from childhood to adolescence.* New York: Basic Books.

Magnusson, D. (1985). Implications of an interactional paradigm for research on human development. *International Journal for Behavioral Development, 8,* 115–137.

Overton, W. F. (1990). Competence and procedures: Constraints on the development of logical reasoning. In W. F. Overton (ed.), *Reasoning, necessity, and logic: Developmental perspectives.* Hillsdale, NJ: Lawrence Erlbaum.

Rudinger, G. (1978). Erfassung von Entwicklungsveränderungen im Lebenslauf (Assessment of developmental change across the life-span). In H. Rauh (ed.), *Jahrbuch für Entwicklungspsychologie* (pp. 157–214). Stuttgart: Klett-Cotta.

Rudinger, G., Chaselon, F., Zimmermann, E. & Henning, H. J. (1985). *Qualitative Daten: Neue Wege sozialwissenschaftlicher Methodik* (Qualitative data: New approaches in the methodology of social sciences). München: Urban & Schwarzenberg.

Schröder, E. (1989). *Vom konkreten zum formalen Denken; Individuelle Entwicklungsverläufe von der Kindheit bis zum Jugendalter* (From concrete to formal thought: Individual developmental trajectories from childhood to adolescence). Bern: Huber.

Staudenmeyer, K. (1976). Understanding conditional reasoning with meaningful propositions. In R. J. Falmagne (ed.), *Reasoning: Representation and process in children and adults* (pp. 55–79). Hillsdale, NJ: Lawrence Erlbaum.

Toulmin, S. (1981). Epistemology and developmental psychology. In E. S. Gollin (ed.), *Developmental plasticity* (pp. 253–267). New York: Academic Press.

von Eye, A. (1985). Structure identification using nonparametric models. In J. R. Nesselroade & A. von Eye (eds.), *Individual development and social change: Explanatory analysis* (pp. 125–154). Orlando: Academic Press.

von Eye, A. & Brandtstädter, J. (1988). Evaluating developmental hypotheses using statement calculus and non-parametric statistics. In P. B. Baltes, D. L. Featherman & R. M. Lerner (eds.), *Life-span development and behavior* (Vol. 8, pp. 61–97). Hillsdale, NJ: Lawrence Erlbaum.

von Eye, A. & Krampen, G. (1987). Basic programs for prediction analysis of cross classification. *Educational and Psychological Measurement, 47,* 141–143.

Winer, G. A. (1980). Class-inclusion reasoning in children: A review of the empirical literature. *Child Development, 51*(2), 309–328.

9 Application of correspondence analysis to a longitudinal study of cognitive development

JACQUES LAUTREY AND PHILIPPE CIBOIS

Our aim in this chapter is to illustrate in what way the constraints inherent in a specific problem motivate the choice of a particular method to analyze longitudinal research data. The problem examined here is the form of intraindividual variability in level of cognitive development, and stability or changes in this form over time. The method is correspondence analysis. The data used for the purposes of illustration chapter are drawn from a longitudinal study by J. Lautrey, A. de Ribaupierre and L. Rieben. This chapter focuses mainly on methodological issues; more detailed information on the study itself can be found elsewhere, for example in Lautrey, de Ribaupierre & Rieben (1985, 1986), de Ribaupierre, Rieben & Lautrey (1985), Rieben, de Ribaupierre & Lautrey (1983). The first main section of the chapter examines methodological constraints related to the theoretical issues and the nature of the data. The second section is devoted to correspondence analysis and presents the features which make it particularly suited to handling these constraints. The third section deals with the results obtained by correspondence analysis and discusses the implications of some methodological choices.

CONSTRAINTS INHERENT TO THE NATURE OF THE PROBLEM

Theoretical issues

The central issue in this study is the form of cognitive development. In other words, does knowledge acquisition adhere to an invariant sequence which is identical for all children, or can cognitive development follow different pathways for different children? In terms of data analysis, such different developmental pathways are inferred from interindividual differences in the form of intraindividual variability. The hypothesis of different pathways refers to the fact that the order of acquisition of two notions, say A and B, can be AB for certain subjects and BA for others. This issue will be examined here by reference to

Piagetian theory, since the postulate of unicity of development is probably formulated most clearly in this view on cognitive development.

According to Piaget, knowledge develops through the construction of mental structures (sensorimotor, concrete, formal) which appear in an invariant sequence. Each of these structures is thought to be general in scope, a feature which is reflected by isomorphism of reasoning across different notional domains at a given point in development. The scope of these structures and their invariant order of construction define a single developmental pathway where the only possible differences between individuals are differences in rate.

The validity of this model has been seriously weakened by the fact that children's level of cognitive development varies widely as a function of the situation in which development is assessed. Showing conclusively that this intraindividual variability corresponds to different pathways in the course of cognitive development rather than to random variations or measurement errors calls for evidence: (1) that intraindividual *décalages* in the order of mastery of various notions do not have the same form (e.g., AB or BA) for different subjects, (2) that they can be accounted for by a meaningful structure at the cross-sectional level, and (3) that such a structure remains stable over time. The third point can only be established through a longitudinal study.

Before presenting a description of this study, the nature of the data calls for discussion.

Nature of the data

Subjects. 154 children were evaluated twice at a three-year interval. They were between the ages of 6 and 12 on the first evaluation (the sample was composed of 22 subjects per age group) and thus between the ages of 9 and 15 on the second evaluation. Since the tasks described below only discriminate ages 6 to 12, only subjects who were between 9 and 12 at the time of the second evaluation (i.e., between the ages of 6 and 9 when tested first) were included in the longitudinal sample. Note, however, that the entire sample was used for the cross-sectional study on the data obtained for the first evaluation. Of the 88 subjects aged 6–9 on the first evaluation, 76 were relocated three years later, thus yielding a 14% loss of subjects.

Variables. Subjects were individually administered eight operational tasks adapted from Piaget and Inhelder. Testing adhered as closely as possible to the 'critical questioning' technique developed by Piaget and colleagues. Limited space prevents us from providing a detailed description of these tasks. A brief description of the material, instructions and scoring criteria can be found in Rieben *et al.* (1983). A more succinct version is included in Lautrey *et al.* (1985) or in de Ribaupierre *et al.* (1985). For the present purposes the names of the tasks are provided and indications as to which of the four broad fields of knowledge they are associated with:

Logicomathematical domain:
- class intersection (6 items)
- quantification of probabilities (7 items)

Physics domain:
- conservation (4 items)
- islands (3 items)

Spatial domain:
- sectioning of volumes (5 items)
- unfolding of volumes (3 items)

Mental imagery:
- folding of lines (4 items)
- folds and holes (6 items)

Each of the eight tasks reflects a cognitive operation, and mastery on the task is considered to be indicative of concrete operations. In addition, however, several items in each task tap a given operation in a variety of situations and are thus measures of potential *décalages* in its construction. In total subjects were tested on 38 items on two occasions. For reasons which are discussed below, the variables for this analysis are the items and not the tasks.

Requirements for data analysis

Classically, relationships between intraindividual variability on a set of variables are analysed by correlational methods and factor analysis. This approach can in principle identify the hierarchy of acquisitions predicted in the case of *universal décalages* (i.e., when the order of mastery is AB for all subjects), which should result in a simplex, and the local orders predicted by *individual décalages* (i.e., the order AB for certain subjects and the order BA for others, corresponding to different developmental pathways), which should result in group factors. A discussion of the relationships between these different types of *décalages* and the different types of factors identified by differentialists can be found in Longeot (1978). Although the present problem clearly calls for a multivariate analysis, classical factor analysis was not used in the present study since it is not the best way to handle the constraints imposed by the nature of the data and the issues at hand.

Constraints arising from the qualitative nature of the data. Most factor-analytic methods use correlations computed on variables assumed to be continuous and to have a normal distribution. These properties cannot be assumed to exist for variables operationalizing a theory which emphasizes structural changes and discontinuities over the course of development. Piagetian tasks are generally designed to induce one form of behavior if the operational structure is present, and another form of behavior if it has not yet emerged (intermediary responses in certain cases form a third form of behavior).

Another constraint in a study which aims at being both developmental and differential is to find a method which can both reveal potential hierarchical relations (associated with universal *décalages*) and potential equivalence relations (associated with individual *décalages*).

These constraints motivated the choice of a multivariate analysis which can handle qualitative data, and can reveal both equivalence and hierarchical relations. As shown below, correspondence analysis is equipped to handle these constraints.

Constraints created by the necessity of establishing correspondence between item grouping and subject grouping. In terms of relationships between variables, a multivariate analysis of interindividual differences in the form of intraindividual variability should result in the grouping of items having similar profiles (i.e., items being passed and failed by the same subjects).

In terms of relationships between subjects, this multivariate analysis should be capable of identifying clusters of subjects whose profiles are similar in terms of performance on items (i.e., subjects who succeed or fail on the same items).

Methods of data analysis can generally deal with one type of clustering or the other, but their simultaneous examination is often problematical. As its name suggests, the method used here preserves the *correspondence* between grouping of variables and grouping of subjects. Because of this feature, the developmental profile of those subjects contributing most to factors accounting for relations between variables can be identified easily.

Constraints imposed by the longitudinal nature of the study. Although correspondence analysis can identify individual *décalages* (i.e., interindividual differences in the form of intraindividual variability) at a given point in development, proof that these *décalages* correspond to developmental trajectories requires showing that they are stable in time. Correspondence analysis is applicable here too. It provides a means of plotting 'supplementary' individuals on the multivariate space defined by one analysis, who were not originally included in it. This feature means that the developmental profile of a subject tested later in time can be plotted on the initial analysis space. Comparing respective coordinate positions of individuals who were part of the analysis on the first occasion and then plotted as supplementary individuals on the second occasion, is one of the ways of testing the stability of a developmental profile.

The next section is devoted to a detailed description of the way in which correspondence analysis takes the constraints inherent in this study into account.

CORRESPONDENCE ANALYSIS

Correspondence analysis has been popularized by Benzecri (1973, 1980), but see also Cibois (1983, 1984), Greenacre (1984), Greenacre & Hastie (1987), Escofier & Pagès (1988), Lebart, Morineau & Warwick (1984), Van der Heijden (1987). In this section a simple example is used to present the principles of correspondence analysis with a minimum of mathematical formulation. Readers familiar with the mathematics can, however, refer to the appendix which summarizes the equations referred to in the description.

Whereas classical factor analysis only accepts symmetric matrices, (correlation matrices), correspondence analysis can also handle non-symmetric matrices. More specifically, correspondence analysis exploits a matrix where the subjects are in rows and the tasks are in columns such that the number of times a subject succeeds on a task is expressed as a score on a row × column cross-tabulation. Since the task is only administered once, the matrix can only contain zeros or ones, which is illustrative of the qualitative nature of the data.

Take, for example, the fictitious matrix T (see Table 9.1), where six individuals (rows) numbered from 1 to 6 were administered five tasks (columns) labelled A to E. The row × column table indicates a 1 if the subject succeeded and a 0 if s/he failed.

Correspondence analysis of this matrix serves a twofold purpose:

1. it decomposes the matrix into the sum of five particularly elementary matrices since they are obtained by simple multiplication of the marginal coefficients (five matrices termed 'one-dimensional' matrices since 5 is the smallest dimensionality of T);
2. it classifies these simplified matrices in descending order so as to be able to discard the latter. The magnitude of each matrix is indicated by the size of chi-square value.

Simply for the purposes of obtaining the above indicator, the initial matrix must be decomposed into the sum of several matrices. This is

Table 9.1. *Matrix T*

	Tasks				
Individuals	A	B	C	D	E
1	0	1	0	1	0
2	1	1	0	1	0
3	1	1	1	0	0
4	0	0	0	0	1
5	0	0	1	0	1
6	0	1	0	1	1

Table 9.2. *Matrix* T_0

	Tasks					
Individuals	A	B	C	D	E	
1	0.2857	0.5714	0.2857	0.4286	0.4286	2
2	0.4286	0.8571	0.4286	0.6429	0.6429	3
3	0.4286	0.8571	0.4286	0.6429	0.6429	3
4	0.1429	0.2857	0.1429	0.2143	0.2143	1
5	0.2857	0.5714	0.2857	0.4286	0.4286	2
6	0.4286	0.8571	0.4286	0.6429	0.6429	3
Total	2	4	2	3	3	14

because calculating the difference between the observed value and the expected value under an independence assumption requires postulating that the original matrix is the sum of the matrix of the expected values and the matrix of the deviations from independence.

To return to our example, under the independence assumption the matrix T_0 is as in Table 9.2.

T_0 is already a simplified (one-dimensional) matrix since it is the product of the margins divided by the total. The matrix of deviations from independence is obtained by subtracting the independence matrix from the observed values. This yields the matrix $R_1 = T - T_0$ (see Table 9.3).

In this deviation from independence matrix R_1, the plus signs indicate success on tasks (scored 1) and the minus signs indicaté failure (scored 0). Thus the same qualitative information as in the initial matrix can be obtained purely by using signs.

Table 9.3. *Matrix R_1*

	Tasks				
Individuals	A	B	C	D	E
1	−0.2857	0.4286	−0.2857	0.5714	−0.4286
2	0.5714	0.1429	−0.4286	0.3571	−0.6429
3	0.5714	0.1429	0.5714	−0.6429	−0.6429
4	−0.1429	−0.2857	−0.1429	−0.2143	0.7857
5	−0.2857	−0.5714	0.7143	−0.4286	0.5714
6	−0.4286	0.1429	−0.4286	0.3571	0.3571

Table 9.4. *Matrix K_0*

	Tasks					
Individuals	A	B	C	D	E	Total
1	0.2857	0.3214	0.2857	0.7619	0.4286	2.0833
2	0.7619	0.0238	0.4286	0.1984	0.6429	2.0556
3	0.7619	0.0238	0.7619	0.6429	0.6429	2.8333
4	0.1429	0.2857	0.1429	0.2143	2.8810	3.6667
5	0.2857	0.5714	1.7857	0.4286	0.7619	3.8333
6	0.4286	0.0238	0.4286	0.1984	0.1984	1.2778
Total	2.6667	1.2500	3.8333	2.4444	5.5556	15.7500

The chi-square value corresponding to these deviations is obtained as follows: the deviation from independence for each cell is squared and the result is weighted by the frequency corresponding to independence. This yields matrix K_0 (see Table 9.4).

In this matrix, the contribution to the chi-square values of the cells corresponding to failure are equal to the expected values, which is always the case when the observed values are null.

Factor decomposition in correspondence analysis is carried out by continuing the decomposing process begun with the independence matrix: the final goal is to find the one-dimensional matrix T_1 that exhibits the best fit with deviation matrix R_1 and at the same time accounts for the greatest contribution to the overall chi-square value.

To obtain the first matrix, the deviation matrix is subjected to an algorithm to search for the pair of eigenvectors defining this matrix (for a sample algorithm, see Cibois (1983)).

Table 9.5. *Matrix* T_1

Individuals	Tasks A	B	C	D	E	*VI*1
1	0.1593	0.2747	−0.1801	0.2425	−0.4964	0.4391
2	0.2442	0.4211	−0.2761	0.3716	−0.7608	0.6730
3	0.0621	0.1071	−0.0702	0.0945	−0.1935	0.1711
4	−0.1763	−0.3041	0.1994	−0.2683	0.5493	−0.4859
5	−0.2723	−0.4696	0.3079	−0.4144	0.8484	−0.7504
6	−0.0170	−0.0293	0.0192	−0.0259	0.0530	−0.0469
*VJ*1	0.3628	0.6258	−0.4103	0.5522	−1.1305	

Let *VJ*1 be the eigenvector corresponding to the columns of the matrix:

*VJ*1	A	B	C	D	E
	0.3628	0.6258	−0.4103	0.5522	−1.1305

and *VI*1 be the eigenvector corresponding to the rows:

*VI*1	1	2	3	4	5	6
	0.4391	0.6730	0.1711	−0.4859	−0.7504	−0.0469

To obtain the first one-dimensional matrix T_1 approaching the deviations from independence matrix R_1, the elements of the eigenvectors are multiplied matricaly. For example, to obtain the value for the individual 1, task A, multiply 0.4391 by 0.3628, which yields 0.1593. In this fashion, matrix T_1 can be entirely reconstituted, which corresponds to this first factor (see Table 9.5).

Since the matrix T_1 covers part of the deviations from independence, it is possible to identify which part of the corresponding chi-square value it accounts for. This is done by calculating the contribution of each cell to the chi-square value of the matrix, and summing the rows, columns and the total.

For example, for reference cell (1, A) the part of the chi-square value is calculated by squaring the part of the deviation taken into account in the matrix and dividing the result by the original expected value. In other words, for this cell of matrix K_1 the values are: $0.1593 \times 0.1593/0.2857 = 0.0888$ (see Table 9.6).

The K_1 matrix is part of the original matrix K_0 which decomposes into $K_0 = K_1 + K_2 + K_3 + K_4$ (there are only four factors which contribute to the chi-square value because T_0, the independence matrix, makes no contribution).

Table 9.6. *Matrix K_1*

Individuals	Tasks A	B	C	D	E	Total
1	0.0888	0.1321	0.1136	0.1372	0.5749	1.0465
2	0.1391	0.2069	0.1779	0.2148	0.9004	1.6391
3	0.0090	0.0134	0.0115	0.0139	0.0582	0.1060
4	0.2176	0.3236	0.2782	0.3360	1.4082	2.5636
5	0.2594	0.3859	0.3317	0.4007	1.6793	3.0570
6	0.0007	0.0010	0.0009	0.0010	0.0044	0.0079
Total	0.7146	1.0628	0.9137	1.1036	4.6254	8.4201

Since this decomposition is additive, it can be seen that the contribution to the chi-square value of this first factor is from 8.4201 (the chi-square value for matrix K_1) to 15.75 (the chi-square value for matrix K_0), or 53%.

The factor decompound is thus still not sufficient since the decomposition of the first factor only accounts for 53% of the total chi-square value, and the procedure is reiterated. For this, matrix T_1 corresponding to the first factor is subtracted from the deviations from independence matrix R_1, and the remainder R_2 (not indicated here) is subjected to the algorithmic search for eigenvectors.

$$R_2 = R_1 - T_1$$

Let *VI*2 and *VJ*2 be the pair of eigenvectors corresponding to the second factor

*VJ*2	A	B	C	D	E	
	−0.5126	0.1241	−0.7497	0.6217	0.5165	
*VI*2	1	2	3	4	5	6
	0.3758	−0.0285	−0.9465	0.2716	−0.3197	0.6473

As was the case for the first factor, matrix T_2 which is the approximation of R_2 is reconstituted by multiplying the elements of the eigenvectors. Similarly, to determine what part of the chi-square value is accounted for by this factor, the chi-square value corresponding to this factor is obtained by squaring each cell and dividing by the initial expected value. The result shows that the sum of the contributions of all the cells of this second factor to the chi-square value is equal to 5.6280 or 36%: the total contribution of these two first factors to the chi-square value when summed is 89%.

Since nine-tenths of the chi-square value can thus be accounted for by the first two factors, the decomposition can stop here (the third factor would yield 99% and the fourth obviously 100%).

Because two factors are sufficient to cover the information contained in the deviation from independence matrix, these deviations can be displayed graphically where the *X* axis gives the coordinates of the first eigenvector for individuals and for tasks, and the *Y* axis indicates the second eigenvector: this yields the factorial graph shown in Figure 9.1.

This graph can be read in terms of angular conjunctions between rows and columns; for example, the vector from the origin to individual 1 who succeeded on tasks B and D is in angular conjunction with the vectors analogous to these tasks. In contrast, task A is in angular conjunction with individuals 2 and 3 who succeeded on this particular task.

This simultaneous representation of individuals and tasks makes it possible to establish correspondences between these two sets (hence the name correspondence analysis) and identify profiles of comparable individuals which can be accounted for by comparable successes. For example, individuals 1 and 2 both succeeded on tasks B and D, as can be seen by the reciprocal angular proximity of these four points.

The graph can also be interpreted globally. For example the first

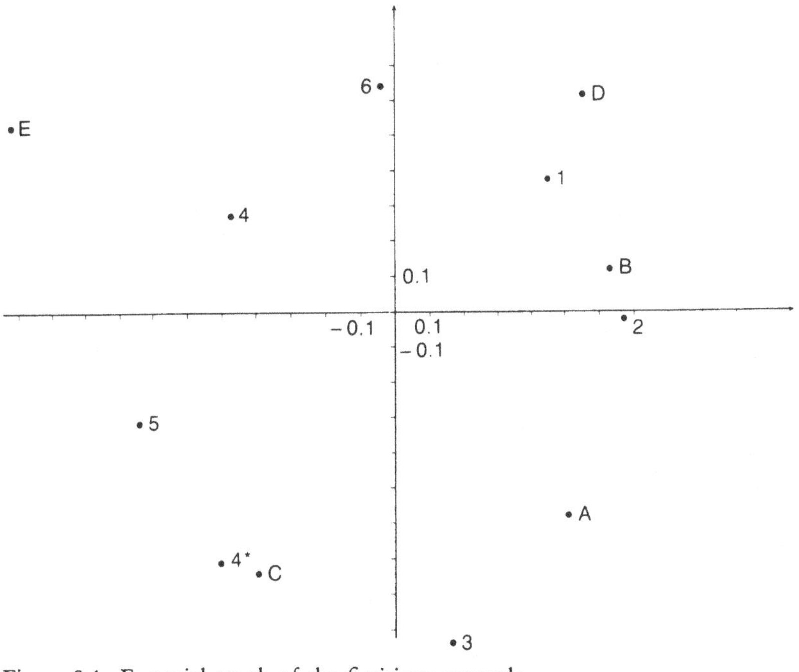

Figure 9.1. Factorial graph of the fictitious example.

(horizontal) axis contrasts success on tasks BDA to tasks EC, since the same individuals succeeded on each of these groups of tasks.

This finding can be verified easily by reclassifying the rows and columns according to the order of first factor: the opposition introduced by this factor is readily apparent.

	B	D	A	C	E
2	1	1	1	0	0
1	1	1	0	0	0
3	1	0	1	1	0
6	1	1	0	0	1
4	0	0	0	0	1
5	0	0	0	1	1

This reconstruction of the matrix clearly indicates the 'pure' individuals, i.e. all the subjects whose successes fall into one group of tasks and their failures into another. For instance individual 2 for BDA and individual 5 for CE are the closest to axis 1 and in addition are the individuals who contributed the most to the construction of this axis. If we return now to the chi-square table for the first factor (K_1) and insert the contributions of each of the rows to the total chi-square according to factor order we obtain:

2	1.6391
1	1.0465
3	0.1060
6	0.0079
4	2.5636
5	3.0570

This arrangement of the data clearly shows that the extremes on either side of the axis contribute the most to the chi-square value. In contrast individuals 3 and 6 who are the 'weakest' in terms of the contrast revealed by the first factor contribute the least.

These individuals who make no contribution to the first factor are however those who contribute the most to the second factor; a similar reconstitution of rows and columns can be obtained by following this factor order.

	D	E	B	A	C
6	1	1	1	0	0
1	1	0	1	0	0
4	0	1	0	0	0
2	1	0	1	1	0
5	0	1	0	0	1
3	0	0	1	1	1

This shows that the contrasts derive from two tasks and not three, which in addition explains why this factor is only in second position. It contrasts success on tasks DE ('pure' individual 6) with success on tasks AC ('pure' individual 3). A similar verification procedure shows that these individuals contribute the most to this factor.

The purpose of this example was to demonstrate that correspondence analysis can (1) treat categorized data in a purely descriptive manner, and (2) identify contrasts (factors) which reveal individual–task hierarchies. As a function of the interpretation assigned to a given factor, one hierarchy rather than another will be exploited. Note that the interpretation of contrasts is facilitated by the simultaneous representation of individuals and tasks. The profiles of individuals who contributed the most to each opposition can be identified.

Another feature of correspondence analysis is that it can be used to compare different kinds of individuals (or tasks): one possible application is longitudinal analysis. To return to the fictitious data, take the case of individual 4 who is retested on the same tasks at a later point in time. The results show greater mastery such that this subject now succeeds on tasks A and D as well as on task E as before. It would be useful to integrate this individual, denoted 4*, into the previous analysis without, however, having the data intervene directly. This is because the difference in time periods between analyses makes it unsound for us to associate these data with data from subjects tested at another time. On the other hand it would be of value to compare the results obtained by the same individuals at different points in time.

Correspondence analysis can be used to incorporate supplementary individuals into a completed analysis by determining the best plot fit to other individuals in the analysis with whom they share the greatest number of features. Individual 4* who succeeded on A, C and E is placed between individual 5 who succeeded on C and E, and individual 3 who succeeded on A and C.

The coordinates for 4* on the graph must be calculated factor by factor. For each factor, the coordinate for the individual is calculated by obtaining the algebraic sum of the factorial coordinates (divided by their marginal sum) and weighting this sum by the square root of the chi-square divided by the overall sum.

For individual 4* who succeeded on A, C and E this yields

	Coordinate for the first factor	Frequency
A	0.3628	2
C	−0.4103	2
E	−1.1305	3

The chi-square value for the first factor is 8.4201, and the overall sum

14. The algebraic sum of the coordinates divided by the sample size yields −0.4006 which is divided by the square root of (8.4201/14). This equals −0.5165 which will be the coordinate on the first factor for supplementary point 4*.

Obviously if a supplementary individual has exactly the same profile as an existing individual, the coordinates will overlay the same points. If we calculate a point for 1* who succeeded as 1 did, on B and C, it can be seen that the result is equal to 0.4391 which is the coordinate for 1 on the first factor. Numerically, this yields

$$\frac{((0.6258/4) + (0.5522/3))}{\sqrt{(8.4201/14)}} = 0.4391$$

Analogous calculations can be performed to plot 4* on the second factor; what changes is the factorial coordinates and the chi-square, the sums remains the same.

This method of calculation for supplementary individuals can also be used for tasks; in this case the coordinates of supplementary tasks are calculated by applying the same rules to the coordinates of individuals who performed on this task.

Other more sophisticated methods have recently been proposed to use correspondence analysis with longitudinal data. They emphasize the fact that correspondence analysis may be considered as a method of representation of residuals from expected values following the independence model.

It is possible to decompose residuals from model other than independence. For longitudinal data, Escofier & Pagès (1988) define the 'intra-analysis': their decomposition, using correspondence analysis, is from a model which suppresses the information that is not concerned with time (the inter-inertia) and shows the intra-inertia.

Van der Heijden (1987) decomposes residuals from log-linear models, from quasi-independence (when tables are incomplete because observations cannot possibly occur on given cells), from symmetry or quasi-symmetry. These methods may be used for contingency tables indexed by time, transition matrices, three and higher-wave univariate categorical panel data, multivariate categorical panel data, event-history data.

RESULTS

Correspondence analysis was applied to the longitudinal data described in the first section. The 154 individuals tested on the first occasion appear in the rows and the 38 items they were administered appear in the columns. For each item, subjects were scored 1 if they succeeded or

0 if they failed (in fact, there are 76 columns, since success and failure are represented as two disjunctive modalities for each item).

Analysis of the first occasion (cross-sectional approach)

Correspondence analysis of this matrix yields three interpretable factors (cf. Lautrey *et al.*, 1986).

First factor. In the plane formed by the first two factors (1 and 1 bis) the items' positions form a horseshoe which, in correspondence analysis, is one possible indication of a hierarchical relationship between variables, as a function of their rank on the first factor (in this configuration, factor 1 bis has a purely technical role and no psychological meaning: this is why this factor is not commented on and is labeled 1 bis). This hierarchical relationship is, however, very approximative and relative. Several groups of items have strong inner hierarchies, but these local hierarchies are only weakly interrelated. The first factor can be interpreted as a general factor of complexity (as regards items) and as a general factor of development (as regards subjects).

Second factor. The next factor contrasts 'logical' and 'infralogical' items. Piaget used the term 'logical' to refer to operations bearing on the relationships between *discrete objects* (the logical domain is hence discontinuous) and the term 'infralogical' to refer to operations bearing on relationships between *parts of objects* (the infralogical domain is continuous, for example space or time; the subject must thus isolate parts from the continuum before operating on them). Nevertheless, aside from this distinction, Piaget considered that logical and infralogical operations were isomorphic and arose from the same overall structure.

The simultaneous representation of items and subjects can be used to locate, on each of the two poles of the axis, the items and the individuals which contributed most to the part of the chi-square value that the axis accounts for. Reading Table 9.7 horizontally shows profiles of some of these individuals for these items, and vertically shows profiles of these items for these individuals.

The items are presented in the columns. Those which contribute most to the definition of the 'logical' pole of axis 2 appear on the left-hand side of the table and are denoted L. These items are tasks of varying difficulty and are about class intersection and quantification of probabilities. The items which contribute the most to the definition of the infralogical pole of axis 2 appear on the right-hand side of the table and have been labelled IL They cover tasks on the sectioning of volume,

Table 9.7. *Success patterns of the five subjects contributing the most to each pole of factor 2*

Subjects			Logical items							Infralogical items					
Sex	Age		L1	L2	L3	L4	L5	L6	L7	IL1	IL2	IL3	IL4	IL5	IL6
		N	100	76	68	44	40	18	18	64	45	32	39	24	19
M	7		1	1	1	1	1	1	0	0	0	0	0	0	0
M	9		1	1	1	1	1	1	1	0	0	0	1	0	0
M	9		1	1	0	1	1	0	1	1	0	0	0	0	0
F	12		1	1	1	1	1	1	0	0	0	0	0	0	0
M	10		1	1	1	1	1	1	0	0	0	0	0	0	0
F	11		0	0	0	0	0	0	0	1	1	1	1	0	0
M	12		1	0	0	0	0	0	0	1	1	1	1	0	1
F	10		0	0	0	0	0	0	0	1	1	0	0	0	0
G	12		1	1	0	0	1	0	0	1	1	1	1	1	1
F	6		0	0	0	0	0	0	0	1	0	0	1	0	0

folding of volumes and mental imagery. As in the fictitious example, the columns were reclassified within each group of items according to the order of the first factor. The numbers of the items (e.g., *L*1, *L*2, . . . , *Ln*) correspond to the order of their coordinates on this factor. The number of subjects *N* (out of 154) who succeeded on them appears below.

The subjects identified by sex (M or F) and age (6 to 12) are presented in the rows. The five subjects contributing the most to the 'logical' pole of axis 2 appear at the top and the five subjects who contributed the most to the 'infralogical' pole appear at the bottom. Within each of these groups the rows were reclassified as a function of the order of the coordinates on axis 2.

The shape of these patterns is entirely characteristic of what was termed 'individual *décalage*' or 'interindividual difference in the form of intraindividual variability' above. Some subjects apparently made progress in the logical domain while stagnating in the infralogical domain, whereas the reverse was observed for other subjects.

Third factor. The infralogical items which contributed most to the definition of the second factor are the tasks where the parts of objects that the individuals had to perform mental actions on were visible. The items contributing most to the third factor were infralogical items where the parts to be manipulated mentally could not be seen. Within this set of items, axis 3 contrasts items from the physical domain (e.g., conservation of volume) with items from the spatial domain (e.g., folds and holes). The table which can be derived from the items and subjects contributing the most to this factor exhibits the same shape as in Table 9.7.

Longitudinal analysis

The correspondence analysis on the first evaluation is informative on the state of intraindividual *décalages* at a given point in development for each subject. However, to determine whether the *décalages* correspond to different trajectories in the course of cognitive development, it must be shown that these remain stable over time.

Method of analysis of the relationships between the two evaluations. The study of stability and changes in success profiles over time exploits the possibility of plotting supplementary individuals onto an analysis that they were not included in. The success profiles of subjects for the same set of items they were tested on three years previously (when they were 9–12 years of age) were plotted as supplementary individuals on the analysis of the first evaluation. The sample used in the first evaluation serves as an appropriate base of reference since it also treats subjects aged 9 to 12 who can be used for purposes of comparison. This procedure also has the additional advantage of situating each subject in terms of his/her own coordinate position three years earlier on an identical axis system.

Stability and changes from evaluation 1 *to evaluation* 2. (a) Stability and change in subject's absolute position. The metric on which correspondence analysis is based can be used to identify the distance between the two points characterizing a given subject on each evaluation, and to decompose this distance along the various axes. The coordinates of these two points are entirely comparable since the axis they are plotted on is the same. Rather than illustrate this feature in terms of subjects, we have opted to represent the coordinates for age groups on axis 1 for the two evaluations. These age groups have been treated here as supplementary individuals. The procedure for plotting the age groups is identical to the one used in the fictitious example for individual 4*, except that the profile for a fictitious individual representing an age group is obtained by averaging over the profiles of the subjects in this group.

Figure 9.2 illustrates axis 1 which is bounded at its extreme left by the coordinate of the easiest item (I_1) and on its extreme right by the most difficult item (I_{39}). The age group coordinates are indicated by arrows located above the axis for the first evaluation (A6 to A12), and below the axis for the second evaluation (A'9 to A'12). Groups A'9 to A'12 are thus made up of the same subjects as groups A6 and A9 three years

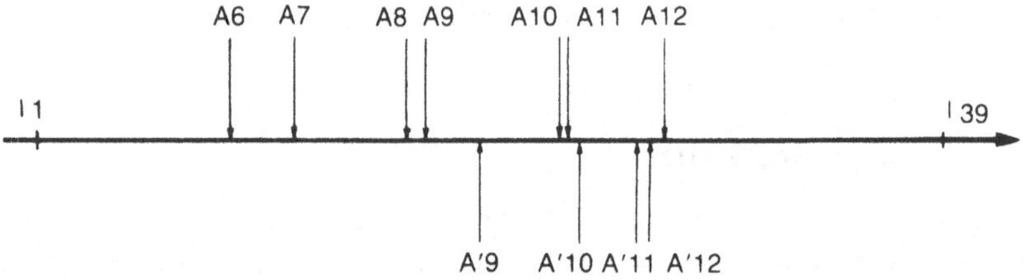

Figure 9.2. Simultaneous projection of items and individuals on the first axis. The 'individuals' are the age groups on the first (A6 to A12) and the second (A'9 to A'12) occasions.

earlier. Inspection of the plots of the age groups on the first occasion and their progress on the second occasion gives additional support to the assumption that the first factor is a general factor of development. The differences between age groups, however, are not all regular. One possible explanation is that development itself is irregular; another is that irregularities are due to problems in sampling subjects or variables. To clarify, changes in the coordinates of the groups over time can be examined. The short distance between groups A8 and A9 recurs three years later between groups A'11 and A'12, whereas the coordinates for groups A11 and A12 are spread normally. Similarly, the normal spread between A7 and A8 recurs between A'10 and A'11 whereas the distance between A10 and A11 is minimal. Thus in all likelihood the irregularities in the distances between age groups on axis 1 are due to problems of subject sampling. Note that the distances between groups are approximately the same from evaluation 1 to 2 along this axis.

(b) Stability and change in subjects' relative position. This aspect of stability and change can be assessed by correlations calculated for each axis between coordinates for individuals on the first evaluation (where they appear as main elements) and on the second evaluation (where they were plotted as supplementary elements). For the first four factors, the correlations are respectively 0.76 (r significant at $p < 0.0001$), 0.35 ($p < 0.001$), 0.34 ($p < 0.002$) and -0.06 (NS).

These figures indicate that during the three-year time period, order of subject coordinates on the first factor remained fairly stable. In addition there is a weaker trend towards stability in intraindividual *décalages* which is accounted for by factors 2 and 3. This is shown by the level of significance but also by the difference in the value of the correlation on axis 2 or 3 and on axis 4 which could not be interpreted.

Advantages and limitations of the 'supplementary individuals' technique. These will be discussed by comparing the correlation values obtained by applying this method with correlations obtained through other methods.

The problems raised by the longitudinal comparison of two occasions can also be handled without resorting to supplementary elements. A second possibility is to perform a correspondence analysis on the matrix containing the profiles of the subjects in groups A6 to A8 and groups A′9 to A′11 (groups A9 and A′12 were dropped to avoid having two groups of nine year olds in the same analysis). In this case the subjects tested on the first and on the second occasion are incorporated in the same analysis. The third possibility is to perform two separate analyses, one on groups A6 to A9 and the second on groups A′9 to A′12. The comments that follow are restricted to the consequences of these choices on correlations between coordinates for the two evaluations on each of the first four factors. These are respectively 0.73 ($p < 0.0001$), 0.26 ($p < 0.05$), 0.21 ($p < 0.10$) and 0.08 (NS) if the second method is applied, and 0.70 ($p < 0.001$), −0.12 (NS), 0.21 ($p < 0.10$) and 0.23 ($p < 0.05$) for the third.

As shown by comparing the correlation values obtained using each of the three techniques, values are the highest when the ‘supplementary individuals’ technique is used to plot the success profiles for the second occasion on the factors identified in the analysis of the first. These correlations drop, mainly for factors 2 and 3, when the successes profiles for occasions 1 and 2 are analyzed together (second solution). They drop further, at least for factor 2, when the analyses are performed separately for occasions 1 and 2. In other words, the correlations between the coordinates on the factors for the two occasions are the highest when the second evaluation contributes the least to determining these factors.

This paradoxical finding suggests that the same meaning cannot be assigned to the factors identified on the first and second occasions. A detailed analysis of the items that contribute the most to the different factors show that this is indeed the case. Separate analyses of the 6–9 and 9–12 age groups on the first evaluation (the subjects used in the cross-sectional analysis) yield the same factors as those identified in the analysis of the entire sample (see Lautrey *et al.*, 1986). However, a separate analysis of the 9–12 age group on the second occasion identifies factors with a slightly different meaning, as indicated by the nature of the items located at each of the poles of the factors. The reason seems to be that the 9–12 age group on the second occasion is more advanced than the 9–12 age group on the first occasion (this can be seen in Figure 9.2, by comparing respectively the positions of groups A′9 and A9, A′10 and A10, A′11 and A11, on the first axis). This difference may be due to sampling fluctuations, or to the fact that subjects on the second occasion were taking the tests for the second time. The consequence is that those logical items in the class intersection task were no longer discriminant among these subjects. When this group is analyzed separately, discriminant logical items are no longer in sufficient number to give rise to a purely logical pole on the second factor. Logical items are thus mixed with infralogical items which were the nearest to them in the analysis of the first occasion. The change in the meaning of the factors between the two occasions is thus apparently due to technical rather than to theoretical reasons. In this case, the technique of plotting subject success profiles on the second evaluation as 'supplementary individuals' provides a means of constraining the factors used to analyze stability over time to conserve the same meaning. In the framework of this interpretation, it is no longer paradoxical that the correlations between the coordinates on the factors for the two occasions are the highest when the second occasion contributes the least to determining these factors. The technique of 'supplementary individuals' may not, however, be optimal in all circumstances: constraining the factors to preserve the meaning that they had on the first occasion only makes sense if the changes between the two occasions can be attributable to some undesirable artefacts.

CONCLUSION

In the specific study which has served as an illustration here, correspondence analysis has been used to investigate individual differences in development as measured by a series of Piagetian tasks. More precisely, the aim was to analyze the structure and stability of interindividual differences in the form of intraindividual variability. The findings show that this variability is not entirely attributable to random fluctuations: the observed variability exhibits an interpretable structure and relative stability over time. This suggests that a multidimensional model of cognitive development may be better adapted than the unidimensional Piagetian model to account for observational data, including those obtained on Piagetian tasks. These data are congruent with the assumption that different trajectories are possible during cognitive development.

This example was selected because the constraints generated by both the theoretical issues and the nature of the data were particularly well suited to illustrating the potential of correspondence analysis for handling categorical data. The method has been shown here to be especially useful in cases where there is a need to perform a multivariate analysis of qualitative data. In this respect, correspondence analysis is comparable to multidimensional scaling. In addition it affords simultaneous representation of variable and individual space on the same axis system, which facilitates the analysis of correspondences between the structures observed in each of these two spaces, and provides complementary information on both. Lastly, correspondence analysis can situate supplementary elements in an analysis in which they were not originally included. This feature is doubtless the most valuable one for longitudinal studies. It can provide a useful solution to methodological problems that occur when the aim is to keep the position of axes constant across time occasions. The rationale for this solution is comparable to constraining the position of factors in the framework of confirmatory factor analysis. This kind of solution is naturally inapplicable when changes in the meaning of factors between two occasions are likely to have theoretical causes. In this case, it is better to compare factors in separate correspondence analyses or to use more sophisticated versions of correspondence analysis designed to handle longitudinal data, such as those suggested by Escofier & Pagès (1987) or by Van der Heijden (1987).

APPENDIX

Number of subjects expressed as:

cell n_{ij}, line total n_i, column total n_j, grand total n

Frequencies: respectively

$$f_{ij} = n_{ij}/n, \quad f_i = n_i/n, \quad f_j = n_j/n$$

Conditional frequencies:

$$f^i_j = n_{ij}/n_i, \quad f^j_i = n_{ij}/n$$

Eigenvalues for a given factor are written:

λ and ξ with $\xi = \sqrt{\lambda}$

Eigenvectors calibrated, weighted: y^i and y^j
Eigenvectors calibrated, unweighted: y_i and y_j where

$$y^j = y_j/f_j \quad \text{and} \quad y^i = y_i/f_i \tag{1}$$

Reconstitution equation for a given factor:

$$f_{ij} = y^i y^j f_i f_j/\sqrt{\lambda} = y_i y_j/\xi = (y_i/\sqrt{\xi})(y_j/\sqrt{\xi})$$

where $y_i/\sqrt{\xi}$ and $y_j/\sqrt{\xi}$ are termed semi-calibrated, unweighted eigenvectors. To reconstitute in terms of number of subjects and not in terms of proportions, the following equation is used:

$$n_{ij} = y_i y_j n/\xi = (y_i\sqrt{n}/\sqrt{\xi})(y_j\sqrt{n}/\sqrt{\xi})$$

The semi-calibrated eigenvectors written in terms of number of subjects are:

$$Y_i = y_i\sqrt{n}/\sqrt{\xi} \quad \text{and} \quad Y_j = y_j\sqrt{n}/\sqrt{\xi} \tag{2}$$

then $n_{ij} = Y_i Y_j$.

Transition equation (supplementary elements):

$$y^i = (1/\xi) \sum_j f^i_j / y^j$$

in a 0/1 matrix,

$$f^i_j = 1/n_i \quad \text{if} \quad n_{ij} = 1$$

and $$f^i_j = 0 \quad \text{if} \quad n_{ij} = 0$$

then $\Sigma_j f^i_j y^j = (1/n)\ \Sigma_j y^j$

and

$$y^i = (1/n_i\xi) \sum_j y^j \qquad (3)$$

Equation (2) yields:

$$y_i = Y_i\sqrt{\xi}/\sqrt{n} \quad \text{and} \quad y_j = Y_j\sqrt{\xi}/\sqrt{n} \qquad (4)$$

Equation (1) yields:

$$y_i = y^i f_i \quad \text{and} \quad y_j = y^j f_j$$

where $f_i = n_i/n$ and $f_j = n_j/n$ which gives $y_i = y^i n_i/n$ and $y_j = y^j n_j/n$. y_i is replaced by its value in (4):

$$Y_i\sqrt{\xi}/\sqrt{n} = y^i n_i/n$$

which yields

$$y^i = (Y_i\sqrt{\xi}/\sqrt{n})(n/n_i) = Y_i\sqrt{\xi}\,\sqrt{n}/n_i$$

and

$$y^j = Y_j\sqrt{\xi}\sqrt{n}/n_j$$

The equations make it possible to go from the results obtained in most programs (y^i and y^j) to semi-calibrated values in terms of number of subjects (Y_i and Y_j).

The values are entered into (3):

$$Y_i\sqrt{\xi}\,\sqrt{n}/n_i = (1/n_i\xi) \sum_j Y_j\sqrt{\xi}\sqrt{n}/n_j$$

which yields

$$Y_i = (1/\xi) \sum_j Y_j/n_j$$

similarly

$$Y_j = (1/\xi) \sum_i Y_i/n_i$$

Since the eigenvectors are expressed in terms of φ^2 and not in terms of χ^2 where $\varphi^2 = \chi^2/n$,

If χ^2 is the chi-square of a given eigenvector:

$$\xi = \sqrt{\chi^2}/\sqrt{n} \quad \text{and} \quad Y_i = (\sqrt{n}/\sqrt{\chi^2}) \sum_j Y_j/n_j$$

REFERENCES

Benzecri, J. P. (1973). *L'analyse des données* (Vol. 2). Paris: Dunod.

Benzecri, J. P. (1980). *Pratique de l'analyse des données* (Vol. 1). Paris: Dunod.

Cibois, P. (1983). *L'analyse factorielle.* Paris: PUF.

Cibois, P. (1984). *L'analyse des données en sociologie.* Paris: PUF.

Escofier, B. & Pagès, J. (1988). *Analyses factorielles simples et multiples.* Paris: Dunod.

Greenacre, M. J. (1984). *Theory and applications of correspondence analysis.* New York: Academic Press.

Greenacre, M. J. & Hastie, P. (1987). The geometric interpretation of correspondence analysis. *Journal of the American Statistical Association, 82,* 437–447.

Lautrey, J., de Ribaupierre, A. & Riben, L. (1985). Intra-individual variability in the development of concrete operations: Relations between logical and infralogical operations. *Genetic, Social, and General Psychological Monographs, 111,* 167–192.

Lautrey, J., de Ribaupierre, A. & Rieben, L. (1986). Les différences dans la forme du développement cognitif évalué avec des épreuves piagétiennes: une application de l'analyse des correspondances. *Cahiers de Psychologie Cognitive, 6,* 575–613.

Lebart, L., Morineau, A. & Warwick, K. (1984). *Multivariate descriptive statistical analysis.* New York: Wiley.

Longeot, F. (1978). *Les stades opératoires de Piaget et les facteurs de l'intelligence.* Grenoble: Presses Universitaires de Grenoble.

de Ribaupierre, A., Rieben, L. & Lautrey, J. (1985). Horizontal decalages and individual differences in the development of concrete operations. In V. L. Shulman, L. C. Restaino-Baumann & L. Butler (eds.), *The future of piagetian theory: the neo-piagetians* (pp. 175–200). New York: Plenum Press.

Rieben, L., de Ribaupierre, A. & Lautrey, J. (1983). *Le développement opératoire de l'enfant entre 6 et 12 ans.* Paris: Editions du CNRS.

Van der Heijden, P. (1987). *Correspondence analysis of longitudinal categorical data.* Leiden: DWSO Press.

10 Event-history models in social mobility research

HANS-PETER BLOSSFELD, ALFRED HAMERLE AND KARL ULRICH MAYER

INTRODUCTION

The analysis of social mobility is probably the field of sociology that has been most affected by methodological and theoretical developments in the period since the 1950s (see, e.g., Sørensen, 1986). In classical mobility studies Rogoff (1953), Glass (1954), Svalastoga (1959), and Carlsson (1958) studied social inequality on the basis of *mobility tables.* These tables were obtained from cross-sectional samples of men who were asked about their current position and about their father's position when they grew up. However, as respondents had different ages at the time of the interview and therefore had different historical experiences, these efforts did not provide very interpretable results (Sørensen, 1986).

Mobility tables were sometimes disaggregated by birth cohorts (Featherman & Hauser, 1978; Goldthorpe, 1980), but this does not alleviate the problem because careers take place in the labor force. This means the relevant period is the amount of time spent in the labor force and not the age of the people (Blossfeld, 1986). Members of the same birth cohort are at different career stages because they spent different times in the educational system. Thus, positions reflected by mobility tables of birth cohorts are observations of locations of people at different stages in their career (Sørensen, 1986).

The typical mobility table not only ignores differences in the historical location of cohorts and the amount of labor force experience of people, but also neglects the fact that job mobility is strongly influenced by education and other background variables of the individual. A first solution to this problem was provided by Blau & Duncan (1967) with the introduction of *path analysis* using linear regressions. This research induced a major change in methodology in the late 1960s and early 1970s. At that time, the use of regression analysis and the formulation of causal models in sociology was synonymous with *status attainment research* (Sørensen, 1986). This research was very successful and employed a richer set of variables than work based on classical mobility tables. But the basic design for collecting the data remained the same. This research was based on cross-sectional surveys. Thus, the defects of the data continued. Status attainment models also ignored the temporal nature of the mobility process. The effects of variables were established whether the current occupation of the respondents was the first or the one they had been holding for 50 years in the labor market (Sørensen, 1986).

Since the late 1970s, *labor market researchers* have increasingly drawn attention to the fact that the observed occupational attainment of an individual at a specific time is the result of a process of change. They have developed continuous-time models to conceptualize individual mobility processes (see, e.g., Sørensen, 1977, 1984; Sørensen & Tuma, 1981; Spilerman, 1977; Tuma, 1985; Carroll & Mayer, 1986; Blossfeld, 1986). The increasing availability of *event history data* on job moves in the 1980s has permitted the application of statistical techniques to estimate such models (Tuma & Hannan, 1984; Blossfeld, Hamerle & Mayer, 1989). Using these methods, substantial progress has been made in understanding the mechanisms of individual career processes, especially in understanding the role played by individual characteristics (e.g., education, labor force experience, etc.) and structural attributes (e.g., occupations, cohorts, etc.) in shaping career trajectories.

In this chapter we give a didactic example of how job mobility can be studied as a continuous process with event-history data. We do this in four steps.

1. We discuss the advantages of the event-oriented collection design for the analysis of job mobility.
2. We describe the German Life History Study which is used as the empirical base of the example.
3. We discuss some statistical aspects of event-history analysis necessary for an adequate understanding of the empirical analysis.
4. We present the results of the analysis of job mobility as a continuous process. The chapter concludes with a short discussion of potentialities and limitations of event-history analysis in social science research.

ADVANTAGES OF EVENT-HISTORY DATA

Compared with cross-sectional or panel data, event-history data have several advantages for studying mobility processes. A simple example may illustrate these advantages. Suppose that data have been collected for an individual with regard to education and occupation with the aid of a cross-sectional sample, a panel, and an event-oriented sample design (Figure 10.1). The individual's career path is differentiated into seven states (training, occupation 1, occupation 2, occupation 3, occupation 4, unemployment, and illness) which the individual may occupy.

First, looking at Figure 10.1 one observes that in a cross-sectional survey the educational and occupational history of a person is only represented by a single point, that being the state at the time of the interview. Somewhat more information is obtained by the four-wave panel in which the circumstances of the respondent can be observed at four different points in time. However, the career between the four waves of the panel remains unclear. It is only in the *event-oriented collection design* that changes in states and their precise times are explored. Such a design allows the educational and occupational career to be reconstructed in detail in its various phases and at any point in time.

This example shows the following.

- As a rule, cross-sectional analysis presupposed a steady state (i.e., the distribution at any given point in time is only informative if the underlying process remains relatively stable over time). In cases of major fluctuations and changes, the 'snapshot' of a cross-section will not be a good picture of the situation because the analysis will depend upon the specific conditions prevailing at the time of survey. In contrast, panel and event-oriented data explicitly take into account change and the dynamics of empirical phenomena.
- Even if empirical conditions are predominantly stable, panel and event-history data are more informative than cross-sections. Cross-sectional data can be regarded as a special case of panel and event-history data because cross-sections can be reconstructed from the latter. Moreover, in cases of empirical application, only the recording of panel or event-history data can demonstrate whether stability really exists over time. Finally, unlike cross-sections, panel and event-history data provide information on prior history which can help to improve the explanatory and prognostic capacity of statistical models.
- Whereas in the panel method the course of events between the individual survey points remains unknown, the event-oriented observation plan permits the reconstruction of the continuous process. The panel method may also be suitable to determine the course of events if the changes take place at clearly defined points in time coinciding with the survey intervals (e.g., the determination of yearly income on a yearly basis) or if a continuous variable (e.g., a person's weight) can only be appropriately observed on the basis of time discrete surveys. Yet, all other changes in qualitative variables that may occur at any point in time can only be fully reconstructed if the states and time of their changes are exactly registered. Therefore, the

event-oriented observation plan proves to be a necessary precondition for the adequate reconstruction of mobility processes.

- Finally, if one considers the dynamic analysis of *complex feedback processes* (e.g., between processes in the family and processes in the labor market), the continuous survey of qualitative variables would seem to be the only adequate method to assess empirical change. This is particularly true if the events of parallel processes occur not only at arbitrary points in time, but also have an interactive effect at a later stage.

In sum, the major advantage of an event-oriented observation plan in mobility research is the fact that it permits an adequate representation of changes in careers which may occur at any point in time.

DATA

As an example of an application of event-history analysis in mobility research, we study the process of job change for men in the Federal Republic of Germany. The analysis is based on data from the German Life History Study (GLHS).

The GHLS (Mayer *et al.*, 1987) is useful for this purpose since it provides detailed data about the life histories of 2171 respondents from the birth cohorts 1929–31, 1939–41, and 1949–51, collected in the years 1981–3. These birth cohorts were chosen so that the respondents' phase of transitions from school to work fell in particularly significant periods in history: for the 1930 cohort, this transition phase lies in the immediate postwar period; those born around 1940 left school in a time of large-scale economic growth, and the cohort 1949–51 entered the labor market during a phase marked by the expansion of the welfare state. The underlying hypothesis is that these specific historic conditions at the point of transition had a substantial impact on the respondents' subsequent careers.

The educational and occupational histories of the GLHS were recorded retrospectively in accordance with the event-oriented observation plan. This method is demonstrated by an extract from the questionnaire where respondents were interviewed about their work careers (Figure 10.2). It is characteristic that apart from collecting theoretically interesting information about the area of employment, number of working hours, income, and so on, the exact beginning and end of each job were recorded on a monthly basis. When this information about the sequence of job episodes is combned with records of periods of training and interruption, the educational and occupational history of an individual can be completely reconstructed. Such an event-oriented observation plan provides detailed information

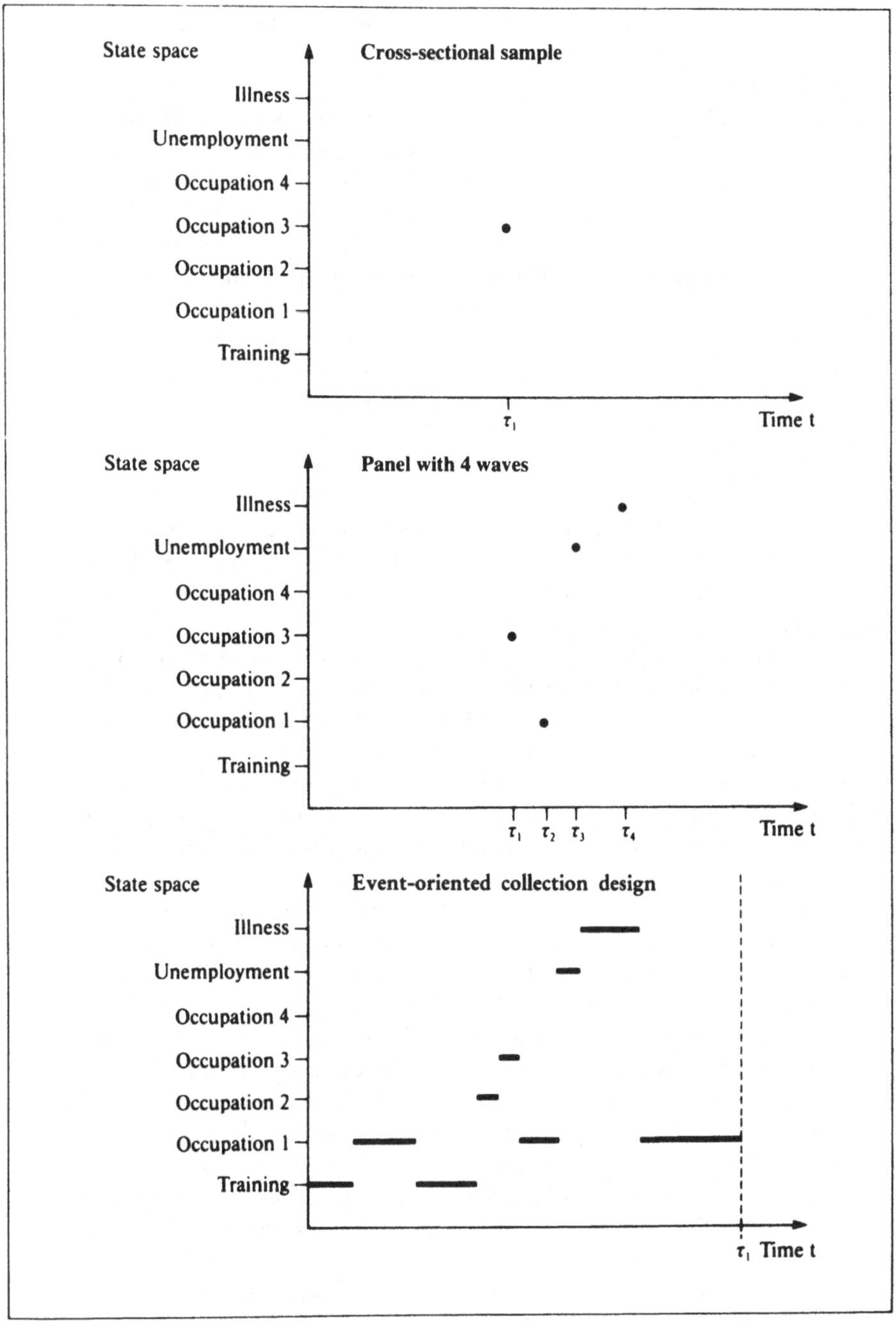

Figure 10.1. Example of an event-oriented observation plan to record work careers.

on the states of a given respondent's career at any point in the period of observation.

A study conducted before the actual drawing of the GLHS sample demonstrated that the reliability of retrospectively recorded data about objective life histories is not systematically affected by a lack of ability to answer questions or deficient memory capacity (Papastefanou, 1980; Tölke, 1980). This study indicated that while the possibility of recall errors was minimal, the form and precision of the survey instrument proved to be of key importance with respect to the quality of the responses. In particular, it was important to divide the life history interview into different spheres of life (education/training, employment, residence, etc.). Lengthy and extensive data editing, data checks, and cross-comparisons also vouched for the quality of the collected information (Mayer & Brückner, 1989). Finally, an examination of the representative quality of the life history data on the basis of census and microcensus surveys shows that the GLHS data provide a reliable picture of sociostructural cross-sections of the past (Blossfeld, 1987).

Because the data cover not only educational and occupational histories, but also provide information on the whole spectrum of the various spheres of life (i.e., information on social background, family history, the spouse's history, residence history, etc.), it is possible to study the effects that events in other parallel processes (e.g., in the case of family history, the event 'marriage') have on occupational careers (e.g., 'stability' of occupational trajectories). Similarly, prior history can be analyzed to examine the extent to which the subsequent career has been predetermined and channelled in certain directions.

A wide range of statistical tools is available today to analyze event-history data. In this chapter we (1) present some fundamental statistical concepts of event history analysis, (2) discuss methods to estimate the unknown parameters, and (3) give an example of the application of event-history analysis to study job changes.

FUNDAMENTAL STATISTICAL CONCEPTS OF EVENT-HISTORY ANALYSIS

The simplest example of an event-history analysis is characterized solely by measurement of the entrance into some initial state until attainment of some final state. The duration of an episode is represented in the statistical model by a nonnegative stochastic variable T. If time is exactly measured, the variable T is a continuous stochastic variable.

Survivor function and hazard rate

The density and distribution function of the duration T ($T \geq 0$) are denoted by $f(t)$ and $F(t)$, respectively. As usual the following relation-

400 Now I want to ask you about your occupation and employment. I shall proceed as I did for the other questions and go through all occupational activities, e.g., including part-time employment or temporary jobs you may have had. Any changes should be recorded as exactly as possible.
INT: If respondent was never employed—go on to Q414, p. 32.

401 Let's begin with your first job.
What occupation did you hold in your first job?
INT: Note exact job title in column 1, continue with Q402

401a What about your next job?
What was your occupation then?
INT: Continue with Q402

402 What was your exact activity at the beginning of this job?
INT: Note below and go on to Q403

403 How did your activity change during this job?—I'm also referring to e.g. changes between full-time and part-time jobs
INT: Let respondent describe the activities and note them down. For each activity go to the next box below. When all activities per page are filled in, go on to Q404

404 In what month and year did the job begin and in what month and year did the job end?

405 *INT: 1st job: Q405a, all subsequent jobs: Q405b*

405a Was this job in the firm in which you did your apprenticeship/vocational training?
INT: Only ask for 1st job

405b Was this the same firm/place of employment as your previous job?

Occupation	Activity at the beginning and changes of activity		M.	Y.	Training establishment
(KA 3)		fr.			yes 1
		to			no 2
(KA 4)		fr.			same firm 1
		to			other firm 2
(KA 5)		fr.			same firm 1
		to			other firm 2
(KA 6)		fr.			same firm 1
		to			other firm 2
(KA 7)		fr.			same firm 1
		to			other firm 2
(KA 8)		fr.			same firm 1
		to			other firm 2
(KA 9)		fr.			same firm 1
		to			other firm 2
(KA 10)		fr.			same firm 1
		to			other firm 2

406 What sector does (did) this firm belong to?
INT: Present blue list 6.

407 How many people are/were employed in the firm you work(ed) for?

408 Did your place of employment belong to the public sector?

409 What was your occupational status at the time? Which of the following applies?
INT: Present white card C.

410 How many hours was your average working week in this job?

411 What about your working hours? Did you work regular hours or, e.g., shiftwork, nightwork, Sundays, etc.?

412 What was your net monthly salary at the beginning and end of your activity as *(INT: name activity)*?

413 Why did your activity then change? / Why did you change jobs?

Sector	Size of firm	yes/no	Occup. status	Hours	Work. hours	Net salary	
		yes 1 no 2			norm. 1 oth. 2	DM at start DM at end	
		yes 1 no 2			norm. 1 oth. 2	DM at start DM at end	
		yes 1 no 2			norm. 1 oth. 2	DM at start DM at end	
		yes 1 no 2			norm. 1 oth. 2	DM at start DM at end	
		yes 1 no 2			norm. 1 oth. 2	DM at start DM at end	
		yes 1 no 2			norm. 1 oth. 2	DM at start DM at end	
		yes 1 no 2			norm. 1 oth. 2	DM at start DM at end	
		yes 1 no 2			norm. 1 oth. 2	DM at start DM at end	

Figure 10.2. Recording of a person's educational and occupational career on the basis of a cross-sectional sample, a panel and an event-oriented collection design.

ship is valid:

$$F(t) = P(T \leqslant t) = \int_0^t f(u)\,\mathrm{d}u, \tag{1}$$

and for all points for which $F(t)$ may be differentiated

$$f(t) = F'(t). \tag{2}$$

The *survivor function*

$$S(t) = P(T \geqslant t) \tag{3}$$

expresses the probability that an individual remains in the state ('survives') until time t, that is, that an event has not yet occurred and the episode is still continuing.

Measuring waiting time continuously, we have

$$S(t) = 1 - F(t). \tag{4}$$

Therefore, the survivor function is a non-increasing function of time, approaching zero as time elapses.

The *hazard rate* (hazard function or failure rate) is defined as

$$\lambda(t) = \lim_{\substack{\Delta t \to 0 \\ \Delta t > 0}} \frac{1}{\Delta t} P(t \leqslant T < t + \Delta t \mid T \geqslant t). \tag{5}$$

The hazard function may be interpreted as the instantaneous probability that episodes in the interval $[t, t + \Delta t]$ are terminating provided that the event has not occurred before the beginning of this interval. Common terminology often found in application of the hazard function are *intensity* or *risk functions, transition* or *mortality rates.*

It is important to note that the values of the hazard function themselves are not (conditional) probabilities. Although they are always nonnegative, they may be greater than one. For a small Δt, $\lambda(t)\Delta t$ can be interpreted as an approximation of the conditional probability $P(t \leqslant T < t + \Delta t \mid T \geqslant t)$.

The *cumulative hazard function* is represented by the integral

$$\Lambda(t) = \int_0^t \lambda(u)\,\mathrm{d}u. \tag{6}$$

From definition (5), one immediately obtains the relationship between the hazard rate and the survivor function

$$\lambda(t) = \frac{f(t)}{S(t)}, \tag{7}$$

and since T has been assumed to be continuous we have

$$\lambda(t) = \frac{f(t)}{1 - F(t)}. \tag{8}$$

Inversely, one may derive the relationship between the survivor function and the hazard function by integration of $\lambda(t)$. From (7) and (8), we have

$$\int_0^t \lambda(u)\,du = \int_0^t \frac{f(u)}{1-F(u)}\,du = -\ln(1-F(u))\Big|_0^t$$
$$= -\ln(1-F(t)) = -\ln S(t). \tag{9}$$

This leads to the important relationship

$$S(t) = \exp\left(-\int_0^t \lambda(u)\,du\right). \tag{10}$$

The density $f(t)$ is obtained from (7) and (10) as a function of the hazard function

$$f(t) = \lambda(t)\cdot S(t) = \lambda(t)\cdot \exp\left(-\int_0^t \lambda(u)\,du\right). \tag{11}$$

If we consider the relationships (1) to (11) it becomes evident that each of the three quantities $f(t)$, $S(t)$, and $\lambda(t)$ may be used to describe the duration of an episode. If one of these functions is known, the derivation of both the other functions is always possible. In particular, if one knows the hazard rate, the probability law of the process is completely characterized.

But the hazard rate approach does not identify new parameters. As we shall see, for estimation of the unknown parameters the likelihood function can be written equivalently in terms of hazard rates of probability density functions, but it is the same likelihood function in either case.

One of the most commonly applied distributions for the waiting time and lifetime is the exponential distribution. It is characterized by a constant hazard rate

$$\lambda(t) = \lambda, \quad t \geqslant 0, \lambda > 0.$$

A generalization of the exponential model is the Weibull model which allows for duration dependence. Its hazard function is

$$\lambda(t) = \lambda\alpha(\lambda t)^{\alpha-1} \quad (t > 0). \tag{12}$$

with the parameters $\lambda > 0$ and $\alpha > 0$. In the special case $\alpha = 1$, equation (12) reduces to the hazard rate of the exponential model.

The hazard or transition function of the Weibull distribution increases monotonically if $\alpha > 1$, decreases if $\alpha < 1$, and is constant if $\alpha = 1$. The Weibull model is quite flexible and therefore adaptable to a wide variety of models of durations and lifetimes.

The hazard rate approach can be readily extended to the multistate–multiepisode case. In this case, the process can be decomposed into two related processes, the transition process and the duration process. The transition process is the stochastic process which governs the transitions between states. The duration process governs the length of stay in a particular state. Both the duration and the transition process can be simultaneously characterized by a transition-specific or cause-specific hazard rate. We do not give the exact definition here.

Introducing covariates: regression models

In addition to the duration or lifetime, generally, various covariates or prognostic factors are collected for each individual or subject, and an important aim of statistical analysis is to ascertain the quantitative influence of these exogenous or endogenous variables on the hazard or transition rate. The covariates may be quantitative or qualitative. Qualitative variables are treated as in analysis of variance by coding categories using dummy variables.

An important difference compared with cross-sectional regression is that in the duration models some covariates may be time dependent. Such is the case, for example, when a specific medical therapy is applied only during a certain time period. The aim of such a study might be to examine the influence of the therapy during the effective application period or to check for possible secondary effects (side-effects). To accomplish this, for example, two dummy variables may be defined, $x_1(t)$ and $x_2(t)$ with (dropping subscript i)

$$x_1(t) = \begin{cases} 1 & \text{during the time period of active participation} \\ & \text{of an individual in a therapy or program,} \\ 0 & \text{otherwise} \end{cases}$$

$$x_2(t) = \begin{cases} 1 & \text{after the individual's termination of the 'medical} \\ & \text{treatment' within a specific therapy or program,} \\ 0 & \text{otherwise.} \end{cases}$$

If the hazard rate depends on the independent variables and given that the corresponding regression coefficients are negatively (positively) significant, a therapy is then effective and lowers (increases) the instantaneous probability of a change of state. Furthermore, if the first coefficient is larger in absolute value than the second, then the effect of the therapy sinks (rises) after termination of the therapy.

One possible method of analyzing the influence of covariates upon the duration times or lifetimes is to formulate a regression model in which the distribution of the duration times or lifetimes are dependent upon the covariates. Designating $\boldsymbol{x}$ as the covariate vector, one has to specify a model for the duration times or lifetimes T under the given covariate vector $\boldsymbol{x}$.

Obviously, an analogous procedure to traditional regression analysis may be chosen and the above introduced distributions, such as the exponential or Weibull distribution, may be generalized such that one or more parameters are assumed to depend on the covariates $\boldsymbol{x}$.

The values of the quantitative covariates of an individual or study subject i, as well as the codings of all main effects and the interaction effects of the qualitative covariates included in the model are then collected in a design vector $\boldsymbol{x}_i$.

Since in the analysis of durations or event histories the hazard rate is the mathematically simpler concept, the hazard rate is modeled depending on the covariates.

For the exponential model the hazard rate is given by

$$\lambda(t \mid \boldsymbol{x}) = \exp(\boldsymbol{x}'\boldsymbol{\beta}). \tag{13}$$

(13) is time invariant provided that the covariates do not depend on time.

The hazard rate of the Weibull regression model is

$$\lambda(t \mid \boldsymbol{x}) = \delta\lambda_0(\lambda_0 t)^{\delta-1} \exp(\boldsymbol{x}'\boldsymbol{\beta}). \tag{14}$$

The Weibull model belongs to the class of proportional hazards models, since the quotient of the hazard rates for two individuals is time invariant.

An extension is the semi-parametric approach originally proposed by Cox (1972). The hazard rate of the Cox model is

$$\lambda(t \mid \boldsymbol{x}) = \lambda_0(t) \exp(\boldsymbol{x}'\boldsymbol{\beta}) \tag{15}$$

where $\lambda_0(t)$ is an unspecified 'baseline' hazard rate. Such modeling achieves more flexibility, but different approaches are required for estimation and testing.

ESTIMATION

After the construction of a statistical model for the event history under discussion, the unknown parameters have to be estimated from the data. In applying an estimation method the problem of possibly censored observation has to be solved.

Since in event-history analysis the termination of the entire observation time period is given, a time interval may not be closed. In such a situation we have right censored data. The sample realization t_i of an individual simply states then that the duration of an episode is of at least t_i time units. Usually the sample consists of some t_i values which are complete durations, whereas the remaining t_i values are right censored. This is expressed with the aid of a *censoring indicator* δ_i as

$$\delta_i = \begin{cases} 1 & \text{if } t_i \text{ is not censored} \\ 0 & \text{if } t_i \text{ is censored}, \quad i = 1, \ldots, n. \end{cases}$$

The possibility of simply ignoring the censored data and thereby reducing the size of the sample is not recommendable since this generally leads to biased estimates.

The maximum likelihood method offers the possibility of considering explicitly right censored data within the estimation procedure. Accordingly, one must analyze in depth the underlying censoring mechanism of the data and formulate a statistical model.

A widely used approach is to assume the durations T_i and the censoring times C_i are independent random variables and, in addition, that the distribution of the censoring time does not depend upon the parameters determining the duration distribution. Then, the likelihood function is

$$L = c \cdot \prod_{i=1}^{n} f_i(t_i / x_1)^{\delta_i} S_i(t_i \mid x_1)^{1-\delta_i}$$

and utilizing the relationship between hazard rate and survivor function, one obtains

$$L = \prod_{i=1}^{n} \lambda_i(t_i \mid x_i)^{\delta_i} \exp\left(-\int_0^{t_i} \lambda_i(u \mid x_i)\, du\right). \qquad (16)$$

Using a special parametric model for the hazard rate, (16) or the log-likelihood function can be maximized with respect to the unknown parameter. Usually this is done by applying an iterative method such as the Newtonian method or a modified Newtonian method.

Hypothesis testing and construction of confidence intervals can be done in the usual way, based on the asymptotic distribution of the maximum likelihood estimator. The asymptotic properties of the maximum likelihood estimator, in particular consistency and asymptotic normality, can be derived elegantly using results from the theory of counting processes (for proportional hazard models). See, for example, Andersen & Gill (1982).

For the Cox model another estimation procedure is necessary, since the likelihood function depends on the unknown 'unisance' function $\lambda_0(t)$. Cox (1972, 1975) proposed a partial likelihood method. For a detailed description of this estimation procedure see, for example, Kalbfleisch and Prentice (1980, Ch. 4), Lawless (1982, Ch. 7), or Blossfeld, Hamerle & Mayer (1989, Section 3.6).

Regressor variables whose values change over the course of time intervals are conceptually straightforward to handle in the hazard rate framework. No analogue in cross-sectional regression is available. Suppose the regressor x is a function of time $x(t)$, where t is measured from the beginning of the time interval. Write the hazard rate as $\lambda(t \mid x(t))$. Using our integration formulas we can write the integrated hazard, survivor, and density functions. These will in general depend on the entire time path of the regressor up to t. Owing to the linearity of the integral, the calculation is simplified if the regressors are step functions over time. An application of this simpler case is presented in the next section.

There are many extensions and generalizations, for example, to the inclusion of several states (competing risks) or multiple time intervals of an individual, or with regard to residual analysis and specification checking. For further details see, for example, Kalbfleisch & Prentice (1980), Cox & Oakes (1974), Blossfeld, Hamerle & Mayer (1989), Anderson & Borgan (1985), Clayton (1988), or Manton & Stallard (1988).

A problem to which recently a lot of attention has been given is unobserved heterogeneity. On this point it has always been assumed that the measured covariates completely determine the hazard rate. But there may be omitted variables which are important and influence the hazard rate as well. In the duration model the unobserved heterogeneity can be represented by a random variable v. A convenient approach is

$$\lambda(t \mid x, y) = \lambda(t \mid x) \cdot v.$$

Since the hazard rate is not negative, v must be limited to positive values. The 'deviation' v varies from individual to individual and is not observable. In demographic and medical studies these models are referred to as 'frailty' models (see Vaupel, Mauton & Stallard, 1979). If a parametric form for the distribution of unobserved heterogeneity is assumed, one can estimate the unknown parameters of this distribution along with the unknown parameters of $\lambda(t \mid x)$ using a 'marginal likelihood' integrating out the heterogeneity. For a more detailed treatment see, for example, Blossfeld, Hamerle & Mayer (1989), Aalen (1988), or Heckman & Singer (1984).

RESULTS

The German Life History Data can be used to estimate the job change among men as being dependent on education (EDU), prestige (PRES), number of previously held jobs (NOJ) labor force experience at the beginnings of each job (LFX), as well as dummy variables for the birth cohorts 1939–41 (COHO2) and 1949–51 (COHO3) (see Appendix) with an exponential model:

$$\lambda(t \mid \boldsymbol{x}_k) = \exp(\boldsymbol{x}'\boldsymbol{\beta}),\ t = \text{duration}.$$

The exponential model rests on the assumption of a constant event risk and thus implies the assumption of proportional risks over the duration. This model lends itself to easy interpretation and is commonly applied as the basic or reference model to which estimates of more complex distribution models are compared. The maximum likelihood estimation for this model is calculated using the program RATE (developed by Nancy Tuma, 1985). The results of this estimation are reported as Model 1 in Table 10.1.

First of all, if one compares this exponential model with the exponential model without covariates, then based upon the likelihood ratio test a chi-square value of 705.90 with six degrees of freedom is obtained. The included covariates thus contribute to explaining the risk of men changing jobs, and the null hypothesis which states that none of the introduced β coefficients is different from zero must be rejected.

A significance test may be implemented for the individual regression parameters by dividing the coefficients $\hat{\beta}_i$ by their estimated asymptotic standard errors $s(\hat{\beta}_i)$. Assuming the hypothesis H_0: $\beta_i = 0$, these test values are approximately characterized by a standard normal distribution. If one uses a 0.05 significance level and a two-sided test, then the covariates have a significant effect if the absolute values of their standardized coefficients satisfy

$$\left| \frac{\hat{\beta}_i}{s(\hat{\beta}_i)} \right| > 1.96.$$

This is the case for the constant β_0 (CONST) as well as for the variables PRES, NOJ, LFX, COHO2, and COHO3. Only education (EDU) does not have a significant influence upon the rate of job change among men.

One can easily interpret the influence of a covariate x_i, given the constancy of the remaining covariates $\boldsymbol{x}'\boldsymbol{\beta}$, by demonstrating the percentage change in the rate given an increase in the covariate x_i by a specific value Δx_i. For example, an increase in the number of previously held jobs (NOJ) of 1 unit results in an increase of the rate equivalent to about 19% $[(\exp(0.171426) - 1) \cdot 100\% = 18.70\%]$. On the other hand, an increase in prestige (M59) of 20 units leads to a decline in the inclination to change jobs of about 10% $[(\exp(-0.00521)^{20} - 1) \cdot 100\% = -9.9\%]$. A simultaneous change of NOJ by 1 unit and prestige (M59) by 20 units, which would represent a career advance, raises the rate by only about 7% $[(\exp(0.171426)^1 \cdot \exp(-0.00521)^{20} - 1) \cdot 100\% = 6.95\%]$ and not of the magnitude of about 9% $[18.70\% - 9.9\% = 8.80\%]$.

Applying the relationship

$$E(T \mid \boldsymbol{x}) = \frac{1}{\lambda(\boldsymbol{x})} = \frac{1}{\exp(\boldsymbol{x}'\boldsymbol{\beta})},$$

given an exponential distribution, one may explicitly state, how, when all other covariates are constant, the average duration $E(T \mid \boldsymbol{x})$ changes if one increases the value of the independent variable x_i by the amount Δx_i:

$$\delta_{\Delta x_i} = \frac{\dfrac{1}{\exp(\boldsymbol{x}'\boldsymbol{\beta} + \beta_i(x_i + \Delta x_i))} - \dfrac{1}{\exp(\boldsymbol{x}'\boldsymbol{\beta} + \beta_i x_i)}}{\dfrac{1}{\exp(\boldsymbol{x}'\boldsymbol{\beta} + \beta_i x_i)}} \cdot 100\%$$

$$\delta_{\Delta x_i} = \left(\frac{1}{\exp(\beta_i)^{\Delta x_i}} - 1\right) \cdot 100\%.$$

Increasing the number of previously held jobs (NOJ) by 1 accordingly results in a decrease in average employment duration by about 16% $[(1/\exp(0.171426) - 1) \cdot 100\% = -15.75\%]$. On the other hand, an increase in prestige (M59) by 20 units results in an increase in employment duration by about 11% $[(1/\exp(-0.00521)^{20} - 1) \cdot 100\% = 10.98\%]$. A simultaneous change of NOJ by 1 unit and prestige (M59) by 20 units, which again would represent a career jump, lowers the average duration by about 7% $[(1/(\exp(0.171426)^{1} \exp(-0.00521)^{20}) - 1) \cdot 100\% = -6.5\%]$ rather than by about 5% $[10.98\% - 15.75\% = -4.77\%]$.

For selected subgroups, prognoses may also be made concerning the average duration, the median of the duration, the average number of events occurring in a given time period, and the probability of remaining in the same state at a given point in time.

For example, if one observes a man from the cohort 1939–41 (COHO2 = 1 and COHO3 = 0) who is employed in an occupation valued at the 50-point prestige level (M59 = 50) and who previously worked in 10 jobs (NOJ = 10) as well as having collected 100 months of labor force experience (LFX = 100), the following forecast equation for the rate of job change is derived:

$$\hat{\lambda} = \exp(-4.338 - 0.005 \cdot 50 + 0.171 \cdot 10 - 0.009 \cdot 100 + 0.180 \cdot 1)$$
$$= 0.0274.$$

Consequently, this person is characterized by an average duration of about 37 months $[1/\lambda = 1/0.0274 = 36.496]$, which is well below the average of about 98 months. Furthermore, one can forecast the median duration of employment as $\hat{M}^* = 0.6934 \cdot 36.5 = 25.31$ months and in one year expect an average of $\hat{\lambda} v = 0.0274 \cdot 12 = 0.3288$ job changes. Finally, the probability that this individual is still employed in the same occupation about eight years is about 7% $[\hat{S}(96) = \exp(-0.0274 \cdot 96) = 0.072]$, whereas the average for all men is about 38%.

By means of further prognoses for additional subgroups, one obtains

Table 10.1. *Estimates of models for the risk of job change*

	Estimates for model:		
	1	2	3
CONST	−4.338*	−4.283*	−3.492*
EDU	0.013	0.025	0.007
PRES	−0.005*	−0.004*	−0.004*
NOJ	0.171*	0.173*	0.160*
LFX	−0.009*	−0.007*	−0.008*
COHO2	0.179*	0.159*	0.124*
COHO3	0.486*	0.415*	0.341*
MAR		−0.714*	
TDEP			0.8266
$\chi^{2'}$	705.9	969.9	868.7
d.f.	6	7	7

* Statistically significant at 0.05 level.

a well-differentiated picture of job changing behavior among men as well as an indication of the significance of varying factors of influence.

Model 1 in Table 10.1 reported the influence of time-independent variables. One speaks of time-independent covariates when they are measured at the beginning of episode k and their values remain unchanged over the duration $v_k = t - t_{k-1}$ (see Figure 10.3c). Time-dependent covariates may, however, change their values within episode k. Given discrete time-dependent covariates, the values remain constant over certain subintervals v_{k_i}, $v_k = \sum_{i=1}^{s} v_{k_i}$ (see Figure 10.3b), whereas continuous time-dependent variables may change continuously.

Time-dependent covariates are especially interesting because one may more realistically formulate the influence of the covariates on hazard rates and combine two or more parallel processes directly with one another (Blossfeld, 1986). It is not uncommon that a duration dependency arises because the observed states are aggregates of unobserved states. This is due to the simple fact that time-dependent covariates are dealt with as time-independent covariates in the model.

In general, economics and the social sciences deal with variables that do not change continuously over time. Such variables are characterized by a step function and influence duration by changing the rate within a given episode. For example, if one assumes that for men the event of marriage has a stabilizing effect on the process of job mobility (see Figure 10.3), then this relationship may be studied by introducing a time-dependent covariate.

If for an individual i, $t_{i,k-1}$ is designated as the beginning of an

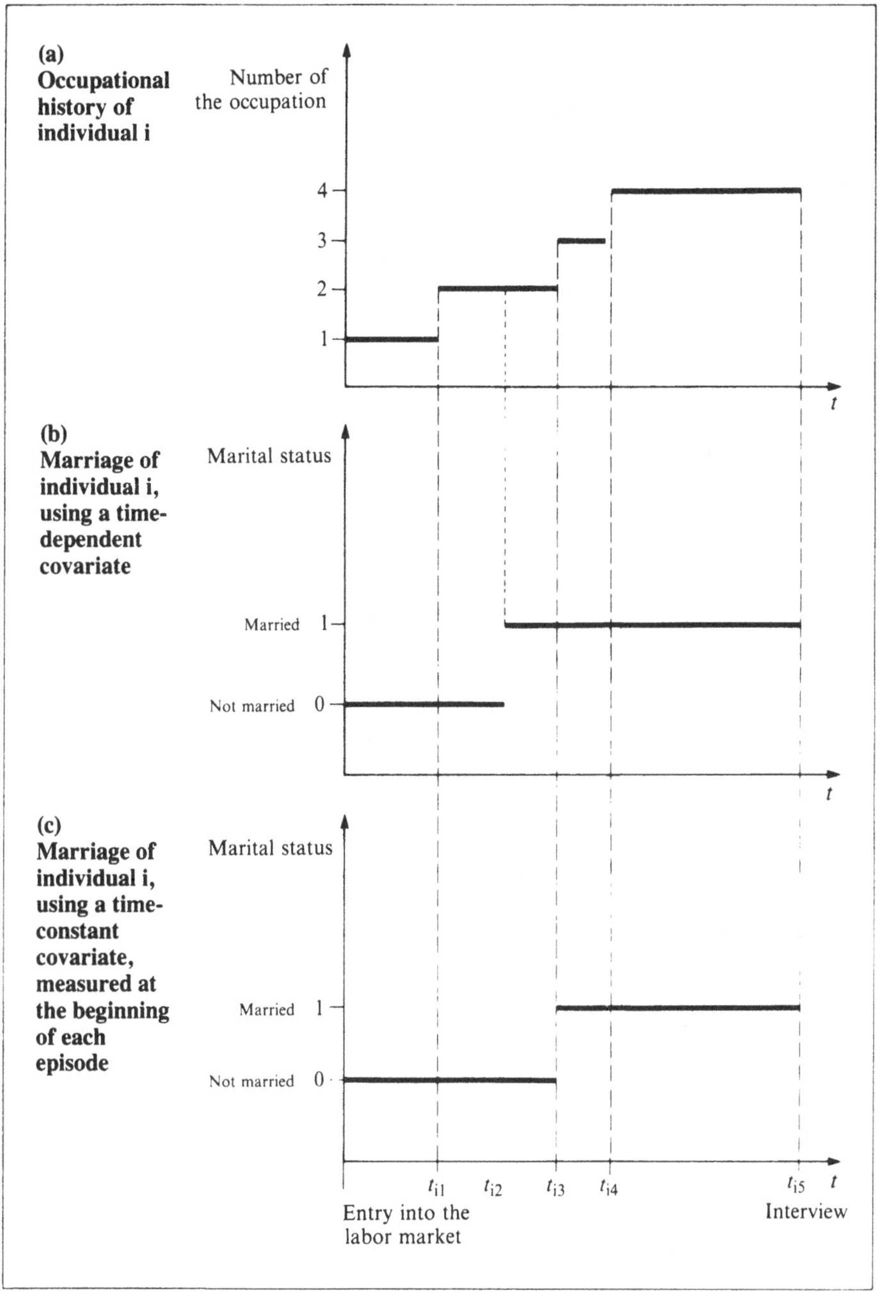

Figure 10.3. Modeling the influence of marriage (a) on the career path, (b) as a time-dependent covariate, and (c) as a time-dependent covariate measured at the beginning of each episode.

occupational episode k, and if v represents the duration of episode k, and t_i^H is the time of marriage of individual i, then the value of the time-dependent dummy variable marriage $x_{ik}^H(v)$ is characterized by:

$$x_{ik}^H(v) = \begin{cases} 0 & \text{for } t_i^H - t_{i,k-1} \geqslant v \\ 1 & \text{for } t_i^H - t_{i,k-1} < v. \end{cases}$$

Including discrete time-dependent covariates within a maximum likelihood estimation procedure is relatively easy. These follow a step function over time and are constant over subepisodes (see Figure 10.3b). Designating $t_0 < t_1 < \ldots < t_s$ as the time points of change of the covariate vector within the duration interval $[0, t)$ and given $t_{s+1} = t$, then the cumulative hazard rate may be decomposed into an integral sum. The probability that no event occurs until the time point t is obtained from the product of the survivor functions of the subepisodes in which the covariate vector remains unchanged:

$$S(t \mid x(t)) = \prod_{r=1}^{s+1} S(t_r \mid t_{r-1}, x(t_{r-1})).$$

The maximum likelihood estimation is gained by splitting the observed duration t_i based upon the s_i time points of change into $s_i + 1$ independent subepisodes. The hazard rate is estimated as in the case of time-constant covariates. Thus, for each of these subepisodes in which the covariate vector remains unchanged, the newly created data record contains the following information:

1. the values of the covariates at the beginning of each subepisode:
2. the duration at the beginning and end of a subepisode (the duration as such is sufficient only for the exponential model);
3. censoring information indicating whether the subepisode ends with an event (CEN = 1) or not (CEN = 0).

The newly created event-history data set which has split episodes according to the time of marriage, may now be treated in the same way as for time-constant covariates. The data set is accessed by the program RATE to estimate the exponential model with the time-dependent marriage variable

$$\lambda(t \mid x(t)) = \exp(x'(t)\boldsymbol{\beta}).$$

The results are presented in model 2 of Table 10.1. The $\hat{\beta}$ coefficient of the time-dependent covariate MAR is significant and negative, which means that the rate of changing occupations after marriage is greatly reduced. Compared with the mobility rate of unmarried men, the mobility rate of married men decreases by about 51%[(0.4897 − 1) · 100% = −51.03%].

Whereas discrete time-dependent covariates can very simply be included in parametric rate models by splitting the original durations into subepisodes characterized by constancy, this simple way does not exist given continuous time-dependent covariates. If the continuous time-dependent covariates are assumed to be a function of the duration then a Weibull, a Gompertz-(Makeham), a log-logistic, a log-normal, or a gamma model may be used to do the estimation.

If job shifts are studied, the duration v in a job may serve as a proxy variable for job-specific knowledge and skills which have to be newly acquired in each occupation. If the hypothesis that the inclination towards changing jobs decreases with increasing accumulation of job-specific knowledge is true, then we expect that the Weibull distribution will possess a significant $\hat{\alpha}$, lying between 0 and 1.

The Weibull model is very flexible and appropriate for a wide variety of situations. Like the Gompertz distribution, the Weibull distribution can also be used to model a monotonically falling ($0<\alpha<1$) or monotonically increasing ($\alpha>1$) risk. For the special case $\alpha=1$ one obtains an exponential distribution, and it is therefore possible to test the null hypothesis of a constant event risk against the alternative $\alpha\neq 1$.

In order to include covariates in the Weibull model, the parameter λ is related to the covariate vector $\boldsymbol{x}$ log-linearly: $\lambda(\boldsymbol{x})=\exp(\boldsymbol{x}'\boldsymbol{\beta}^*)$. The Weibull model is then expressed as:

$$\begin{aligned}\lambda(v \mid \boldsymbol{x}) &= \exp(\boldsymbol{x}'\boldsymbol{\beta})^{\alpha}\alpha v^{\alpha-1}\\ &= \exp(\boldsymbol{x}'\boldsymbol{\beta})\alpha v^{\alpha-1}\end{aligned}$$

with

$$\boldsymbol{\beta}=\alpha\boldsymbol{\beta}^*.$$

The parameter estimations are carried out with the program system GLIM (Roger & Peacock, 1983) and presented as model 3 in Table 10.1.

The estimated coefficients for EDU, PRES, NOJ, LFX, COHO2, and COHO3 of model 3 are relatively consistent with those of models 1 and 2. A test of the null hypothesis $H_0:\alpha\geqslant 1$ against the alternative hypothesis $H_1:\alpha<1$ gives a monotonically decreasing inclination to change jobs:

$$z=\frac{\hat{\alpha}-1}{s(\hat{\alpha})}=\frac{0.8266-1}{0.1293}=-13.41.$$

This means that the inclination to change jobs decreases monotonically with increasing job-specific knowledge.

CONCLUDING REMARKS

The major advantage of event-history data is the fact that they permit an adequate representation of changes in qualitative variables which may occur at any point in time. The question nevertheless remains: Why has the event-oriented observation plan thus far only seldom been used in economic and social science research?

One explanation can certainly be found in the extensive and costly observation procedures necessary to record event histories. One way of doing this is to observe the process and follow the development of the characteristics of individuals with the survey instrument over a lengthy period of time. However, if then often takes a long time before the data are finally available and theory has sometimes developed in a different direction. Event-history data are therefore often collected retrospectively. As was also the case in the GLHS, the history of events is thus reconstructed over a long period of time. This type of data collection is sometimes the only way of obtaining event-oriented information (e.g., today, the educational and occupational careers of the 1929–31, 1939–41, and 1949–51 birth cohorts can only be recorded on a retrospective basis). However, such data are often criticized as being unreliable, in particular when the events to be recalled took place in the distant past. Retrospective recording of event-history data therefore requires a greater degree of care and control and this can generally only be achieved by extensive data checking and time-consuming data editing. Moreover, if the data are retrospectively recorded on only one occasion or for only one birth cohort, there is a considerable risk of the data base becoming obsolete relatively quickly.

This is why in the case of the socioeconomic panel (Hanefeld, 1987), the advantages of the traditional panel are combined with the retrospective recording of event-history data. Thus each new panel wave provides not only up-to-date information for the time of survey, but by retrospective questions one also records the most important changes and their precise point of time between these waves (for comparison of panel and retrospective studies see Featherman, 1979–80).

Regardless which of the described procedures to record event-history data is selected, it is always an *extensive and costly exercise.* But there exists a potentially strong demand for dynamic analysis of processes and courses in the fields of economics and the social sciences. This growing demand should lead to an increased supply of event-history oriented data structure in these fields in the future.

APPENDIX

List of variable names used in the example

Variable name	Definition
NOJ	Number of previously held jobs
LFX	Labor force experience in months
EDU	Education, measured in years:
	9 years Lower secondary school qualification (completion of compulsory education)

	10 years	Middle School qualification (certificate from *Realschule*)
	11 years	Lower secondary school qualification with additional vocational training (apprenticeship or certificate from specialized vocational school)
	12 years	Middle school qualification with additional vocational training degree (apprenticeship or certificate from specialized vocational school)
	13 years	*Abitur* (included in this category are certificates from a *Gymnasium, Kolleg* or *Wirtschaftsgymnasium*; also certificates from a secondary technical school, the *Fachoberschule* or the *Höhere Berufsfachschule*)
	17 years	Professional college qualification (certificate from a higher technical college or a professional college, the *Fachhochschule, Ingenieurschule* or *Höhere Fachschule*)
	19 years	University degree (from all institutions of higher education)
COHO2	Dummy variable for cohort 1939–41: 1 cohort 1939–41 0 other	
COHO3	Dummy variable for cohort 1949–51: 1 cohort 1949–51 0 other	
PRES	Wegener's (1985) prestige score for job i	
MAR	Marital status: 0 not married 1 married	
TDEP	Time dependence in parametric models	
CONST	Intercept	

REFERENCES

Aalen, O. O. (1988). Heterogeneity in survival analysis. *Statistics in Medicine, 7,* 1121–1137.

Andersen, P. K. & Borgan, Ø. (1985). Counting process models for life history data: A review (with discussion). *Scandinavian Journal of Statistics, 12,* 97–158.

Andersen, P. K. & Gill, R. D. (1982). Cox's regression model for counting processes: A large sample study. *Annals of Statistics, 10,* 1100–1120.

Blau, P. M. & Duncan, O. D. (1967). *The American occupational structure.* New York: Wiley.

Blossfeld, H.-P. (1986). Career opportunities in the Federal Republic of Germany: A dynamic approach to the study of life course, cohort, and period effects. *European Sociological Review, 2,* 208–225.

Blossfeld, H.-P. (1987). Zur Repräsentativität der SfB-3-Lebensverlaufsstudie: Ein Vergleich mit Daten aus der amtlichen Statistik. *Allgemeines Statistisches Archiv, 71,* 126–144.

Blossfeld, H.-P., Hamerle, A. & Mayer, K. U. (1989). *Event history analysis.* Hillsdale, NJ: Lawrence Erlbaum.

Carlsson, G. (1958). *Social mobility and class structure.* Lund: C. W. K. Gleerup.

Carroll, G. & Meyer, K. U. (1986). Job shift patterns in the Federal Republic of Germany: The effects of class, industrial sector, and organizational size. *American Sociological Review, 51,* 323–347.

Clayton, D. (1988). The analysis of event-history data: A review of progress and outstanding problems. *Statistics in Medicine, 7,* 819–841.

Cox, D. R. (1972). Regression models and life-tables (with discussion). *Journal of the Royal Statistical Society B, 34,* 187–220.

Cox, D. R. (1975). Partial likelihood. *Biometrika, 62,* 269–276.

Cox, D. R. & Hinkley, D. V. (1974). *Theoretical statistics.* London: Chapman & Hall.

Cox, D. R. & Oakes, D. (1974). *Analysis of survival data.* London: Chapman & Hall.

Featherman, D. I. & Hauser, R. M. (1978). *Opportunity and change.* New York: Academic Press.

Glass, D. V. (ed.) (1954). *Social mobility in Britain.* London: Routledge & Kegan Paul.

Goldthorpe, J. H. (1980). *Social mobility and class structure in modern Britain.* London: Routledge & Kegan Paul.

Hanefeld, U. (1987). *Das Sozio-ökonomische Panel. Grundlagen und Konzeption.* Frankfurt an Main and New York: Campus.

Heckman, J. J. & Singer, B. (1984). Econometric duration analysis. *Journal of Econometrics, 24,* 63–132.

Kalbfleisch, J. D. & Prentice, R. L. (1980). *The statistical analysis of failure time data.* New York: Wiley.

Lawless, J. F. (1982). *Statistical models and methods for life-time data.* New York: Wiley.

Manton, K. G. & Stallard, E. (1988). *Chronic disease modelling: Measurement and evaluation of the risks of chronic disease processes.* London: Griffin.

Mayer, K. U. *et al.* (1987). Lebensverläufe und Wohlfahrtsentwicklung. Materialien zur Konzeption, Design und Methodik der Hauptuntersuchung 1981/82. Max Planck Institute for Human Development and Education, Berlin.

Mayer, K. U. & Brückner, E. (1989). *Lebensverläufe und Wohlfahrtsentwicklung* (Materialien aus der Bildungsforschung Nr. 35). Berlin: Max-Planck-Institut für Bildungsforschung.

Papastefanou, G. (1980). Zur Güte von retrospektiven Daten – Eine Anwendung gedächtnispsychologischer Theorie und Ergebnisse einer Nachbefragung. Working paper No. 29 of the SfB 3 'Mikroanalytische Grundlagen der Gesellschaftspolitik'. Frankfurt am Main and Mannheim.

Roger, J. H. & Peacock, S. D. (1983). Fitting the scale as a GLIM parameter for Weibull, extreme value, logistic and log-logistic regression models with censored data. *GLIM-Newsletter, 6,* 30–37.

Rogoff, N. (1953). *Recent trends in occupational mobility.* New York: Free Press.

Sørensen, A. B. (1977). The structure of inequality and the process of attainment. *American Sociological Review, 42,* 965–978.
Sørensen, A. B. (1984). Interpreting time dependency in career processes. In A. Diekmann & P. Mitter (eds.), *Progress in stochastic modeling of social processes.* New York: Academic Press.
Sørensen, A. B. (1986). Theory and methodology in stratification research. In U. Himmelstrand (ed.), *The sociology of structure and action.* New York: Sage Publications.
Sørensen, A. B. & Tuma, N. B. (1981). Labor market structures and job mobility. *Research in Social Stratification and Mobility, 1,* 67–94.
Spilerman, S. (1977). Careers, labor market structure and socioeconomic achievement. *American Journal of Sociology, 83,* 551–593.
Svalastoga, K. (1959). *Prestige, class and mobility.* Copenhagen: Scandinavian University Books.
Töike, A. (1980). Zuverlässigkeit retrospektiver Verlaufsdaten – Qualitative Ergebnisse einer Nachbefragung. Working paper No. 30 of the SfB 3 'Mikroanalytische Grundlagen der Gesellschaftspolitik'. Frankfurt am Main and Mannheim.
Tuma, N. B. (1985). Effects of labor market structure on job-shift patterns. In J. J. Heckman & B. Singer (eds.), *Longitudinal analysis of labor market data.* Cambridge, MA: Cambridge University Press.
Tuma, N. B. & Hannan, M. T. (1984). *Social dynamics: models and methods.* New York: Academic Press.
Vaupel, J. W., Mauton, U. G. & Stallard, E. (1979). The impact of heterogeneity in individual frailty on the dynamics of morality. *Demography, 16,* 439–454.
Wegener, B. (1985). Gibt es Sozialprestige? *Zeitschrift für Soziologie, 14,* 209–235.

11 Behavioral genetic concepts in longitudinal analyses

NANCY L. PEDERSEN

The purpose of this chapter is to give a short description of some of the parameters of interest when behavioral genetic methods are applied to longitudinal designs. In order to make this clear, some examples will be provided from the ongoing Swedish Adoption/Twin Study of Aging (SATSA). Finally, several of the models currently being used will be presented and discussed.

PARAMETERS OF INTEREST OR WHAT DO WE WANT TO ASSESS?

To understand the application of behavioral genetic models to longitudinal designs, one must first be aware of the essential parameters in the simple univariate, one-occasion case. Unlike normative studies in which the primary emphasis is on mean levels of a behavior or phenotype, behavioral genetic studies focus on describing interindividual differences by partitioning phenotypic variance (P) into genetic (G) and environmental (E) sources of variation.[1]

The relationship of these parameters can be described in an equation, the simplest of which is $P = G + E$, or in a path diagram (Figure 11.1). Regardless of form of presentation or number of parameters included, the main idea is to determine to what extent interindividual differences are due to genetic and environmental differences in the population. Behavioral genetic methodology applies the principles of quantitative genetics to the study of subjects with differing degrees of relatedness and varying similarities in their environments to partition variation. (For further descriptions of basic behavioral genetic techniques and their application to a variety of phenotypes, see Plomin, DeFries & McClearn, 1990.)

A general longitudinal model

The simple univariate, one-occasion model can be expanded to a longitudinal design, different versions of which are depicted in Figures

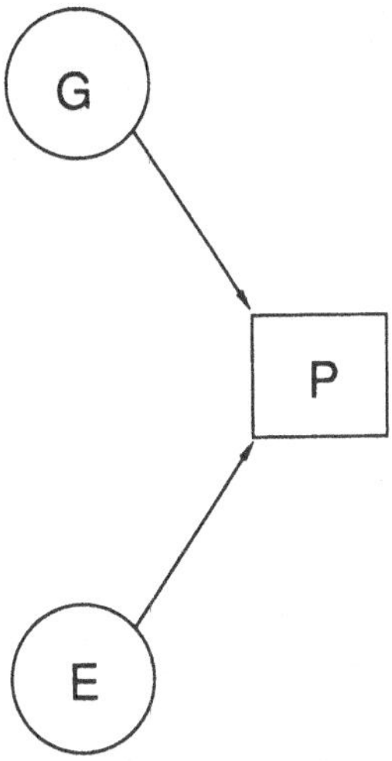

Figure 11.1. Simplest path diagram representing the contribution of genetic (G) and environmental (E) effects to phenotypic variation (P).

11.2–11.6. At each time of measurement, genetic (G_1, G_2, G_N) and environmental (E_1, E_2, E_N) influences may be important for expression of the measure of interest. As discussed below, a number of models are available which describe the relationship of the parameters at time 1 to those at subsequent time points. Each model, however, makes it possible to determine the relative importance of genetic and environmental effects for interindividual differences at each time point. The models differ primarily in whether or not causality is modeled between parameters, higher-order factors are included in the models, and whether means as well as covariances are structured.

The models are all based on quantitative genetic expectations of factors contributing to the similarity and differences of biologically related individuals. There are a number of standard assumptions which are made, or can be tested for, including the absence of interactions and correlations between genetic and environmental influences, lack of assortative mating for the phenotype of interest, and, in the case of twins, equality in the similarity of environments for identical and fraternal twins. The extent to which these assumptions are fulfilled is phenotype specific. This topic is further described in most behavioral genetic textbooks (e.g., Plomin, DeFries & McClearn, 1990) or discussions of model fitting (see, e.g., Eaves, Last, Young & Martin, 1978).

All of the models allow us to assess the relative importance of G and E at each time point. Some of the models can further decompose the variance at one occasion into that which is unique to that point and that which is in common with other time points. The models can also measure the degree of genetic and environmental stability, i.e. the degree to which the same genetic and environmental effects contribute to variability across occasions. Furthermore, the phenotypic stability can be partitioned into genetic and environmental components. Finally, some of the models assess the importance of genes and environments for average growth curves.

An example from the Swedish Adoption/Twin Study of Aging (SATSA)

SATSA is an ongoing study in gerontological genetics based on a subsample of adult twins, reared apart and reared together, from the Swedish Twin Registry. Mailout questionnaires covering health, personality and aspects of the environment were sent to the SATSA sample in 1984 (time 1) and 1987 (time 2). For the present purposes, results on extraversion and neuroticism from the 518 pairs in which both members of the pair responded to both questionnaires will be reported. Further details concerning the design of the study and the nature of the sample are reported by Pedersen *et al.* (1984) and McClearn *et al.* (in press). Results from the first occasion of measure for extraversion and neuroticism are reported in detail by Pedersen, Plomin, McClearn & Friberg (1988).

Partitioning the variation at each time point

The first concept mentioned above was partitioning the variation at each time point into genetic and environmental sources. The proportions of total variation due to genetic variance (heritabilities) for both neuroticism and extraversion are very similar in 1984 and in 1987 (Table 11.1). At both times, genetic factors account for approximately 37% of the variance in neuroticism. Heritability decreases from 42% in 1984 to 35% in 1987 for extraversion (Figure 11.2a).

The next feature of these models is that the genetic and environmental components can be broken down further into those which are unique to that occasion and those in common with other occasions. In SATSA, no new genetic effects came into play at T_2 for neuroticism, thus all the genetic variance at T_2 was in common with that at T_1. For extraversion, most of the genetic variance at T_2 was in common with that at T_1 (27% of the total variance at T_2) but some genetic innovations unique to T_2, which account for 8% of the total variance at that time point, were also operating (Figure 11.2b).

The distinction between effects unique to an occasion and those in common with the previous time point may be seen more clearly for the

Table 11.1. *Comparison of estimates for time 1 and time 2 from longitudinal model*

	Percentage of variance			
	Genetic		Environmental	
Measure	Ga (*c*, *u*)	Gd (*c*, *u*)	Ens (*c*, *u*)	Es (*c*, *u*)
Neuroticism				
*T*1	37	—	60	3
*T*2	37	—	63	0
	(37, 0)		(17, 46)	
Extraversion				
*T*1	—	42	51	6
*T*2	—	35	60	5
		(27, 8)	(20, 40)	(3, 2)

Note: Ga and Gd are proportions of total variation due to additive and non-additive sources of variation, respectively; Ens and Es are proportions of total variation due to nonshared and shared environmental variance, respectively.
c is the percentage of total variation at time 2 in common with time 1.
u is the percentage of total variation unique to time 2.

non-shared environmental parameter. Even though non-shared environmental effects account for 63% of the total variation at T_2 for neuroticism, only 17% of the total variation at T_2 is a result of the direct path between T_1 and T_2 (in common with T_1). Most of the non-shared environmental variance (46% of the total variance) is unique to T_2. A similar pattern (20% common, 40% unique or innovative) can be seen for extraversion.

Genetic and environmental stability or change

Other than studying the relative importance of G and E at different occasions, behavioral genetic models can also assess stability or change in genetic and environmental factors. The genetic correlation (r_G) and environmental correlation (r_E) describe the extent to which there is stability in the genetic and environmental effects, respectively, operating at two time points (Plomin & DeFries, 1981). For example, the genetic correlation between time 1 and time 2 for extraversion in SATSA is 0.88, indicating that there is considerable overlap in the genetic influences operating at each of the two time points. The environmental correlation of about 0.58 indicates that slightly more than half of the

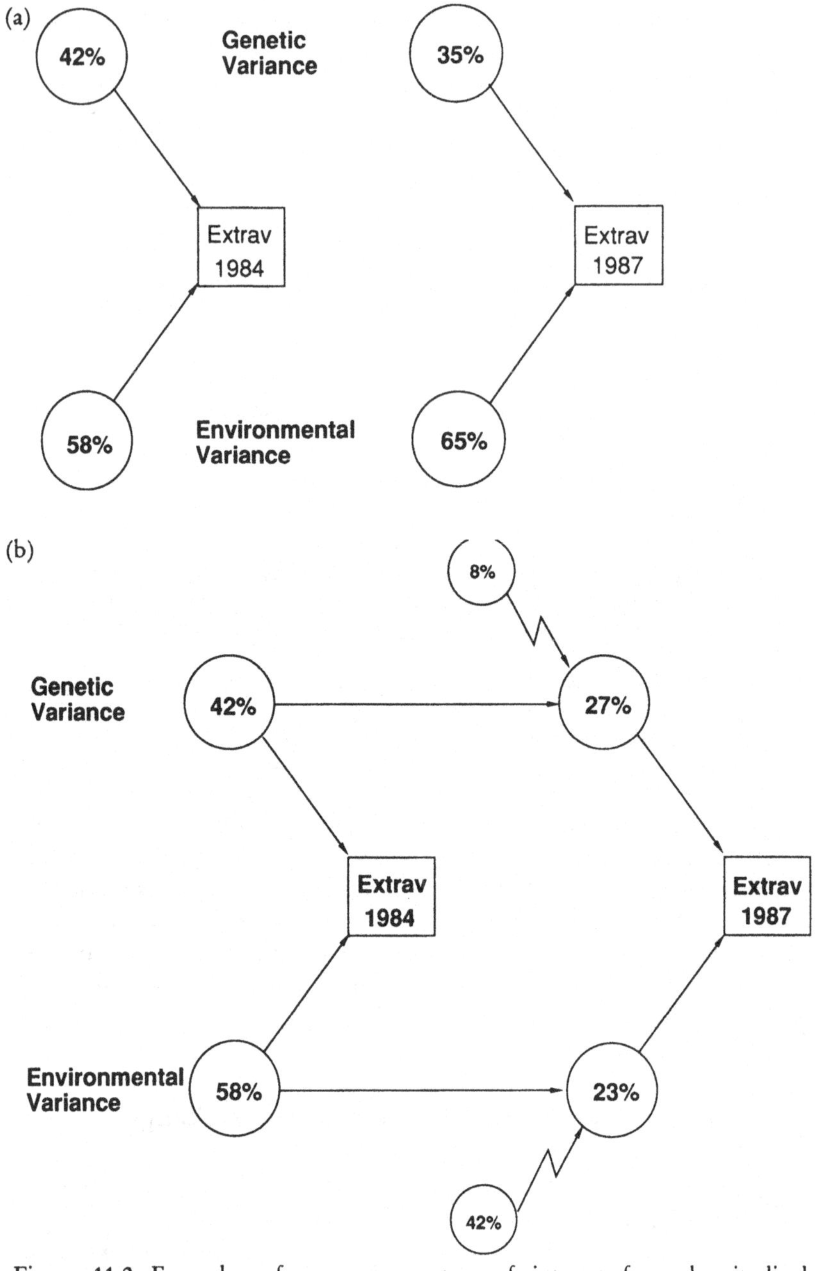

Figure 11.2. Examples of some parameters of interest from longitudinal behavioral genetic models.
(a) Genetic and environmental proportions of variation for extraversion in 1984 and in 1987.
(b) Variation at time 2 (1987) is further partitioned into that unique to that time (circle with jagged arrow; 8% genetic and 42% environmental) and in common with previous occasion (27% genetic and 23% environmental).
(c) Genetic and environmental paths in non-causal longitudinal model.

(c)

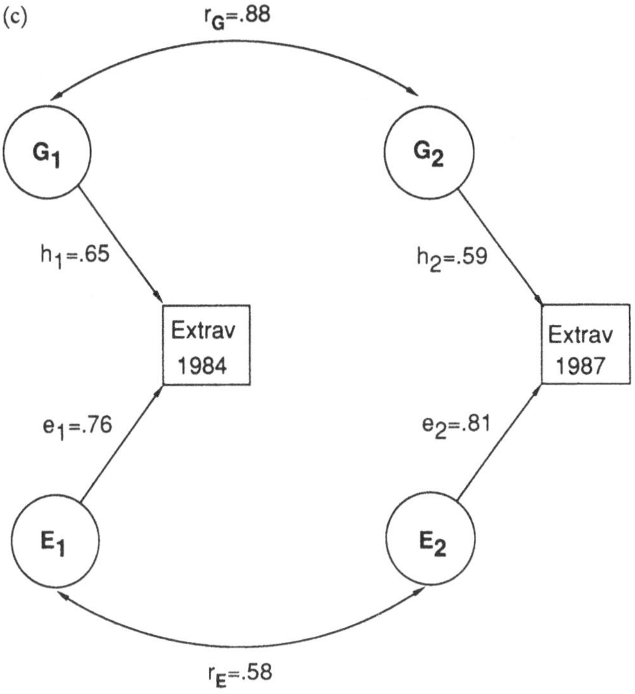

Figure 11.2. (*cont.*)

non-shared environmental influences operating at T_1 are the same as those operating at T_2. Another way of thinking about these correlations is in terms of unique and common variance. If the correlation is 1.0, all the variance is in common. If the correlation is less than 1.0, some innovative variance (unique) must be operating at subsequent time points. These correlations, which are equivalent to double headed arrows between G_1 and G_2 or between E_1 and E_2, can be computed from most developmental behavioral genetic models (see, e.g., Figure 11.2c).

Genetic and environmental contributions to stability and change

A very different concept is the contribution of genes and environments to stability or change. In this case, the emphasis is on the extent to which the phenotypic correlation can be explained by genetic or environmental effects. If we return to Figure 11.2c, the question now is what proportion of the phenotypic correlation is due to the genetic chain of paths ($h_1 r_G h_2$) and to the environmental chain of paths ($e_1 r_E e_2$)? The path coefficients h_1, h_2, e_1, and e_2 represent the square roots of the heritabilities and 'environmentalities' at T_1 and T_2. From the example on extraversion provided above, we know that the heritabilities at time 1 and time 2 are 0.42 and 0.35, respectively, which give path coefficients $h_1 = 0.648$ and $h_2 = 0.592$. The genetic chain of paths (phenotypically standardized covariances) is thus $0.648 \times 0.88 \times 0.592 = 0.34$. The genetic contribution to stability is computed by dividing the 'genetic chain' by the phenotypic correlation (stability), i.e., $0.34/0.71 = 48\%$. Thus, although there is considerable stability in genetic effects across the two time points ($r_G = 0.88$), genetic factors account for only 48% of the phenotypic stability.

WHAT MODELS ARE AVAILABLE?

There are a number of ways to model longitudinal changes within developmental behavioral genetic designs. One of the earliest path models, described by Plomin & DeFries (1981), was the two-occasion model depicted in Figure 11.2c. As discussed above, this model highlights the importance of G and E at the two time points, the genetic and environmental stabilities (r_G and r_E), and the genetic and environmental contributions to stability. The model does not posit that effects at time 1 are causal to time 2, but by including double-headed arrows between G_1 and G_2 or between E_1 and E_2, concentrates on the associations between effects at the two occasions. As the model is presented, it is not possible to distinguish between unique variance at one time point and variance in common with the previous time point.

The genetic simplex model

The *genetic simplex model* (Figure 11.3), presented in detail by Molenaar, Boomsma and Dolan in Chapter 12 of this volume, is basically the same as the model discussed in conjunction with Figure 11.2b. In contrast to the Plomin & DeFries model, simplex designs include causal pathways between effects at adjacent occasions. Thus, G_1 is causal to G_2 and E_1 is causal to E_2. Furthermore, the 'innovations' discussed above which represent residual variance at T_2 and each subsequent time point are included. Including the residuals enables calculation of percentages of variation unique to each occasion and in common with the previous occasion. The genetic and environmental correlations (r_G and r_E) may also be derived from the simplex model. When modeled using LISREL (Jöreskog & Sörbom, 1986), these correlations are the same as the beta values in the standardized solution. Because the genetic and environmental correlations and the path

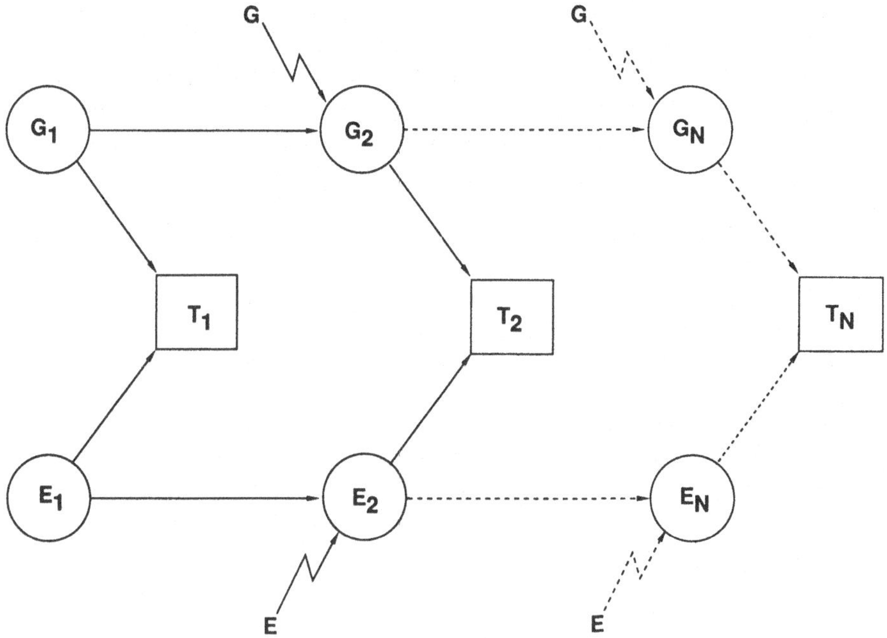

Figure 11.3. The genetic simplex model.

coefficients are available, one can also assess the contribution of genetic and environmental factors to stability and change. Molenaar and colleagues (Chapter 12 of this volume; Boomsma, Molenaar & Orlebeke, in press) point out that individual 'genetic and environmental scores' may also be derived in applications of the genetic simplex model. These individual scores are much like factor scores, and indicate how much an individual's phenotypic level (or pattern across time) is due to genetic and environmental factors, respectively.

Molenaar and colleagues have extended the genetic simplex model to include the simultaneous analysis of the phenotypic means and covariance structures (Chapter 12 of this volume; Dolan, Molenaar & Boomsma, in press). The model thereby addresses both the trend of the average growth curve as well as the stability of individual differences. The objective is to test the hypothesis that there is a common underlying process influencing changes in average response and the stability of individual differences. This model differs from the latent growth curve model (McArdle & Epstein, 1987) in that it is based on the simplex model rather than the traditional common factor model (see a discussion of the latent growth curve model below). It is limited to data in which the number of observed variables exceed by one the number of factors related to the means. In the double simplex model in which both genetic and environmental effects are included, there are four parameters associated with the mean trend: E[G(1)] and E[E(1)], the latent genetic and environmental means, respectively; and G_Δ and E_Δ, which correspond to the innovative genetic and environmental effects at each occasion associated with the mean. The consequence of this limitation is that, when one observed variable is measured at each time point, data from at least five occasions must be available for analysis. Criticisms and a defense of the simplex model are discussed by Molenaar *et al.* (Chapter 12 of this volume).

The extension of the genetic simplex model to analysis of the structure of the means represents an exciting and important breakthrough. Perhaps the greatest difference between behavioral genetics and other behavioral fields has been the emphasis on variation rather than the means. The relationship between the mean and variance, however, is a central issue in life-span development and one which can now be addressed by behavioral genetic models. This extended model bridges the gap between normative and differential approaches to the study of human development.

Common factor model

Whereas the simplex model is particularly well suited to longitudinal series in which there is occasion-to-occasion transmission and correlations decrease with increasing distances between time points, a *common-factor model* may be used to describe pleiotropic influences which affect a trait at all occasions. One example of such a mechanism, presented by Hewitt, Eaves, Neale & Meyer (1988) is for blood pressure.

> For example, we may suppose that throughout early adulthood the constitutional properties of an individual's cardiovascular system give rise to consistently high or low blood pressure. The perturbations around this mean level, perhaps associated with an illness or an especially stressful period for the individual, are transient and whatever caused this perturbation has no effect on later occasions. We can call this a common-factor mechanism or pleiotropy. (p. 134)

The common-factor model, presented in Figure 11.4, includes one genetic and one environmental factor on which the phenotypic values at all time points load. It is possible to assess the degree of genetic and environmental stability as well as the contribution of genes and environments to phenotypic stability from the parameter estimates in this model. Causality (transmission) is not testable, however unique variances at the separate occasions may be included. The 'common' variances differ from those in the simplex model in that they are

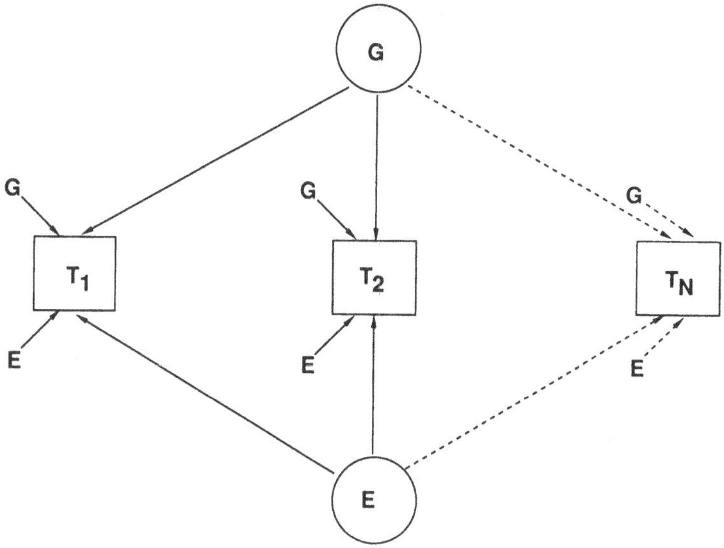

Figure 11.4. The common-factor model.

common to all points of measurement rather than sequential. Boomsma & Molenaar (1987) have demonstrated that a simplex model is more appropriate than a common-factor model when there is occasion-to-occasion transmission.

Transmission-factor models

Eaves, Long & Heath (1986) and Hewitt *et al.* (1988) have incorporated aspects of both the simplex and the common-factor models into the same model (Figure 11.5). By fixing certain parameters, the relative fit of the common-factor model versus a 'transmission' model may be determined. With three or fewer measurement occasions, there can be no unambiguous resolution of which model is more appropriate. All of the parameters of interest discussed above, with the exception of genetic and environmental influences on the structure of the means, may be addressed in the transmission-factor model.

Latent growth curve model

In the *latent growth curve model* described by McArdle (1986) and McArdle & Epstein (1987), means and covariances are modeled simultaneously within a traditional common-factor model. Two latent factors, level and shape, 'represent dimensions of individual differences in growth over time or, simply, latent curves' (McArdle, 1986) (simplified in Figure 11.6). While this model provides valuable informa-

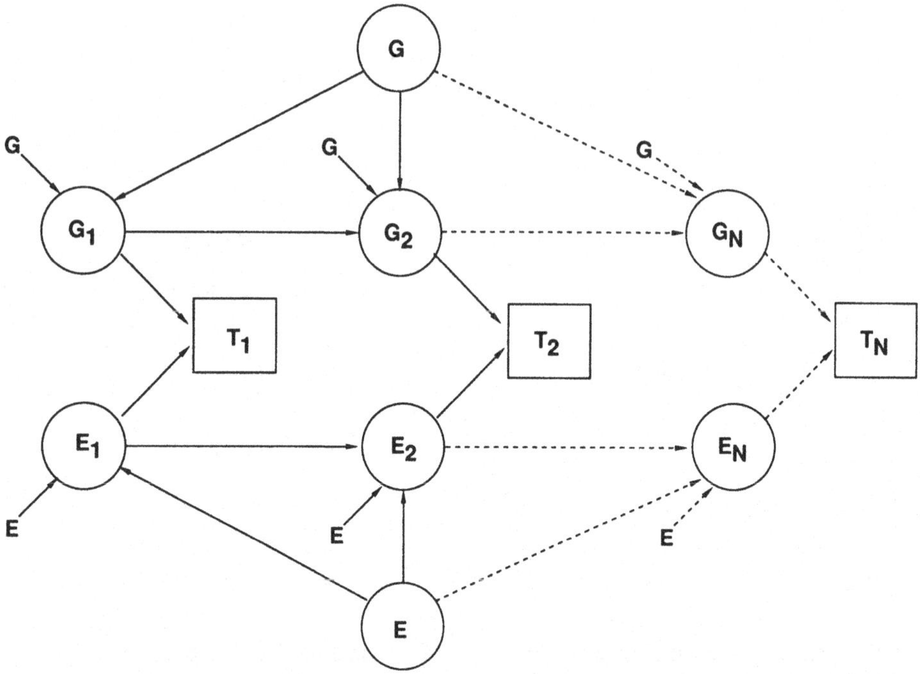

Figure 11.5. The transmission-factor model.

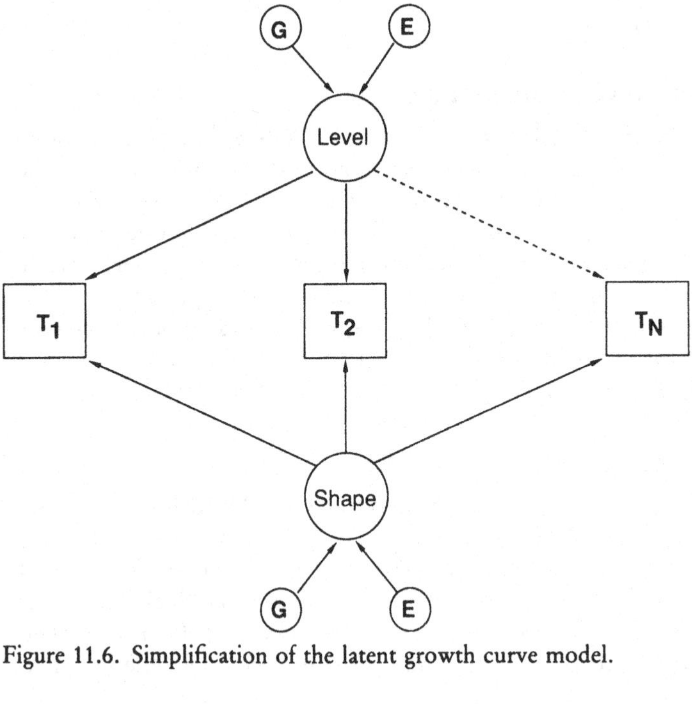

Figure 11.6. Simplification of the latent growth curve model.

tion about genetic and environmental influences for mean changes in growth, it is susceptible to the problems inherent in applying common-factor models to longitudinal data which are better represented by the simplex model.

FUTURE DIRECTIONS

Each of the models presented above has obvious advantages and disadvantages. Hybrid models such as the transmission-factor model presented by Hewitt *et al.* (1988) and the genetic simplex model which includes structuring of the means (Molenaar *et al.*, Chapter 12 of this volume) represent exciting and powerful extensions of developmental behavioral genetic principles. Comparison of the fit of nested models enables testing of competing hypotheses concerning the structure of genetic and environmental influences in a longitudinal framework. Until recently, few data have been available on which these models can be applied. Notable exceptions are the height and weight data from adolescent Swedish twins (Fischbein, Molenaar & Boomsma, 1990), an extension of these models which includes both twin and parent-offspring data from the Louisville Twin Study (Phillips & Matheny, 1990), and a test of the transmission-factor model on adoptive-sibling and twin data from the Colorado Adoption project (Fulker & Cardon, in press).

A number of interesting concepts within longitudinal research have yet to be addressed by these developmental behavioral genetic models. Some of the key words mentioned at this workshop, such as rates and velocities (Lindgren) 'turning points' (Pickles), and intraindividual variability versus intraindividual change (Nesselroade) have not been specifically addressed. A twin study with P-technique data would contribute to our understanding of the etiology of intraindividual variability versus intraindividual change. The applications alluded to by Molenaar and colleagues (Chapter 12 of this volume; Molenaar & Boomsma, 1987; Boomsma, Molenaar & Orlebeke, in press) indicate that the genetic simplex model may be adaptable to rates and velocities, and nonlinear trends; however, it is likely that hybrid models, such as the transmission-factor model, are necessary for analyzing the consequences of major events or turning points (such as puberty, menopause or significant life events). Surely as some genes are 'turned off' and others 'turned on', the variance architecture must change.

Other issues central to life-span developmental research, such as the triangulation of age, period, and cohort effects should be next on the agenda for refinements in developmental behavioral genetic modeling. Still in its infancy, this exciting field promises to be a powerful and productive addition to the arsenal of methodologies available for the study of human development.

ACKNOWLEDGEMENTS

This chapter was written under support from the MacArthur Foundation Research Network on Successful Aging and from the National Institute of Aging (AG-04563). SATSA is an ongoing study performed at the Department of Environmental Hygiene of the Karolinska Institute in collaboration with the Research Center for Developmental and Health Genetics in the College of Health and Human Development at the Pennsylvania State University. Co-investigators are G. E. McClearn, Robert Plomin and J. R. Nesselroade (USA) and Nancy L. Pedersen, Lars Friberg, U. DeFaire and Stig Berg (Sweden).

NOTE

1. The genetic parameter can be further subdivided into additive (Ga) and non-additive (Gd) genetic variance (which describe whether the effects of genes add up linearly in their effects or whether they interact between or within loci). Three types of environmental variance may be of interest: non-shared environmental variance unique to the individual (Ens), shared rearing environment (Es), or correlated environments (Ec). Genetic and environmental factors may be correlated (GE), i.e. some genotypes may be more often found in certain environments, or they may be differentially expressed in certain environments (genotype by environment interaction or GXE).

REFERENCES

Boomsma, D. I. & Molenaar, P. C. M. (1987). The genetic analysis of repeated measures. I. Simplex models. *Behavior Genetics, 17,* 111–123.

Boomsma, D. I., Molenaar, P. C. M. & Orlebeke, J. F. (in press). Estimation of individual genetic and environmental factor scores. *Genetic Epidemiology.*

Dolan, C. V., Molenaar, P. C. M. & Boomsma, D. I. (in press) Simultaneous causal modeling of longitudinal covariance and means structure using the simplex model.

Eaves, L. J., Long, J. & Heath, A. C. (1986). A theory of developmental change in quantitative phenotypes applied to cognitive development. *Behavior Genetics, 16,* 143–162.

Eaves, L. J., Last, K. A., Young, P. A. & Martin, N. G. (1978). Model-fitting approaches to the analysis of human behaviour. *Heredity, 41,* 249–320.

Fischbein, S., Molenaar, P. C. M. & Boomsma, D. I. (1990). Simultaneous genetic analysis of longitudinal means and covariance structure using the simplex model: Application to repeatedly measured weight in a sample of 164 female twins. *Acta Geneticae Medicae et Gemellologiae, 39,* 165–172.

Fulker, D. W. & Cardon, L. (in press). Developmental trends in IQs of twins and siblings aged one to seven years.

Hewitt, J. K., Eaves, L. J., Neale, M. C. & Meyer, J. M. (1988). Resolving causes of developmental continuity or 'tracking'. I. Longitudinal twin studies during growth. *Behavior Genetics, 18,* 133–151.

Jöreskog, K. G. & Sörbom, D. (1986). *LISREL VI: Analysis of linear structural relationships by the method of maximum-likelihood.* Chicago: International Educational Services.

McArdle, J. J. (1986). Latent variable growth within behavior genetic models. *Behavior Genetics, 16,* 163–200.

McArdle, J. J. & Epstein, D. (1987). Latent growth curves within developmental structural equation models. *Child Development, 58,* 110–133.

McClearn, G. E., Pedersen, N. L., Plomin, R., Nesselroade, J. R., Friberg, L. & DeFaire, U. (in press). Age and gender effects for individual differences in behavioral aging: The Swedish Adoption/Twin Study of Aging.

Molenaar, P. C. M. & Boomsma, D. I. (1987). The genetic analysis of repeated measures II. Karhunen-Loeve transformation. *Behavior Genetics, 17,* 229–242.

Pedersen, N. L., Floderus-Myrhed, B., Friberg, L., McClearn, G. E. & Plomin, R. (1984). Swedish early separated twins: Identification and characterization. *Acta Geneticae Medicae et Gemellologiae, 33,* 243–250.

Pedersen, N. L., Plomin, R., McClearn, G. E. & Friberg, L. (1988). Neuroticism, extraversion and related traits in adult twins reared apart and reared together. *Journal of Personality Social Psychology, 55,* 950–957.

Phillips, K. & Matheny, A. P. (1990). Quantitative genetic analysis of longitudinal trends in height: Preliminary results from the Louisville Twin Study. *Acta Geneticae Medicae et Gemellologiae, 39,* 143–163.

Plomin, R. (1986). *Development, genetics, and psychology.* Hillsdale, New Jersey: Lawrence Erlbaum Associates.

Plomin, R. & DeFries, J. C. (1981). Multivariate behavioral genetics and development: Twin studies. In L. Gedda, P. Parisi & W. E. Nance (eds). *Twin research 3: Part B* (pp. 25–33). New York: Alan R. Liss.

Plomin, R., DeFries, J. C. & McClearn, G. E. (1990). *Behavior genetics: A primer.* (2nd edn). New York: W. H. Freeman.

12 Genetic and environmental factors in a developmental perspective

PETER C. M. MOLENAAR, DORRET I. BOOMSMA AND CONOR V. DOLAN

INTRODUCTION

Developmental behavior genetics is concerned with the diverse ways in which genetic and environmental processes are involved in changes as well as continuity in development (Plomin, 1986; DeFries & Fulker, 1986). During ontogenesis, observed (phenotypic) change of a quantitative character may be due to distinct subsets of genes turning on and off, whereas continuity, on the other hand, may be caused by stable environmental causes. In contrast to the popular point of view, then, genetically determined characters are not always stable, nor are longitudinally stable characters always due to hereditary influences. Only through carefully designed longitudinal investigation of phenotypic changes in genetically related individuals can the dynamic patterns of genetic and environmental influences be disentangled.

In the following we shall mainly be concerned with a particular type of genetic model for the analysis of longitudinal phenotypic data, namely the simplex model (Jöreskog, 1970). The genetic simplex model is a genuine time series model and therefore can explain the characteristic time-dependent patternings of serial correlation (autocorrelation) as observed in longitudinal studies. It was already shown by Cronbach (1967) that common factor analysis of autocorrelation matrices will yield spurious, i.e. invalid, results. Consequently, recent efforts in the genetic modeling of longitudinal data have put particular emphasis on the elaboration of simplex models in this context (Boomsma & Molenaar, 1987*a*; Eaves, Hewitt & Heath, 1988).

Presently, we will introduce two important generalizations of the genetic simplex model. Firstly, we will consider the estimation of latent time-dependent profiles of genetic and environmental influences for each individual subject. Behavior geneticists never considered the genetic and environmental scores of single subjects. Yet in a mathematical–statistical sense, genetic single-subject scores are similar to factor scores and therefore can be obtained by means of standard techniques for the estimation of factor scores. This approach would seem particularly worthwhile for genetic research into deviances and the consequent possibilities of carrying out preventive interventions (cf. Mednick *et al.*, 1983). In fact, Boomsma, Molenaar & Orlebeke (in press) show that for two subjects with the same phenotypic pattern of high blood pressure, the high blood-pressure of one subject is associated with a high genetic score, whereas the blood pressure of the other subject is associated with a high environmental score. Given such information, any interventions aimed at normalizing blood pressure could be entirely different for each of these subjects. We will show that the estimation of single-subject scores can be extended to the genetic simplex model, thus yielding longitudinal trajectories of intraindividual variation of genetic and environmental scores. This will be shown for the most difficult case in which only univariate phenotypic measurements are available at each time point. Not only is this the more relevant case from the application-oriented point of view, but its success will guarantee the success of analogous multivariate cases because the availability of multivariate phenotypic measurements at each time point will always yield much better conditioned estimates of the latent time-dependent profiles concerned.

Secondly, the simplex model will be generalized to include latent genetic and environmental trends. Behavior geneticists do not usually consider the role of genetic and environmental influences on both the stability and change of individual differences as well as the species-specific developmental function or average growth curve. Yet, these two aspects of longitudinal data are complementary and not necessarily independent in understanding development. This approach would seem particularly useful for genetic analyses of unstandardized longitudinal data pertaining to, for example biological or ability development. In particular when multivariate phenotypic measurements are available at each time point, this combined analysis of interindividual and intraindividual changes in the means and variation of genetic and environmental scores can yield important explanatory evidence concerning the maturational and learning processes underlying developmental trait patterns (Baltes, personal communication; see Baltes & Nesselroade, 1973). For the same reasons alluded to earlier, we will show that the simplex model for univariate phenotypic measurements can be reliably generalized to include latent genetic and environmental trends.

In the following, the validity of both the estimation of individual genetic and environmental profiles as well as the analysis of the genetic simplex model with structured means will be shown by means of simulation studies. In this way one can directly compare the results obtained with a finite sample of longitudinal data and the true model used in the simulation of the data. In the closing section, we will present the results of an illustrative application of the genetic simplex model, including the proposed generalizations, to real data.

THE GENETIC SIMPLEX

In this section we will discuss the basic genetic simplex model for univariate repeated measurements in a heuristic, application-oriented way. After the presentation of the defining equations, the genetic simplex model for monozygotic (MZ) and dizygotic (DZ) twin data will be reformulated as a particular multigroup LISREL model (see Jöreskog & Sörbom, 1986). As the LISREL program is now widely available, this will facilitate regular applications of the proposed approaches. For ease of presentation, several simplifying assumptions will be made that enable concentration on the main issues. Specifically, interactions and covariances between genetic and environmental influences are assumed to be absent, as are interactions between alleles at loci (i.e., no genetic dominance effects) and interactions between loci (i.e., no epistasis). In addition, it is assumed that assortative mating does not occur, while only one particular type of environmental influences will be considered, namely those influences that are not shared by members of a family. These assumptions do not imply that the effects concerned cannot be detected or modeled: the analysis of genotype–environment interactions and correlations when environmental measures are available is presented in, for example, Plomin, DeFries & Fulker (1988), the application of nonlinear factor analysis to genotype–environment interaction is discussed in Molenaar & Boomsma (1987*a*) and Molenaar, Boomsma, Neeleman & Dolan (in press), a theoretical model of assortative mating and cultural transmission is given in Fulker (1988), while shared environmental influences and dominance can straightforwardly be included in the basic genetic model. Only some of the effects (e.g., epistasis) may be difficult to quantify in human research (Eaves, 1977) and represent cases where theory outruns the available data (Eaves and Young, 1981).

Before presenting our basic model we will briefly discuss its underlying assumptions. The genetic simplex model is a particular instance of the general covariance structure model (Jöreskog & Sörbom, 1986) and therefore obeys the same assumptions as the latter model. That is, for maximum likelihood (ML) estimation to apply it is assumed that the vector of repeated phenotypic observations has a multivariate normal distribution. Browne & Shapiro (1988) show that ML estimation in covariance structure models is quite robust against departures from multivariate normality. A similar result regarding the robustness of ML estimation in structural models of both covariances and means has been obtained by Gourieroux, Monfort & Trognon (1984): if the distribution of the observed phenotypes belongs to the general class of linear exponential distributions and if the model for the means is correctly specified, then ML estimates are consistent and asymptotically normally distributed. The latter result bears on the genetic simplex model including latent genetic and environmental trends.

Another issue concerns the number of MZ or DZ twin pairs, or more generally the number of pedigrees, which is required. The minimum number of pedigrees is directly related to the number of repeated phenotypic measurements. If the number of repeated measurements increases, the dimension of the estimated matrices of mean cross-products (see below) also increases. In order to guarantee the required positive-definiteness of the latter matrices, the number of pedigrees then also has to increase to a value that is strictly larger than the number of repeated measurements. Specifically, if we have T univariate phenotypic measurements then the number of MZ twin pairs and the number of DZ twin pairs each have to be larger than T.

Turning to our basic model, if in a longitudinal design a univariate phenotype P is observed at $t = 1, \ldots, T$ time points, the following dynamic genetic model can be considered:

$$P(t) = G(t) + E(t) + e(t), \quad t = 1, \ldots, T, \tag{1}$$

where $P(t)$, $G(t)$ and $E(t)$ represent phenotypic, genetic and (non-shared) environmental time series, respectively, while $e(t)$ denotes a residual series. An advantageous parametric time series model for the genetic and environmental influences is then given by a first-order autoregression:

$$G(t) = \beta_{\mathrm{G}}(t)G(t-1) + \zeta_{\mathrm{G}}(t). \tag{2}$$

$$E(t) = \beta_{\mathrm{E}}(t)E(t-1) + \zeta_{\mathrm{E}}(t). \tag{3}$$

The autoregressive coefficient $\beta_{\mathrm{G}}(t)$ (similar remarks apply to $\beta_{\mathrm{E}}(t)$) is a measure of the amount of genetic variation at time point $t-1$ that is transmitted to time point t and therefore is associated with the stability (cf. Rudinger, Andres and Rietz, Chapter 13 of this volume) or, stated otherwise, the memory of the genetic process between $t-1$ and t. The so-called innovation $\zeta_{\mathrm{G}}(t)$ (similar remarks apply to $\zeta_{\mathrm{E}}(t)$) denotes the effects of new genes turned on at time point t and will therefore lower the stability of the genetic process between $t-1$ and t.

Identification of the genetic simplex model defined by equations (1)–(3) requires data from genetically related individuals, such as twins. The genetic relations between family members provide information with respect to the latent factor series $G(t)$ and $E(t)$. In particular, monozygotic (MZ) twin pairs have all their genetic material in common and hence $\mathrm{cor}[G_1(t), G_2(t)] = 1$. The instantaneous genetic correlation for dizygotic (DZ) twins is 0.5 on average, i.e. $\mathrm{cor}[G_1(t), G_2(t)] = 0.5$, as is the genetic correlation among ordinary siblings. This information can be used to arrive at an identified model with more than one latent process, even if the observed phenotypic time series is univariate. Specifically, longitudinal data from twins open up the possibility of decomposing a univariate phenotypic series into a genetic and an environmental series which may each behave quite differently in time. This may not always be immediately evident from the observed series (cf. Heath, Jardine, Eaves & Martin, 1988). For example, variance due to $G(t)$ may increase over time, while variance due to $E(t)$ may decrease. Increased genetic variance could be due to the amplification of existing genetic differences, as expressed by large values of $\beta_G(t)$, or to new genetic variance coming into play (new genes 'turned on'), as expressed by large values of $\zeta_G(t)$.

We will now reformulate the genetic simplex model defined by equations (1)–(3) as a LISREL model, while restricting attention to longitudinal MZ and DZ twin data. Furthermore, it is assumed for ease of presentation that the residual series $e(t)$ in equation (1) is absent. First we introduce the $(T \times T)$ diagonal matrices Ψ_G and Ψ_E with time-dependent variances $\Psi_G(t, t) = \mathrm{var}[\zeta_G(t)]$ and $\Psi_E(t, t) = \mathrm{var}[\zeta_E(t)]$ as the tth diagonal elements, respectively ($t = 1, \ldots, T$). Notice that the first diagonal elements of Ψ_G (similar remarks apply to Ψ_E) is special in that no autoregression for $G(1)$ can be formulated at time point 1. Consequently, at $t = 1$ equation (2) becomes simply $G(1) = \zeta_G(1)$, and $\Psi_G(1, 1) = \mathrm{var}[\zeta_G(1)]$ now denotes the genetic variance at time point 1. Only for $t > 1$ do the diagonal elements of $\Psi_G(t, t)$ denote the variances of the genetic innovations. Next, the $T \times T$ matrices $\boldsymbol{B}_G^*$ and $\boldsymbol{B}_E^*$ are introduced. For instance, $\boldsymbol{B}_G^*$ has the following pattern:

$$\boldsymbol{B}_G^* = \begin{bmatrix} 0 & & \cdots & & 0 & 0 \\ \beta_G(2) & 0 & \cdots & & 0 & 0 \\ 0 & \beta_G(3) & 0 & \cdots & & \\ \vdots & 0 & & \ddots & & \vdots \\ & \vdots & \vdots & & 0 & \\ 0 & 0 & \cdots & 0 & \beta_G(T) & 0 \end{bmatrix}$$

where $\beta_G(2), \ldots, \beta_G(T)$ are the autoregressive coefficients in equation (2) $\boldsymbol{B}_E^*$ has the same pattern. Reformulation of the genetic simplex model for MZ and DZ twin pairs is now accomplished by specification of the expected structure of the $(T \times T)$ matrices of mean cross-products between and within these twin pairs. Let Σ_{MZB} and Σ_{MZW} denote the expected structure of the matrices of mean cross-products between and within MZ pairs, respectively. Before specifying the expected structure concerned, we will first consider their respective estimates S_{MZB} and S_{MZM} in order to elucidate the nature of these matrices of mean cross-products. For example, S_{MZB} is obtained as the hypothesis matrix from a one-way multivariate analysis of variance, where the factor has as many levels as there are MZ twin pairs and where the $(T \times 1)$ vector $\boldsymbol{P} = [(P(1), \ldots, P(T)]'$ derived from equation (1) is the dependent variable (the prime $'$ denotes the transpose). S_{MZB} is obtained as the error matrix from the same multivariate analysis of variance. Accordingly, the longitudinal data from the MZ and DZ twin groups are summarized in the four matrices S_{MZB}, S_{MZW}, S_{DZB} and S_{DZW}. The expected structure of these matrices for the genetic simplex model is:

$$\left.\begin{aligned} \Sigma_{\mathrm{MZB}} &= \Lambda_{\mathrm{MZ}B}\boldsymbol{B}_{\mathrm{G}}\Psi_{\mathrm{G}}\boldsymbol{B}'_{\mathrm{G}}\Lambda'_{\mathrm{MZB}} + \boldsymbol{B}_{\mathrm{E}}\Psi_{\mathrm{E}}\boldsymbol{B}'_{\mathrm{E}} \\ \Sigma_{\mathrm{MZW}} &= \boldsymbol{B}_{\mathrm{E}}\Psi_{\mathrm{E}}\boldsymbol{B}'_{\mathrm{E}} \\ \Sigma_{\mathrm{DZB}} &= \Lambda_{\mathrm{DZB}}\boldsymbol{B}_{\mathrm{G}}\Psi_{\mathrm{G}}\boldsymbol{B}'_{\mathrm{G}}\Lambda'_{\mathrm{DZB}} + \boldsymbol{B}_{\mathrm{E}}\Psi_{\mathrm{E}}\boldsymbol{B}'_{\mathrm{E}} \\ \Sigma_{\mathrm{DZW}} &= \Lambda_{\mathrm{DZW}}\boldsymbol{B}_{\mathrm{G}}\Psi_{\mathrm{G}}\boldsymbol{B}'_{\mathrm{G}}\Lambda'_{\mathrm{DZW}} + \boldsymbol{B}_{\mathrm{E}}\Psi_{\mathrm{E}}\boldsymbol{B}'_{\mathrm{E}} \end{aligned}\right\} \quad (4)$$

In these expressions, $\boldsymbol{B}_{\mathrm{G}} = (\boldsymbol{I} - \boldsymbol{B}^{*}_{\mathrm{G}})^{-1}$, where $\boldsymbol{I}$ denotes the $(T \times T)$ unity matrix. The general structure of the above expectations is firmly based on the genetical foundation underlying the biometric model of continuous variation (Mather & Jinks, 1977). In particular, the $(T \times T)$ matrices Λ_{MZB}, Λ_{DZB} and Λ_{DZW} are diagonal matrices with fixed loadings derived from the biometrical model: $\sqrt{2}$ for Λ_{MZB}, $\sqrt{1.5}$ for Λ_{DZB}, and $\sqrt{0.5}$ for Λ_{DZW}. In view of the absence of genetic influences within MZ twins, Λ_{MZW} is a zero matrix.

The four matrix equations given in (4) are fitted to the associated estimates of the matrices of mean cross-products using a four-group LISREL design with parameters to be estimated invariant across groups (for further details, see Boomsma & Molenaar, 1987*a*). In addition to the estimates of all the parameters in Ψ_{G}, $\boldsymbol{B}^{*}_{\mathrm{G}}$, Ψ_{E} and $\boldsymbol{B}^{*}_{\mathrm{E}}$, the standard LISREL solution also gives the matrices of genetic and environmental correlations between time points. Moreover, LISREL supplies the so-called factor scores regression matrix which can be used to estimate the latent $G(t)$ and $E(t)$ time series for each individual subject. In the next section we will discuss a simulation study of the validity of individual $G(t)$ and $E(t)$ trajectories thus obtained.

A SIMULATION STUDY OF INDIVIDUAL GENETIC PROFILES

In order to study the validity and reliability of estimates of the $G(t)$ and $E(t)$ time series for individual subjects, the genetic simplex model will be applied to four sets of simulated data. Each of the factor scores regression matrices thus obtained will be applied to the corresponding data set and the estimated individual $G(t)$ and $E(t)$ trajectories will then be compared with the associated 'true' trajectories used in the simulation. Each longitudinal data set comprises univariate phenotypic observations at $T = 10$ time points for $N = 100$ MZ twin pairs and $N = 100$ DZ twin pairs. At each time point the variance of $G(t)$ as well as that of $E(t)$ was fixed at $\text{var}[G(t)] = \text{var}[E(t)] = 100$, whence the heritability at each point equals $h^2(t) = 0.5$, $t = 1, \ldots, T$. The four data sets are further characterized as follows:

1. $\beta_G(t) = 0$ and $\beta_E(t) = 0$; consequently, the phenotypic series $P(t)$ lacks autocorrelation.
2. $\beta_G(t) = 0.8$ and $\beta_E(t) = 0$; the genetic series $G(t)$ is autocorrelated, whereas $E(t)$ is not autocorrelated.
3. $\beta_G(t) = 0$ and $\beta_E(t) = 0.8$; $G(t)$ is not autocorrelated whereas $E(t)$ is autocorrelated.
4. $\beta_G(t) = 0.8$ and $\beta_E(t) = 0.8$; both $G(t)$ and $E(t)$ are autocorrelated.

A detailed description of the simulation algorithm is given in Molenaar & Boomsma (1987*b*).

The fit of the genetic simplex model to each of the longitudinal data sets is good: chi-squared goodness-of-fit is 190.37 ($p = 0.320$) for data set 1, 171.07 ($p = 0.709$) for data set 2, 187.70 ($p = 0.370$) for data set 3, and 182.41 ($p = 0.477$) for data set 4 (d.f. = 182 in each case). As the combination of an autocorrelated series and an uncorrelated series yields a phenotypic series that has an intricate pattern of autocorrelation (cf. Granger & Morris, 1976), and because this particular combination has been the subject of many theoretical approaches in mathematical signal analysis, we will present more detailed results for data set 2. Table 12.1(a) shows the estimates of $\beta_G(t)$, $\beta_E(t)$, $\Psi_G(t, t)$ and $\Psi_E(t, t)$ for each time point t. Notice that the true values are: $\beta_G(t) = 0.8$, $\beta_E(t) = 0$, $\Psi_G(1, 1) = 100$ at $t = 1$, $\Psi_G(t, t) = 36$ for $t > 1$, and $\Psi_E(t, t) = 100$ for each t. The associated standard errors are, on the average 0.117 for $\beta_G(t)$, 0.72 for $\beta_E(t)$, 12.143 for $\Psi_G(t, t)$ and 11.925 for $\Psi_E(t, t)$.

Using the factor scores regression matrices for data set 2, the $G(t)$ and $E(t)$ time series for each of the 400 individuals subjects in this sample can be estimated and compared with the true individual series used in the simulation. We can now answer several important questions. Firstly, what is the reliability of the estimates of individual $G(t)$ and $E(t)$ series? The answer can be obtained from Table 12.1(b) which shows the standard errors of the estimated $G(t)$ and $E(t)$ series for MZ and DZ twins. Remember that the variance of the true $G(t)$ and $E(t)$ scores is: $\text{var}[G(t)] = \text{var}[E(t)] = 100$. As the standard error of estimated $G(t)$ scores of MZ twins at each time point is about 5, this implies that $G(t)$ scores which differ by at least 1 standard deviation in the original metric can be reliably distinguished at usual significance levels. Similar remarks apply to the reliability of the $E(t)$ scores of the MZ twins as well as the scores of DZ twins (the standard errors with the DZ twins are only slightly larger). Secondly, we can answer the question whether estimated $G(t)$ and $E(t)$ scores are valid indicators of the associated true scores. The answer can be obtained from Table 12.1(c) which shows for each time point t the correlation between estimated and true $G(t)$ scores as well as $E(t)$ scores for both MZ and DZ twins. It turns out that these correlations all lie in the neighbourhood of 0.8 and therefore estimated scores can be considered to yield valid indications of the corresponding true scores at each time point. Thirdly, we can answer the question whether the dynamic structure of the true $G(t)$ and $E(t)$ series is faithfully reflected by the estimated individual trajectories. The answer to this question can be obtained from Table 12.1(d) which shows the autocorrelation between times 1 and 2, times 2 and 3, etc., of the estimated individual $G(t)$ and $E(t)$ trajectories of MZ and DZ twins. The true autocorrelation between these pairs of neighboring time points is 0.8 for the $G(t)$ series and 0 for the $E(t)$ series. Table 12.1(d) shows that this dynamic structure is indeed recovered by the estimated individual trajectories. Finally, we would like to know the cross-correlation between estimated $G(t)$ and $E(t)$ scores. According to the genetic simplex model this cross-correlation is expected to be zero. On the other hand, however, each *uni*variate $P(t)$ series is decomposed into two trajectories: an estimated $G(t)$ and $E(t)$ series. Consequently, the effective cross-correlation between the latter series will deviate from zero. Indeed, it is found that the cross-correlation between estimated $G(t)$ and $E(t)$ series, averaged over 10 time points, is 0.35 for MZ twins and 0.58 for DZ twins.

In conclusion, the results of our simulation study show that on the basis of the genetic simplex model for univariate phenotypic time series, the latent genetic and environmental series of each individual subject can be reliably and validly estimated. The detailed results for data sets 1, 3 and 4 are similar to the results presented above for data set 2. The genetic simplex model has been fitted by means of the LISREL program, which also yields the factor scores regression matrices used in the estimation of the individual genetic and environmental trajectories. Hence, the proposed approach can be readily implemented for the kinds of longitudinal research purposes alluded to earlier.

BEHAVIOR GENETIC SIMPLEX WITH STRUCTURED MEANS

So far the focus has been on detecting the genetic and environmental influences on the stability and change of inter-individual differences during development. The role of genetic and environmental influences on the species-specific function or average growth curve does not

Table 12.1. *Results with data set 2*

(a) *Parameter estimates*

t(ime):	1	2	3	4	5	6	7	8	9	10
$\beta_g(t)$		0.799	0.879	0.778	0.843	0.784	0.839	0.879	0.771	0.727
$\beta_E(t)$		0.040	0.034	0.079	0.079	0.096	0.157	0.090	−0.104	0.090
$\Psi_G(t,t)$	99.89	33.22	40.16	33.72	25.59	30.36	53.83	31.12	17.74	31.52
$\Psi_E(t,t)$	102.0	86.28	104.42	98.89	95.76	113.1	92.4	114.1	107.3	106.9

(b) *Standard errors of estimated $G(t)$ and $E(t)$*

t(ime):	1	2	3	4	5	6	7	8	9	10
MZ	5.81	4.96	5.30	5.09	4.88	5.09	5.48	5.39	4.48	4.92
DZ	6.86	5.98	6.32	6.02	5.77	5.91	6.53	6.42	5.31	5.64

(c) *MZ and DZ correlations true-estimated*

t(ime):	1	2	3	4	5	6	7	8	9	10
MZ										
$G(t)$	0.783	0.879	0.851	0.847	0.868	0.858	0.848	0.832	0.815	0.822
$E(t)$	0.783	0.826	0.852	0.837	0.831	0.857	0.838	0.835	0.854	0.798
DZ										
$G(t)$	0.759	0.813	0.832	0.813	0.834	0.780	0.807	0.813	0.789	0.776
$E(t)$	0.734	0.747	0.809	0.793	0.780	0.777	0.806	0.835	0.753	0.781

(d) *Recovered lag 1 autocorrelations of $G(t)$ and $E(t)$*

lag:	$t1-t2$	$t2-t3$	$t3-t4$	$t4-t5$	$t5-t6$	$t6-t7$	$t7-t8$	$t8-t9$	$t9-t10$
MZ twins									
$G(t)$	0.763	0.788	0.828	0.858	0.845	0.730	0.855	0.894	0.831
$E(t)$	−0.021	0.002	0.088	0.051	0.131	0.176	0.153	−0.140	0.073
DZ twins									
$G(t)$	0.755	0.788	0.832	0.864	0.859	0.729	0.838	0.886	0.835
$E(t)$	0.089	−0.013	0.056	0.116	0.048	0.206	0.039	−0.109	0.119

usually feature in behavior genetic studies of development (see McArdle, 1986, for one attempt to analyze such influences by means of a common-factor model). These two aspects of longitudinal data, however, are complementary and not necessarily independent in understanding development (McCall, 1981). Indeed, Thomas (1980) has noted strikingly large (usually positive) correlations between repeatedly measured means and standard deviations indicating that changes in one are usually accompanied by similar changes in the other. These correlations, which are observed for a variety of physical and psychological variables, encourage the idea that means and variances may in some fashion be related.

In the present section an extension of the genetic simplex model is presented to analyze phenotypic means and covariance structure simultaneously within the context of developmental behavior genetics. The extended simplex is suggested as a way to examine the relationship between means and covariance structure by modeling these with a common set of parameters. This implies that the objective of the simultaneous analysis of means and covariance structure is to test the hypothesis that they can be attributed to a common underlying process. The extension of the double simplex can be detailed briefly as follows: let $E[P(t)]$ denote the expectation of the phenotypic mean at occasion t ($t = 1$ to T) which is, as a basic assumption of the twin method, assumed to be identical for MZ and DZ twins (Mather & Jinks, 1977). $E[P(t)]$ at occasion t is the sum of the latent genetic and environmental means:

$$E[P(t)] = E[G(t)] + E[E(t)], \quad (t = 1 \text{ to } T). \tag{5}$$

The latent means at each occasion t ($t \neq 1$) are in part attributable to the immediately preceding occasion $t-1$ and in part independent thereof:

$$E[G(t)] = \beta_G(t)E[G(t-1)] + G_\Delta \quad (t = 2 \text{ to } T) \tag{6}$$

$$E[E(t)] = \beta_E(t)E[E(t-1)] + E_\Delta \quad (t = 2 \text{ to } T). \tag{7}$$

The autoregressive coefficients $\beta_G(t)$ and $\beta_E(t)$ now account for both the stability of individual differences and the continuity in the mean. The terms G_Δ and E_Δ represent a time-invariant (hence unsubscripted) independent input at each occasion analogous to random innovation terms ζ (see equations (2) and (3)). The latent means ($E[G(1)]$, $E[E(1)]$) are estimated independently at the start of the time series. The addition of structured means does not alter the simplex model for the covariance structure. However, this extension may result in a rejection of the model whenever the continuity in the mean and the stability of individual differences can not both be explained by the common set of autoregressive coefficients.

It can be shown (cf. Dolan, Molenaar & Boomsma, submitted) that the identification of the parameters associated with the mean trend, $E[G(1)]$, $E[E(1)]$, G_Δ and E_Δ, requires longitudinal data for at least at $T = 5$ time points. That is, T must be greater than the number of parameters associated with the means.

Specification as a LISREL VI model

In specifying the extended simplex model as a LISREL model the following has to be taken into account. Firstly we require a method to estimate factor means. Usually this is accomplished by introducing a unit variable and a dummy factor. The parameters of the latent means are then estimated by regressing the latent factors on this dummy factor. As can be seen in Figure 12.1, the unit variable loads on the dummy factor with a fixed loading equal to 1.0 so that the dummy factor ξ, has a mean equal to 1.0. The latent means at the first occasion and the subsequent means innovations are estimated by regressing the first latent variables $G(1)$ and $E(1)$ and the subsequent $G(t)$ and $E(t)$ on the dummy factor.

Secondly, the data have to be summarized in a fashion that retains the phenotypic means. Generally simultaneous structural equation modeling of means and covariance structure is carried out over the so-called augmented (AM) moment matrix, i.e. the matrix of the uncentered moments when a variable equaling one for every sample unit has been added as the last variable (see Jöreskog & Sörbom, 1986). The addition of the phenotypic means to the cross-product matrices is done as follows. Let $S_B(T \times T)$ represent the between cross-product matrix and let $\boldsymbol{m}(T \times 1)$ be the vector of phenotypic means. Then the augmented matrix, $S_{AM}(T+1, T+1)$, is:

$$S_{AM} = \begin{bmatrix} (S_B + \boldsymbol{mm}') & \boldsymbol{m} \\ \boldsymbol{m}' & 1.0 \end{bmatrix}$$

where 1.0 is the variance of the unit variable which will be specified to load with a fixed loading of 1.0 on the dummy factor. Although there are two (between and within) input matrices for MZ and DZ twins, it is sufficient to add the means to just one matrix associated with each zygosity. As the factor loadings of the phenotypic variables on the genetic series are zero in the MZ within-matrix, the means are added to the between-matrices.

A complicating aspect of the genetic simplex in the present context is the presence of the fixed genetic weights in the matrices of factor loadings (see equation (4)). Because these weights are different for each group, it is necessary to introduce a second dummy factor to compensate for the effect of these weights on the estimation of the genetic mean trend. Figure 12.1 shows how the presence of the genetic weights (w) as fixed loadings would weight the contributions of G_Δ at each occasion. As these weights differ across groups it is not possible to constrain the estimates of the latent mean parameters across groups in accordance with the assumption of equal MZ and DZ means. The second dummy factor, denoted D in Figure 12.1, allows one to weigh the latent means parameters with the inverse of the genetic weight in each group, thus canceling out the effect of the genetic weights.

The phenotypic mean at the first occasion is then modeled as:

$$E[P(1)] = wE[G(1)] + E[E(1)], \tag{8}$$

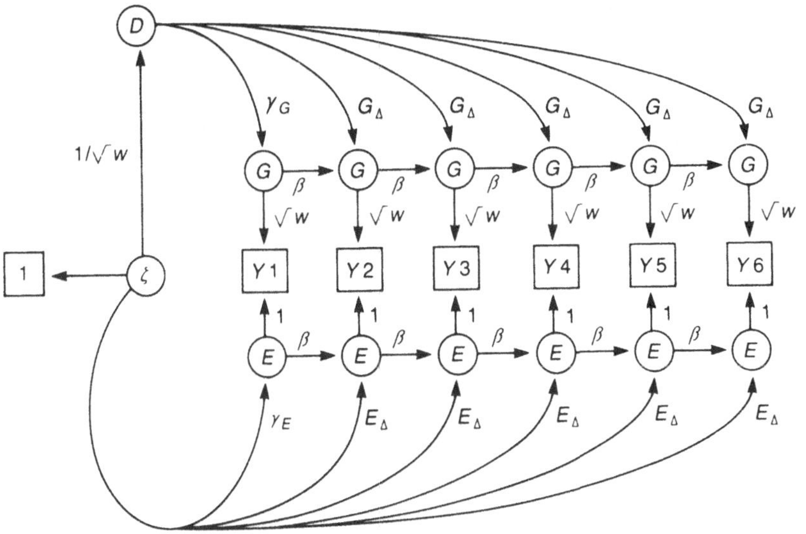

Figure 12.1. The genetic simplex with structured means. γ_G is the estimate of $E[G(1)]$. γ_E is the estimate of $E[E(1)]$. G_Δ and E_Δ are the time invariant means innovations terms.

where

$$E[G(1)] = \gamma_G(1/w) \tag{9}$$

and

$$E[E(1)] = \gamma_E. \tag{10}$$

The subsequent phenotypic means are modeled as:

$$E[P(t)] = wE[G(t)] + E[E(t)] \quad (t = 2 \text{ to } T), \tag{11}$$

where

$$E[G(t)] = (\beta_G(t)E[G(t-1)] + G_\Delta)(1/w) \tag{12}$$

and

$$E[E(t)] = \beta_E(t)E[E(t-1)] + E_\Delta. \tag{13}$$

The terms G_Δ and E_Δ are the fixed innovation terms.

Illustration

The extended double simplex model will be demonstrated with simulated data. To this end $T = 6$ repeated measures were simulated for 100 MZ and 100 DZ twin pairs according to the model described above with an additive genetic and a (specific or non-shared) environmental series.

Table 12.2. *Analysis of cross-product structure with structured means*

	t:2	3	4	5	6
True	0.9	0.8	0.5	0.4	0.3
Est.	0.920(0.038)	0.810(0.054)	0.403(0.073)	0.275(0.087)	0.261(0.092)
$\beta_G(t)$					
True	0.5	0.5	0.5	0.5	0.5
Est.	0.550(0.082)	0.552(0.071)	0.696(0.095)	0.634(0.078)	0.584(0.058)
	$E[G(1)]$	G_Δ	$E[E(1)]$	E_Δ	
True	25	21	35	12	
Est.	22.89(10.5)	19.99(5.2)	36.08(10.6)	10.82(7.3)	
$\chi^2(71) = 79.25(p = 0.23)$					

The true parameter values pertaining to the means structure are given in Table 12.2. The simultaneous analysis of means and covariance structure yielded a chi-square value of 79.25 (d.f. = 71, $p = 0.21$). The parameter estimates and standard errors are given in Table 12.2. It can be seen that the latent means at the first occasion and the fixed means innovation terms are correctly recovered.

Using the factor scores regression matrices associated with the augmented moment matrices for MZ and DZ twins, it is possible to estimate the individual $G(t)$ and $E(t)$ trajectories. Notice that, for example, the estimated $G(t)$ trajectory for each single subject consists of a stochastic (autocorrelated) series, specific to this subject, superimposed on the genetic mean trend common to all subjects. Hence it is possible to estimate the mean genetic and environmental trends by averaging the respective individual trajectories of all twins. Figure 12.2 shows the true and estimated mean genetic and environmental trends thus obtained. It can be seen that the estimated mean trends closely correspond to the true trends used in the simulation.

To demonstrate briefly the discriminatory ability of the model with regard to the relationship between the means and cross-product structure, the analysis was repeated after a constant of 10 had been alternately added to and subtracted from phenotypic means at successive time points. The chi-square value increased considerably to 112.29 which is, given 71 degrees of freedom, significant ($p < 0.01$). This result indicates that the extended simplex model adequately discriminates between means structures which can and cannot be explained by the same parameters as the cross-product structure.

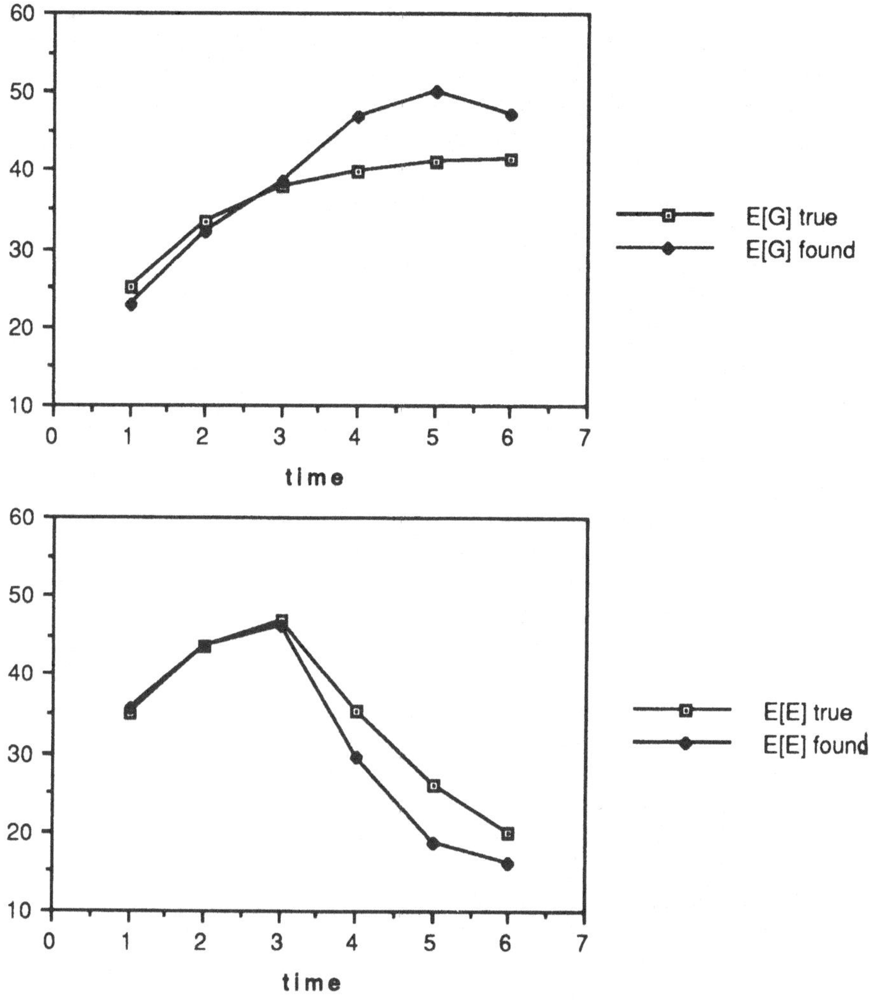

Figure 12.2. Top: the true and estimated mean trend of the genetic series. Bottom: the true and estimated mean trend of the environmental series.

AN APPLICATION TO REAL DATA

In this section we will present some results of an application of the genetic simplex model, including the extensions described earlier, to part of a longitudinal data set provided by Dr Siv Fischbein of the Stockholm Institute of Education. The analysis of the complete data set, involving longitudinal measurements of height and weight of MZ and DZ twins of both sexes at 13 equidistant time points covering seven years, will be presented elsewhere (Fischbein, Dolan, Molenaar &

Boomsma, in preparation). Here, we will restrict attention to the weight data of girls only, at $T = 6$ time points covering three years. At $t = 1$, the mean age of the girls is 11.5 years; at $t = 6$ the mean age is 14 years (standard deviation (s.d.) = 0.37). The means and variances of weight at each time point for MZ (32 pairs) and DZ (100 pairs) twins are presented in Table 12.3(a). Formal tests of the equality of variances between MZ and DZ groups at each time point are not significant at alpha = 0.01.

Firstly, the genetic simplex model is fitted to the matrices of mean cross-products (see equation (4)), thus discarding information concerning the phenotypic mean trend. It turns out that the model fits well (chi-square = 65.97, d.f. = 62, $p = 0.34$). The parameter estimates in this model, presented in Table 12.3(b), indicate the presence of an invariantly high transmission of genetic and environmental information between consecutive time points: all estimates of the autoregressive coefficients lie in the neighbourhood of 1.0. Furthermore, the estimates of the variances of genetic and environmental innovations (reflecting the inception of the effects of new genes or influences) all differ significantly from zero and do not show a decreasing trend with time. Taken together, the parameter estimates in Table 12.3 imply that (a) the stability of intraindividual differences in weight is height, (b) the variance of the genetic series is a nonstationary, almost linearly increasing function of time, (c) the variance of the environmental series shows the same nonstationary pattern as the genetic series, but is much smaller, hence (d) the heritability is high and almost constant across time points. Interestingly, both the $G(t)$ and the $E(t)$ series have the characteristic of Brownian motion, a well-known physical process (cf. Cox & Miller, 1965) that could be employed to interpret further the dynamic influences at hand.

To illustrate the estimation of individual latent trajectories in the genetic simplex model, we selected a single MZ twin pair and estimated the $G(t)$ and $E(t)$ series for each member of this pair by means of the factor scores regression matrix. The obtained trajectories, together with the associated phenotypic series of each girl, are shown in Figure 12.3. It can be seen that for one girl the environmental influences have an augmenting effect that decreases with time, whereas for the other girl the environmental influences have a suppressing effect that also decreases with time.

Secondly, the extended genetic simplex is fitted to the augmented moment matrices, thus including information concerning the phenotypic mean trend. The parameter estimates thus obtained for the structured means model are presented in Table 12.4. Estimates of $\beta_G(t)$, $\beta_E(t)$, var[$\zeta_G(t)$] and var[$\zeta_E(t)$] are almost equal to those presented in Table 12.3. If the complete structured means model is fitted, including

Table 12.3(a). *Means and variances of the monozygotic and dizygotic twin samples*

t	1	2	3	4	5	6
Mean of age (in years) at time of measurement (s.d. = 0.37)						
	11.5	12.0	12.5	13	13.5	14
Covariance matrix DZ twins (N of pairs = 50)						
	24.27					
	24.68	26.61				
	26.25	28.13	32.96			
	26.17	28.20	32.17	34.03		
	26.17	28.18	32.55	33.69	36.13	
	25.93	27.62	31.98	33.25	35.42	37.52
Mean:	35.4	37.6	40.3	42.6	45.2	47.4
Covariance matriz MZ twins (N of pairs = 32)						
	36.77					
	38.80	42.74				
	39.58	43.16	46.52			
	40.32	44.30	48.38	52.42		
	40.75	44.78	48.78	53.12	56.14	
	40.09	43.63	46.99	50.81	53.77	54.35
Mean:	36.4	38.7	41.4	43.7	46.0	48.1

Table 12.3(b). *Results with mean cross-products of weight data (standard errors in parentheses)*

t:	2	3	4	5	6	
Autoregressive coefficients						
$\beta_G(t)$	1.05(0.027)	1.04(0.033)	1.02(0.028)	1.02(0.027)	0.99(0.027)	
$\beta_E(t)$	0.91(0.053)	1.05(0.090)	0.82(0.074)	0.82(0.073)	0.99(0.090)	
Variances of $G(1)$ and $E(1)$ and of innovations at $t > 1$						
var[$G(1)$]	23.41(3.46)					
var[$E(1)$]	3.44(0.82)					
var[$\zeta_G(t)$]	1.33(0.23)	2.27(0.44)	1.36(0.35)	1.80(0.37)	1.97(0.41)	
var[$\zeta_E(t)$]	0.33(0.08)	0.93(0.22)	0.93(0.21)	0.72(0.17)	0.93(0.22)	
Overall goodness-of-fit						
$\chi^2(62) = 65.97$ ($p = 0.341$)						
Derived statistics at each time						
var[$G(t)$]	23.41	27.59	32.12	35.04	38.26	38.49
var[$E(t)$]	3.44	3.20	4.48	4.01	3.43	4.30
$h^2(t)$	0.87	0.89	0.87	0.89	0.91	0.89

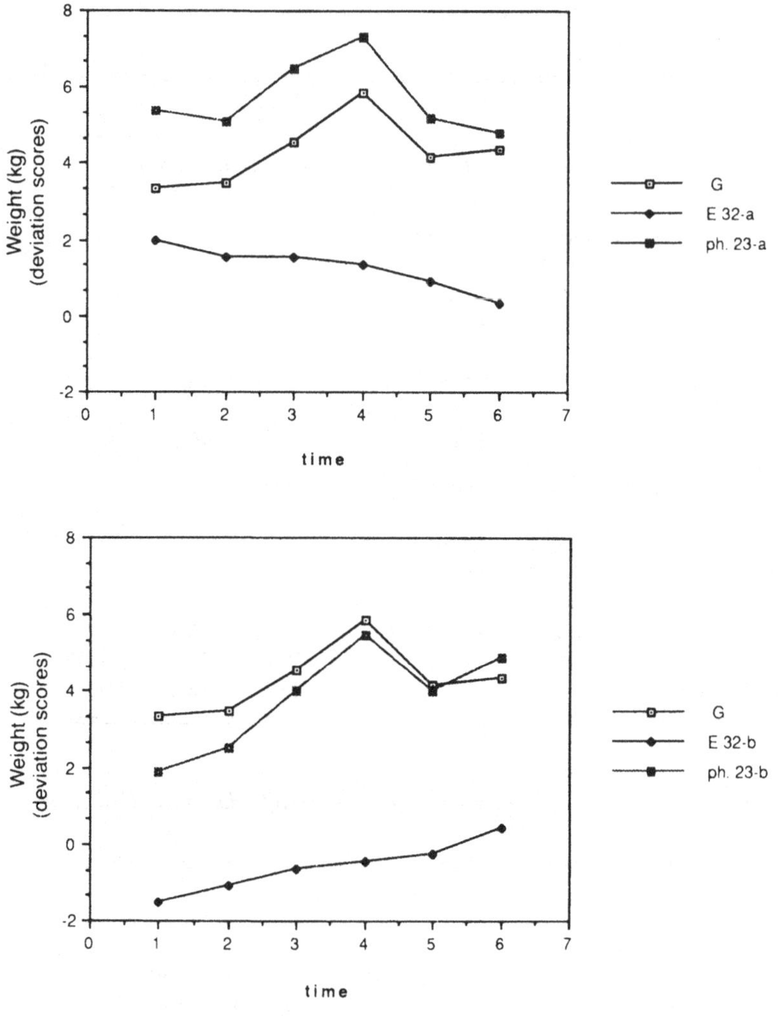

Figure 12.3. Individual phenotypic, genetic and environmental series of two monozygotic twins obtained with mean cross-products.

the parameters $E[G(1)]$, G_Δ, $E[E(1)]$, E_Δ, then the fit of the genetic simplex model thus extended is good: chi-square = 67.33, d.f. = 71, $p = 0.63$. It turns out, however, that the estimate of E_Δ and $E[E(1)]$ are not significant and therefore a restricted model is fitted in which first E_Δ is fixed at zero. It then appears that the restricted model still fits well (chi-square = 69.65, d.f. = 72, $p = 0.56$), while the estimate of $E[E(1)]$ still does not differ significantly from zero. Consequently, a second restriction was introduced by fixing $E[E(1)]$ at zero. Again the fit of this

Table 12.4. *Results with augmented moments of weight data (standard errors in parentheses)*

Model 1 means estimated in E and G series	
$E[G(1)] = 25.84(7.48)$	$G_{\Delta} = 5.59\ (2.78)$
$E[E(1)] = 9.95(7.45)$	$E_{\Delta} = -4.064\ (2.71)$
Chi-square (71) = 67.33 ($p = 0.63$)	
Model 2 means estimated at E(1) and in G series	
$E[G(1)] = 32.34\ (6.23)$	$G_{\Delta} = 1.68(0.77)$
$E[E(1)] = 3.45\ (6.19)$	$E_{\Delta} = 0.0(0.0)$
Chi-square (72) = 69.65 ($p = 0.56$)	
Model 3 means estimated in G series	
$E[G(1)] = 35.76\ (1.07)$	$G_{\Delta} = 1.34\ (0.507)$
Chi-square (73) = 69.79 ($p = 0.59$)	

model is good: chi-square = 69.79, d.f. = 73, $p = 0.59$. In sum, these results suggest that in the present sample of Swedish twins (a) both the stability and the change of the interindividual and intraindividual differences in weight as well as the average growth curve can be explained by the same simplex model involving genetic and non-shared environmental influences, while (b) the average growth curve appears to be solely under genetic control.

Using the factor scores regression matrix, we estimated the individual $G(t)$ and $E(t)$ trajectories. As was pointed out earlier, it is then possible to estimate the mean genetic trend by averaging the individual genetic trajectories of all twins. Figure 12.4 shows the estimated mean genetic

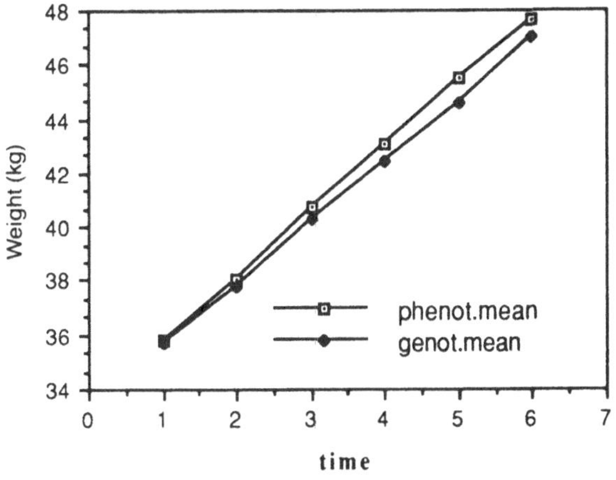

Figure 12.4. Phenotypic and estimated genetic mean trends.

trend thus obtained, together with the phenotypic mean trend. This figure reinforces our conclusion that the average phenotypic growth curve appears to be solely under genetic control.

To illustrate further the estimation of individual latent trajectories in the extended simplex model under consideration, we selected the same MZ twin pair for which the results were shown in Figure 12.3 and again estimated the $G(t)$ and $E(t)$ series for each member of this pair. Figure 12.5 shows the effect of including information concerning the

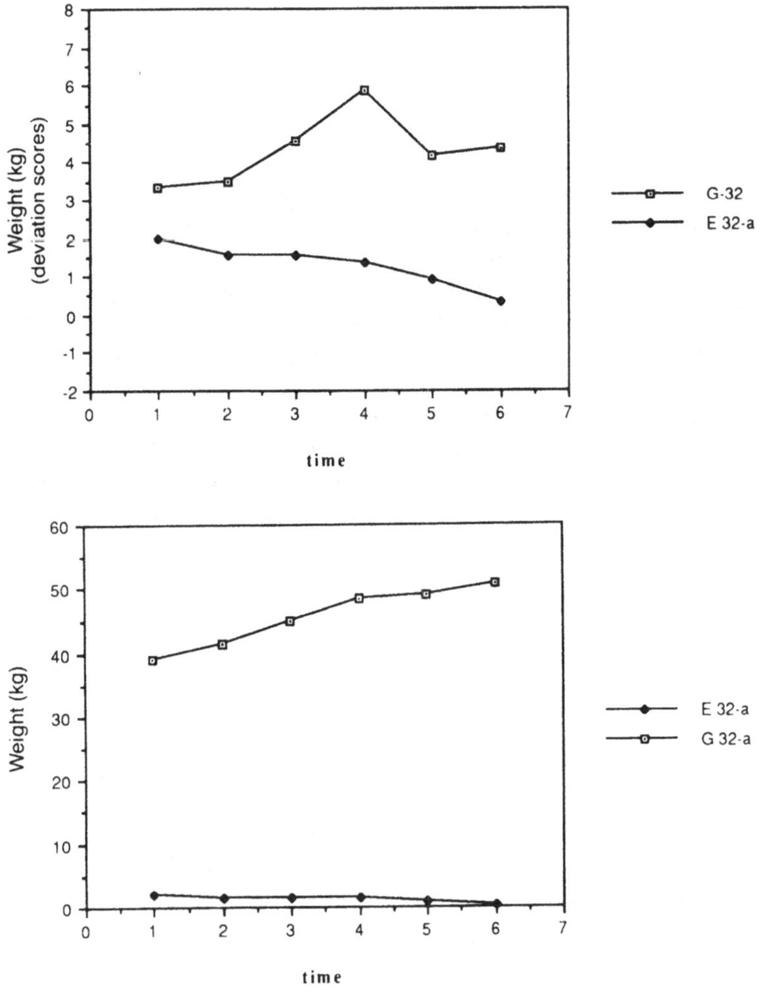

Figure 12.5. Individual genetic and environmental series of one monozygotic twin obtained with mean cross-products and augmented moments.

phenotypic mean trend on these estimates. The first graph of Figure 12.5 is a replica of the $G(t)$ and $E(t)$ series of one of the girls already shown in Figure 12.3, i.e., as determined on the basis of the covariance structure. The second graph depicts the estimated $G(t)$ and $E(t)$ series of this same girl, now determined on the basis of both the phenotypic mean trend as well as the covariance structure. Clearly, the raw longitudinal weight series of this girl appears to be almost completely due to genetic influences; a conclusion that might be missed if information concerning mean trends is not considered. Of course, this conclusion can only be drawn because both interindividual and intraindividual variation as well as mean growth can be explained by the same genetic simplex model.

DISCUSSION AND CONCLUSION

The genetic simplex model for longitudinal phenotypic data can be generalized in a number of ways. Firstly, the order of the autoregression describing $G(t)$ and/or $E(t)$ may be increased, for instance to accommodate the presence of time-dependent oscillations. Secondly, the random innovations $\zeta_G(t)$ and/or $\zeta_E(t)$ can be taken to be autocorrelated, thus leading to a consideration of more involved latent process models of autoregressive-moving average type. Thirdly, the genetic time-series model given by equation (1) can be extended by the inclusion of a common environmental process which is shared by members of the same family. Fourthly, the simplex model can be generalized to enable the decomposition of a multivariate phenotypic series into common and specific genetic and environmental processes. In a way, however, these generalizations turn out to be straightforward extensions of the genetic simplex model discussed earlier.

There have been some criticisms of simplex modeling in the recent literature. Notwithstanding the fundamental critique of applying common-factor analysis techniques to autocorrelated matrices of longitudinal data (see Wohlwill, 1973: 270–272), it has been suggested that both simplex and common-factor models are equivalent models in case variances and means are included in the analysis or a confirmatory analysis is carried out. A definite refutation of such suggestions, however, can be given on the basis of the following mathematical–statistical result: the spectrum of a Toeplitz (autocorrelation) matrix is continuous, whereas a factor model presupposes a discrete or at least mixed spectrum (cf. Grenander & Szegö, 1958). This implies, among other things, that when the number T of time points increases, an increasing number of common factors is needed in order to describe the autocorrelation structure of a univariate simplex. Cronbach (1967) already showed that the common factors so obtained are spurious. Another criticism of simplex modeling has been raised by Rogosa &

Willett (1985), who showed by means of a simulation experiment that a simplex model may yield a satisfactory fit to a covariance structure associated with an entirely different (linear random coefficient) growth model. However, we repeated this simulation experiment and found that the results of Rogosa & Willett are related to a particular instance of the linear random coefficient growth model. Specifically, if the number of time points ($T = 5$ in the original simulation experiment) is slightly increased (e.g. $T > 6$) then the simplex model no longer fits the obtained covariance structure. A full discussion of these new results will be given in a separate publication. It is concluded that the mentioned criticisms of simplex modeling of longitudinal data do not appear to be serious. This conclusion is reinforced by the fact that autoregressive models such as those considered in this chapter occupy a very prominent place in the mathematical–statistical theory of time-dependent processes (Hannan & Deistler, 1988).

Whereas the genetic simplex model can be conceived as a parametric model, there now exist non-parametric approaches to the genetic analysis of stretches of time-dependent data of arbitrary length (Molenaar & Boomsma, 1987*b*,*c*). In these non-parametric approaches, each autocorrelated phenotypic series is transformed into a sequence of uncorrelated variables, either in the time domain (Karhunen–Loève transformation) or in the frequency domain (Fourier transformation), thus enabling the application of standard biometrical analysis techniques to each transformed variable separately. These approaches, called genetic signal analyses, can lead to interesting applications in, for example, psychophysiological studies.

The possibility of estimating the time course of $G(t)$ and $E(t)$ for each individual subject can also lead to interesting applications in genetic counseling and epidemiology. In particular, this enables one to determine the impact of genetic and environmental processes on specific subjects or on groups of subjects who suffer from deviant development. Estimation of individual $G(t)$ and $E(t)$ trajectories is also possible in genetic signal analysis. Of course, these possibilities may provide important information concerning the ways in which remedial treatment is to be carried out.

The inclusion of mean genetic and environmental trend functions in a single simplex process model for the analysis of phenotypic cross-products has important theoretical implications. It is now possible to test whether genetic processes underlying individual differences can also account for mean phenotypic growth within a particular population. A sufficient number of constraints has to be imposed on the structured means model to ensure its identifiability. Here we considered a constrained means model given by equations (6) and (7) which closely resembles a first-order autoregression. In contrast, we could have derived a means model from theoretical considerations concerning behavioral growth (Guire & Kowalski, 1979). In general, such theoretical growth models are nonlinear and can only be identified through the imposition of nonlinear constraints. A general LISREL model for the analysis of structural models with nonlinear constraints is presented in Boomsma & Molenaar (1987*b*).

In conclusion we have indicated the potential of genetic simplex models for the analysis of longitudinal data. It can be expected that regular application of this type of models will lead to significant progress in the field of developmental behavior genetics.

ACKNOWLEDGEMENTS

We wish to thank Professors P. B. Baltes, J. de Leeuw, and D. Magnusson, who provided valuable comments that led to this formulation. We also wish to thank Dr S. Fischbein for generously providing her longitudinal twin data.

REFERENCES

Baltes, P. B. & Nesselroade, J. R. (1973). The developmental analysis of individual differences on multiple measures. In J. R. Nesselroade & H. W. Reese (eds.), *Life-span developmental psychology: Methodological issues.* New York: Academic Press.

Boomsma, D. I. & Molenaar, P. C. M. (1987*a*). The genetic analysis of repeated measures. I. Simplex models. *Behavior Genetics, 17,* 111–123.

Boomsma, D. I. & Molenaar, P. C. M. (1987*b*). Constrained maximum likelihood analysis of familial resemblance of twins and their parents. *Acta Geneticae Medicae Gemellologicae, 36,* 29–39.

Boomsma, D. I., Molenaar, P. C. M. & Orlebeke, J. F. (in press). Estimation of individual genetic and environmental factor scores. *Genetic Epidemiology.*

Browne, M. W. & Shapiro, A. (1988). Robustness of normal theory methods in the analysis linear latent variable models. *British Journal of Mathematical and Statistical Psychology, 41,* 193–208.

Cox, D. R. & Miller, H. D. (1965). *The theory of stochastic processes.* London: Methuen.

Cronbach, L. J. (1967). Year-to-year correlations of mental tests: A review of the Hofstaetter analysis. *Child Development, 38,* 283–289.

DeFries, J. C. & Fulker, D. W. (1986). Multivariate behavioral genetics and development. *Behavior Genetics, 16,* 1–10.

Dolan, C. V., Molenaar, P. C. M. & Boomsma, D. I. (Submitted) Simultaneous genetic analyis of longitudinal means and covariance structure in the simplex model. *Behavior Genetics.*

Eaves, L. J. (1977). Inferring the causes of human variation. *Journal of the Royal Statistical Society A, 140,* 324–355.

Eaves, L. J. & Young, P. A. (1981). Genetical theory and personality differences. In R. Lynn (ed.), *Dimensions of personality*. Oxford: Pergamon Press.

Eaves, L. J., Hewitt, J. K. & Heath, A. C. (1988). The quantitative genetic study of human development change: A model and its limitations. In B. S. Weir, E. J. Eisen, M. M. Goodman & G. Namkoong (eds.), *Proceedings of the second international conference on quantitative genetics* (pp. 297–311). Sunderland, Mass: Sinauer Associates, Inc.

Fischbein, S., Dolan, C. V., Molenaar, P. C. M. & Boomsma, D. I. (in preparation) Analysis of repeatedly measured height and weight in a sample of Swedish twins.

Fulker, D. W. (1988). Genetic and cultural transmission in human behavior. In B. S. Weir, E. J. Eisen, M. M. Goodman & G. Namkoong (eds.), *Proceedings of the second international conference on quantitative genetics* (pp. 297–311). Sunderland, Mass.: Sinauer Associates, Inc.

Granger, C. W. J. & Morris, M. S. (1976). Time series modelling and interpretation. *Journal of the Royal Statistical Society A, 139*, (2), 246–257.

Grenander, U. & Szegö, G. (1958). *Toeplitz forms and their applications*. Berkeley: University of California Press.

Gourieroux, C., Monfort, A. & Trognon, A. (1984). Pseudo maximum likelihood methods: Theory. *Econometrica, 17*, 287–304.

Guire, K. E. & Kowalski, C. J. (1979). Mathematical description and representation of developmental change functions on the intra- and interindividual levels. In J. R. Nesselroade & P. B. Baltes (eds.). *Longitudinal research in the study of behavior and development*. New York: Academic Press.

Hannan, E. J. & Deistler, M. (1988). *The statistical theory of linear systems*. New York: Wiley.

Heath, A. C., Jardine, R., Eaves, L. J. & Martin, N. G. (1988). The genetic structure of personality I. Phenotypic factor structure of the EPQ in an Australian sample. *Personality and Individual Differences, 9*, 59–67.

Jöreskog, K. G. (1970). Estimation and testing of simplex models. *British Journal of Mathematical and Statistical Psychology, 26*, 121–145.

Jöreskog, K. G. & Sörbom, D. (1986). LISREL VI: Analysis of linear structural relationships by maximum likelihood, instrumental variables and least squares methods, University of Uppsala, Department of Statistics, PO Box 513, s-751 20 Uppsala, Sweden.

Mather, K. & Jinks, J. L. (1977). *Introduction to biometrical genetics*. London: Chapman and Hall.

McArdle, J. J. (1986). Latent-variable growth within behavior genetic models. *Behavior Genetics, 16*, 79–95.

McCall, R. B. (1981). Nature-nurture and the two realms of development: A proposed integration with respect to mental development. *Child Development, 5*, 1–12.

Mednick, S. A., Moffitt, T. E., Pollock, V., Talovic, S., Gabrielli, W. F. & van Dusen, K. T. (1983). The inheritance of human deviance. In D. Magnusson & V. L. Allen (eds.), *Human development: An interactional perspective*. New York: Academic Press.

Molenaar, P. C. M. & Boomsma, D. I. (1987*a*). Application of nonlinear factor analysis to genotype-environment interaction. *Behavior Genetics, 17*, 71–80.

Molenaar, P. C. M. & Boomsma, D. I. (1987*b*). The genetic analysis of repeated measures II. Karhunen–Loève transformation. *Behavior Genetics, 17,* 229–242.

Molenaar, P. C. M. & Boomsma, D. I. (1987*c*). Spectral analysis of twin time series designs. *Acta Geneticae Medicae Gemellologicae, 36,* 51–59.

Molenaar, P. C. M., Boomsma, D. I., Neeleman, D. & Dolan, C. (in press). Using factor scores to detect $G \times E$ interactive origin of 'pure' genetic or environmental factors obtained in genetic covariance structure analysis. *Genetic Epidemiology.*

Plomin, R. (1986). *Development, genetics and psychology.* Hillsdale, New Jersey: Lawrence Erlbaum Associates.

Plomin, R., DeFries, J. C. & Fulker, D. W. (1988). *Nature and nurture during infancy and early childhood.* Cambridge University Press.

Rogosa, D. & Willett, J. B. (1985). Satisfying a simplex structure is simpler than it should be. *Journal of Educational Statistics, 10* (2), 99–107.

Thomas, H. (1980). A theory of growth. In R. H. Kluwe & H. Spada (eds.) *Developmental models of thinking.* New York: Academic Press.

Wohlwill, J. F. (1973). *The study of behavioral development.* New York: Academic Press.

13 Structural equation models for studying intellectual development

GEORG RUDINGER, JOHANNES ANDRES AND CHRISTIAN RIETZ

INTRODUCTION

In this chapter we investigate in turn the following issues.

1. We test systematically hypotheses concerning the conceptual differentiation of reliability of intelligence measures and stability of intelligence constructs as a feature of the developmental process itself.
2. We test hypotheses about longitudinal changes in structure of the intelligence constructs over time indicated by sets of observables. This is of general interest in intelligence longitudinal research, particulary concerning the differentiation/reintegration hypothesis of intelligence.

We study both problems with intelligence data from the Bonn Longitudinal Study of Aging (BOLSA).

The Bonn Longitudinal Study of Aging (BOLSA) was started in 1965 with a sample of 222 women and men born in 1890–5/1900–5. The younger cohort (1900–5) consisted of 114 persons and the older one (1890–5) of 108. Of the 114 younger subjects, 55 were women and 59 men and in the older cohort there were 49 women and 59 men. Each measurement period took five days; during this period three semi-structured interviews were administered, each of which focused on different sections of our subjects' lives. Furthermore, subjects underwent a series of *intelligence tests* (WAIS/HAWIE, Raven test), psychomotoric, and personality tests, and were examined by a specialist for internal medicine.

As an inevitable fact in every gerontological longitudinal study the sample is subject to attrition. In BOLSA this attrition process reduced the sample from the first to the eighth measurement point in the following way: first measurement in 1965/66 ($N = 222$), second in 1966/67 ($N = 202$), third in 1967/68 ($N = 184$), fourth in 1969/70 ($N = 146$), fifth in 1972/73 ($N = 121$), sixth in 1976/77 ($N = 81$), seventh in 1980/81 ($N = 48$), eighth in 1983/84 ($N = 34$; 25 women, 9 men). Attrition was due to death or poor health in about 95% of the cases. In the following analyses we refer in the first main section to the longitudinal sample available at the fifth measurement (1972/73, $N = 121$), and in the second main section to the longitudinal sample at the sixth measurement (1976/77, $N = 81$).

STABILITY OF INTELLECTUAL DEVELOPMENT AND RELIABILITY OF ASSESSMENT

Theory and data

Stability has proved to be a central concept in the description of development. According to Buss (1979), the multivariate developmental situation can mean stability or differences either between or within subjects over time. An excellent discussion for the various meanings of stability can be found in Wohlwill (1973). The numerous attempts to establish '*developmental functions*' and *growth curves*, especially in the area of cognitive functions, make clear the dominance of this concept (stability as regularity and predictability).

The measurement of intraindividual change over time is a critical aspect of determining the nature and determinants of development. Developmental psychologists are very often interested in determining the stability of interindividual differences over time or, more precisely, in determining the consistency of interindividual differences in intraindividual change. This type of stability implies high correlations of the same variable across occasions. High correlation of an observed variable with itself over time is considered indicative of high stability, i.e., preservation of individual differences and constancy of the relative position across time within the sample. Instability in individual differences, however, will reduce the correlation of a variable (with itself) at a later longitudinal occasion. Thus, given a low or medium test–retest correlation for a single observed variable, it is not known whether this correlation is a function of a high proportion of measurement error (unreliability), low stability of interindividual differences over time, or both. Thus, our general *theoretical* interest aims at the measurement of a developmental construct, such as crystallized intelligence, on the one hand (measurement model), and at the stability of this *theoretical* construct as a relevant feature of the developmental process on the other hand (structural model). Additionally we are interested in the *variances* of the latent constructs. The variances indicate whether the interindividual differences increase over time (e.g. fan spread trajectories), or decrease, or remain stable (see Rogosa, Brandt & Zimowski, 1982). Consequently, the analyses have to turn to the covariance matrix (see the top right part, above the diagonal, of Table 13.1).

Table 13.1. *Four successive intelligence tests in a gerontological study (BOLSA): diagonal, variances; above diagonal, covariances; below diagonal, correlations*

	1965 y_1	1967 y_2	1969 y_3	1972 y_4
1965:y_1	**4.861**	3.093	3.807	3.195
1967:y_2	0.659	**4.537**	3.564	3.154
1969:y_3	0.629	0.643	**6.765**	4.285
1972:y_4	0.564	0.577	0.642	**6.592**

Conceptual issues

Stability and the simplex property. Suppose we measured a particular behavior (intelligence) across several occasions. We have several individuals observed on several occasions with regard to one variable. We then proceed to calculate correlation coefficients between each and every occasion. These coefficients may be summarized in a correlation matrix in which the rows and columns represent occasions (see bottom left part, below the diagonal, of Table 13.1). In the matrix of 'stability coefficients' (such as the bottom left of Table 13.1) we often discover that two occasions which are closer in time have higher correlations than occasions which are further apart in time: the correlation coefficients between the first measurement (1965) and that of the second (1967) is 0.659 while it drops to 0.629, between the first and third (1969), and finally to 0.564 between the first and the fourth (1972) measurement. At a descriptive level, this property in essence represents a simple ordering scheme. Suppose we had observations i, j, k, where i is closer in time to j than to k. Then, we may state for the general case:

$$r_{ij} \text{ is greater than } r_{ik}, \text{ where } |j-i| \text{ is smaller than } |k-i|; \quad j>i,\ k>j.$$

In longitudinal methodology this *simplex property* has led to severe problems in statistical analysis. Guttman (1954, 1955) pointed out that this multioccasion matrix in its raw form should not be used in a classical factor analysis. A classic example of the misunderstandings derived from the factor analysis of a correlation matrix containing the simplex structure is provided in an analysis with Cattell's T-technique carried out by Hofstätter (1954) and subsequenly criticized by Cronbach (1967). Roskam (1976) also notes that classical factor analysis is

Table 13.2. *Perfect simplex correlation matrix (Jöreskog & Sörbom, 1981)*

Occasion	1	2	3	4
1	1.000			
2	0.838	1.000		
3	0.812	0.969	1.000	
4	0.724	0.865	0.892	1.000

insufficient in dealing with longitudinal designs. 'T-technique assumes fixed non-stochastic growth processes, in the same way as factor analysis assumes fixed non-stochastic factor loadings and factor scores, which are fixed non-stochastic within subjects' (Roskam, 1976: 114); see also the discussion on this topic presented by Nesselroade (1977).

However, the simplex implies structure, and structure contains information. It is, therefore, quite worth while finding some approach which will (possibly) come to grips with this problem. The first to formulate a mathematical representation of the simplex property was T. W. Anderson (1960). He considered data from intelligence scores. As already indicated by Roskam's critique, the main thrust of this approach rests on considering the simplex from longitudinal data as a stochastic process: that is to say, that the observation at time 2 depends on the observation made at time 1, and in turn, the observation at time 3 depends on the observation at time 2, and so forth. This represents the notion of a first-order autoregressive process. Anderson proposed treating these processes within the framework of the Markov simplex. Guire & Kowalski (1979: 93) formulate the general Markov process, 'in which . . . the value of the observation at time t is a simple linear function of the measurement made at the preceding time point'. Consider the example (taken from Jöreskog & Sörbom, 1988) shown in Table 13.2 where a correlation matrix adheres to the perfect simplex property. 'Here every correlation ρ_{ij} with $|i-j|>1$ is the product of the correlations just below the diagonal. For example, $\rho_{41} = 0.838 \times 0.969 \times 0.892 = 0.724$' (Jöreskog & Sörbom, 1988).

The quasi Markov simplex. However, it was soon recognized that the perfect Markov simplex was simply too restrictive in psychological measurement, since it maintains that there are no errors of measurement in the manifest variables. In the behavioral sciences this is certainly very seldom the case. Thus, the actual Markov simplex property was shifted to the latent level, where by definition measurement error is removed. This position was termed the 'quasi Markov simplex'.

Jöreskog (1970) formulated the quasi Markov simplex model in the general framework of structural equation models. The model has since often been discussed and refined in the literature (Jöreskog, 1974, 1979; Jöreskog & Sörbom, 1976, 1977, 1988; Sörbom, 1976).

Structural equation models for covariance matrices can represent hypotheses about the underlying relationships among constructs that determine the empirically observed covariance structure (Andres, 1986, 1990; Long, 1983*a*, *b*; Hayduk, 1988). In these models, the covariance structure of the observed variables is a function of other parameters. The distinction between (observed) measures and (theoretical) concepts leads to a corresponding distinction between theoretical models and measurement models. Theoretical models specify structural relations hypothesized to be present in a set of theoretical constructs. Measurement models denote the relation of these concepts to a set of observed variables. This is the theoretical distinction we have in mind throughout the chapter when talking about testable models for these two sets of relations. Inferences about structural relations cannot be made without assumptions about one's measures and the concept of interest. There is need for considerable interplay between theoretical notions of change and the development and refinement of measurement devices. These models, like any other *model*, map relations among variables according to the theoretical notions, in this case of autoregressive structure. *If* the *hypothesized* relational structure is correct, the *observed data* (i.e., covariance matrix) can be 'reconstructed' by the estimated parameters of the *model*, for example estimated variances, such as variances of the latent variables and residual variances, and regression coefficients (β). In case the 'reconstructed' data are consistent with the observed data, the theoretical assumptions regarding both developmental processes *and* quality of measurement can be considered plausible. The use of the confirmatory framework enables models to be tested against each other in a predetermined sequence in order to arrive at the most concise model, within a given specification of alternatives, which is consistent with the data. This is not primarily a matter of data analysis, but influences data analysis heavily. Estimations of model parameters and model tests can be obtained by structural equation modeling techniques (LISREL, EQS, COSAN, etc.) using a variety of estimation procedures (maximum likelihood, unweighted least squares, etc.). For further details see Bentler (1986*a*, *b*, 1988), Ecob (1987*a*, *b*), Hertzog (1987), Jöreskog (1979), Jöreskog & Sörbom (1985), Rogosa (1979), Rudinger (1985*a*, *b*) Saris & Stronkhorst (1984), Schaie & Hertzog (1983).

Structural equation modeling of longitudinal data is modeling of change processes and their determinants (Bentler, 1980, 1984; Jöreskog

& Sörbom, 1976; Sörbom, 1976). This can be done by structural regression models, which involve the estimation of regression coefficients representing sequences of time ordered direct relationships between antecedent and consequent variables. Jöreskog & Sörbom (1977) distinguish in their longitudinal models endogenous and exogenous latent variables. The endogenous latent variables are the constructs that have been measured across time. In our modelling presented in this chapter we confine ourselves to the endogenous variables, i.e., no background variables etc. are employed. Our models are basically autoregressive models for endogenous variables, such as intelligence constructs across longitudinal occasions. In other words, in these models, the variable under study predicts itself at later points in time. A first-order autoregressive sequence models individual differences at time t as a function of individual differences at time $t - 1$. The application of the general model has come into wide use (Dommel & Rudinger, 1986; Heise, 1969; Humphreys & Parsons, 1979; Jagodzinski & Kühnel, 1987; Rudinger & Rietz, 1987; Werts & Hilton, 1977; Werts & Linn, 1970; Werts, Jöreskog & Linn, 1971; Werts, Linn & Jöreskog, 1977, 1978; Wheaton, Muthén, Alwin & Summers, 1978; Wiley & Wiley, 1970).

Since the examples of the present chapter involve longitudinal studies of at maximum four occasions, the outline refers to this case, although generalizations to more than four measurement points will be obvious to the reader. Figure 13.1 summarizes the model in a path diagram.

We have administered a particular intelligence test four times, denoted by y_1, y_2, y_3, y_4. The reader will note that y_i represents the same variable over separate occasions. The administered test generally contains measurement error (ε_i). Thus, each of the manifest variables is considered to be a fallible measure of an underlying hypothetical construct or latent variable. The corresponding latent variables are denoted by η_i. A problem lies in determining the unit of measurement for the latent variables. A natural way of doing this is to assume the same unit of measurement for the latent variables as for the manifest variables ($\lambda_i = 1$). It assumed that the ε_i are uncorrelated with each other, a standard assumption in classical test theory. In the structural equation model, we must consider the feature outlined in the discussion above, namely the stochastic property. This is conceptualized in a first-order autoregressive process. The latent variable η_i depends on the previous observation of η_{i-1}. The residuals of the latent variables (ζ_i) are considered to be uncorrelated with η_j ($j < i$). Furthermore, the ε_i are also uncorrelated with η_i.

After specifying the model in terms of mathematical equations, one has to consider which parameters have to be estimated and whether or not all the parameters can be identified. The parameters of the model are: variance of $\eta_1[V(\eta_1)]$, residual variances of the latent variables, i.e.

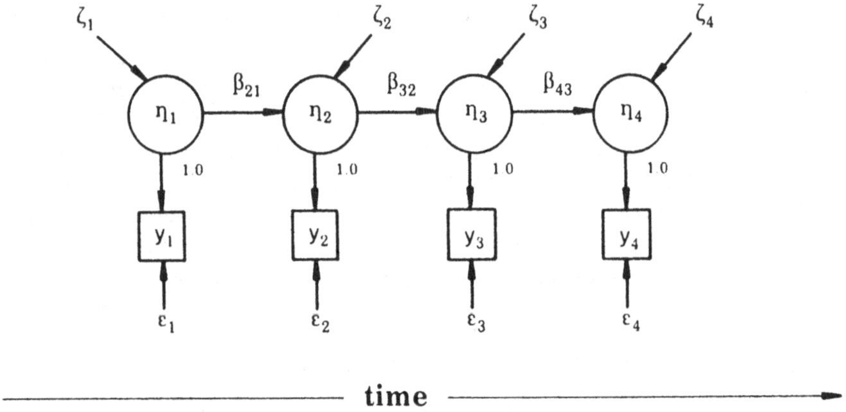

ζ = residuals of latent variables
η = latent variables
β = structural regression coefficients (unstandardized)
y = measured variables, e. g. intelligence test scores
ε = residuals of measured variables ("error")

measurement equations

$$y_1 = \eta_1 + \varepsilon_1$$
$$y_2 = \eta_2 + \varepsilon_2$$
$$y_3 = \eta_3 + \varepsilon_3$$
$$y_4 = \eta_4 + \varepsilon_4$$

structural equations

$$\eta_1 = \zeta_1$$
$$\eta_2 = \beta_{21}\eta 1 + \zeta_2$$
$$\eta_3 = \beta_{32}\eta_2 + \zeta_3$$
$$\eta_4 = \beta_{43}\eta_3 + \zeta_4$$

variances

$$V(y_1) = \psi_{11} + V(\varepsilon_1)$$
$$V(y_2) = V(\eta_2) + V(\varepsilon_2)$$
$$V(y_3) = V(\eta_3) + V(\varepsilon_3)$$
$$V(y_4) = V(\eta_4) + V(\varepsilon_4)$$

$$V(\eta_1) = \psi_{11}$$
$$V(\eta_2) = \beta^2{}_{21}\psi_{11} + \psi_{22}$$
$$V(\eta_3) = \beta^2{}_{32}V(\eta_2) + \psi_{33}$$
$$V(\eta_3) = \beta^2{}_{32}(\beta^2{}_{21}\psi_{11} + \psi_{22}) + \psi_{33}$$
$$V(\eta_4) = \beta^2{}_{43}v(\eta_3) + \psi_{44}$$
$$V(\eta_4) = \beta^2{}_{43}[\beta^2{}_{32}(\beta^2{}_{21}\psi_{11} + \psi_{22}) + \psi_{33}] + \psi_{44}$$

covariances (crucial for stability)

$$cov(\eta_1\eta_2) = \beta_{21}\psi_{11}$$
$$cov(\eta_2\eta_3) = \beta_{32}\beta^2{}_{21}\psi_{11} + \beta_{32}\psi_{22}$$
$$cov(\eta_3\eta_4) = \beta_{43}\beta^2{}_{32}\beta^2{}_{21}\psi_{11} + \beta_{43}\beta^2{}_{32}\psi_{22} + \beta_{43}\psi_{33}$$

Figure 13.1. The 'classic' model for analyzing stability and reliability of longitudinal data: the quasi Markov simplex.

variances of $\zeta_i[\Psi_i]$, residual variances of the observed variables $[V(\varepsilon_i)$ or $\Theta_{\varepsilon i}]$, and the structural regression coefficients (β). These need to be estimated. A detailed analysis of the identification problem involved in this model is provided by Jöreskog & Sörbom (1988).

Reliability and stability. The conceptual distinction emphasized in the quasi Markov simplex, is the distinction between observed measures (y) and theoretical concepts (η) as well as between *measurement* models and *structural* models. Measurement models denote the *assumptions* about relations of theoretical concepts to a set of measured variables (y). The definition of *reliability* refers to this part of the model. Reliability is 'operationalized' as a proportion of the variance of the latent variable (η) and the variance of the observed variable (y):

$$\text{rel}_i = \frac{V(\eta_i)}{V(\eta_i) + V(\varepsilon_i)}$$

In the 'structural part' of the model, relations are *hypothesized* to be present in the set of theoretical concepts (η), such as *stability* over time: stability is 'operationalized' as correlation between latent variables adjacent in time:

$$\rho_{ij} = \frac{\text{Cov}(\eta_i \eta_j)}{\sqrt{V(\eta_i)V(\eta_j)}}$$

Thus we will use the term *stability,* whenever we refer to the consistency of interindividual differences at the level of the construct itself. Stability refers more closely to theoretical assumptions about the developmental process, whereas reliability refers to the quality of measurement of the developmental phenomena.

The empirical study

Hypotheses. We want to test a very strict combined hypothesis of

- equal reliabilities of the assessments across time, i.e.,

  $\text{rel}_1 = \text{rel}_2 = \text{rel}_3 = \text{rel}_4$;

- equal stabilities per time unit (1 year), i.e.,

  $\rho_{jk} = \rho_{kl}$, $j = 1965, \ldots, 1970$, $k = j + 1$, $l = k + 1$; and

- equal variances of the latent variables, i.e.,

  $V(\eta_1) = V(\eta_2) = V(\eta_3) = V(\eta_4)$.

Modeling issues. Within the context of the classical autoregressive quasi Markov simplex model these hypotheses are mirrored by statistical hypotheses about parameters, such as residual variances [$V(\varepsilon)$] of the observed variables, and about the structural regression coefficients (β) between the latent variables. In order to obtain equal reliabilities as well as equal stabilities, it is intuitive to constrain the residual variances [$V(\varepsilon)$] to equality as well as the structural regression coefficients (β).

A word about the quality of structural regression coefficients: within our gerontological longitudinal study (BOLSA) the spacing of the first four measurements is unbalanced: 1st 1965, 2nd 1967, 3rd 1969, 4th 1972, i.e. 2–3 years differences between adjacent assessments. To overcome this incommensurability problem, we introduce some 'phantom' variables: between 1965 and 1967 one phantom variable, between 1967 and 1969 another one, and between 1969 and 1972 two phantom variables. They 'slice' the stream of time into equal (virtually discrete) units of 1 year. Now the 'β' can be constrained to equality for identical time units (e.g.: $\beta_{ji} = \beta_{kj}$; $\text{time}_j - \text{time}_i = \text{time}_k - \text{time}_j$). The technicalities are presented elsewhere (Rindskopf, 1983, 1984; Rudinger & Rietz, 1987).

The purpose of this equality constraint is the specification of the hypothesis that the one-year stabilities are equal. This reflects the assumption of stationarity, i.e. invariant *change* process over time. It implies the assumption that stability from 1965 to 1967 (β^2) is equal to stability from 1967 to 1969, and that stability from 1969 to 1972 is β^3, i.e. one-year stability to the power of 3. It follows for this type of model that *n* years' stability is *one*-year stability to the *power n*, given that the variances of the latent variables are equal to 1 [$V(\eta_i) = 1.0$].

However, the classic quasi Markov simplex model applied to covariances is not suitable for reflecting and *testing* the hypotheses we actually had in mind. The equality constraints of the residual variances [$V(\varepsilon)$] fail, and so do the equality contraints of the structural regression cofficients (β). The reason, why it *has* to fail can easily be derived from Figure 13.1: because of the obviously unequal variances

$$V(\eta_1) \neq V(\eta_2) \neq V(\eta_3) \neq V(\eta_4),$$

and the unequal covariances, consequently the reliabilities and the stabilities are in general also unequal, i.e.:

$$\text{rel}_1 \neq \text{rel}_2 \neq \text{rel}_3 \neq \text{rel}_4, \quad \text{and} \quad \rho_{12} \neq \rho_{23} \neq \rho_{34}.$$

Thus, the problem arises of creating an autoregressive model which satisfies the condition of (a) equal reliabilities (e.g., $\text{rel}_1 = \text{rel}_4$) and (b) equal stabilities (e.g., $\rho_{12} = \rho_{14}$). These two hypotheses are equivalent to the following equations:

$$\frac{\Psi_{11}}{\Psi_{11}+\Theta_{\varepsilon 11}} \stackrel{!}{=} \frac{\beta_{43}^2(\beta_{32}^2(\beta_{21}^2\Psi_{11}+\Psi_{22})+\Psi_{33})+\Psi_{44}}{\beta_{43}^2(\beta_{32}^2(\beta_{21}^2\Psi_{11}+\Psi_{22})+\Psi_{33})+\Psi_{44}+\Theta_{\varepsilon 44}} \qquad \text{(a)}$$

$$\frac{\beta_{21}\Psi_{11}}{\sqrt{(\Psi_{11}(\beta_{21}^2\Psi_{11}+\Psi_{22}))}}$$

$$\stackrel{!}{=} \frac{\beta_{43}\beta_{32}^2\beta_{21}^2\Psi_{11}+\beta_{43}\beta_{32}^2\Psi_{22}+\beta_{43}\psi_{33}}{\sqrt{(\beta_{32}^2(\beta_{21}^2\Psi_{11}+\Psi_{22})+\Psi_{33})(\beta_{43}^2(\beta_{32}^2(\beta_{21}^2\Psi_{11}+\Psi_{22})+\Psi_{33})+\Psi_{44})}} \qquad \text{(b)}$$

These equations make clear that for testing hypotheses about reliability and stability, such as equality, it is necessary to specify *a priori* assumptions about *variances and covariances*. However, the classic model displayed in Figure 13.1 offers no chance to constrain the co/variances to equality, because these constraints lead to nonlinear equations, such as

$$\Psi_{11}=\beta_{21}^2\Psi_{11}+\Psi_{22}=\ldots=\beta_{43}^2(\beta_{32}^2(\beta_{21}^2\Psi_{11}+\Psi_{22})+\Psi_{33})+\Psi_{44}$$

(see Rudinger, Andres & Rietz, 1986). Therefore, in an analysis of covariance matrices with the classic quasi Markov simplex model, it makes no sense to put equality constraints only on the residual variances and the structural regression coefficients. Rudinger & Rietz (1988*a*, *b*) developed a new autoregressive model which is suitable for superimposing *nonlinear* constraints (see the Technical appendix, p. 301). Then equality of covariances is automatically obtained from the equality of variances together with the equality constraint of the structural regression coefficients.

The new model applied to intelligence data in old age. The new model was set up to test simultaneously the hypotheses of:

- equal reliabilities
- equal stabilities, and
- equal variances of the latent constructs across time.

The results are presented in Figure 13.2. The parameters of the standardized solution are exactly the parameters with characteristics as expected from an algebraic point of view: the reliabilities as well as the stabilities are estimated as equal. This is because of the successfully superimposed equality constraints on the variances of the latent variables. So, the equalities of $V(\varepsilon_i)$ and β work in the expected way only in connection with the constraints of the crucial variances $V(\eta_i)$.

Nothing had been said up to now about the fit of the model. In this chapter, fitting models is not so much our primary concern as the

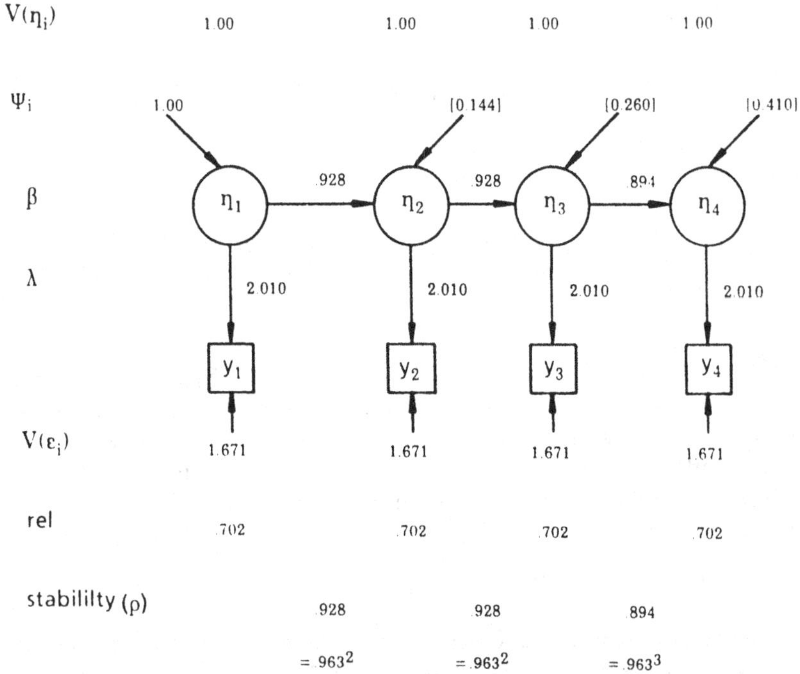

Figure 13.2 Results for the four waves autoregressive model: one variable (y) across time $(1, \ldots, 4)$, with constrained latent variances, and equal residual variances of the observed variables structural regression coefficients per unit of time (1 year) in order to specify and to test the hypotheses of equal reliabilities and invariant stabilities. Standardized solutions. Input: covariance matrix.

mapping of hypotheses onto model structures. However, the chi-square goodness-of-fit index might be of some interest:

$$\text{chi-square} = 10.79, \quad \text{d.f.} = 7, \quad p = 0.148.$$

This model can be compared with a model with unconstrained latent variances, i.e. with the classic quasi Markov simplex analysis:

$$\text{chi-square} = 3.75, \quad \text{d.f.} = 4, \quad p = 0.441.$$

The chi-square difference between these models is nonsignificant: 7.04 with d.f. = 3, $p > 0.05$. The interpretation is as follows: the new model leads to equal reliabilities over time, because of the hypothesis of equal variances of the latent variables over time on the one hand and of the equality of the residual variances on the other hand. This model cannot be significantly improved by *dropping* the assumption of *equal* latent variances. Thus, we stay with the more parsimonious model.

Some perspectives

Before going on to present more complex models in the next section it seems appropriate to discuss some of the implications inherent in the quasi Markov simplex. First, if we can fit the data with a stochastic process of this type, then we deduce that the quality or property which we are measuring follows some systematic developmental function. Second, from a psychometric point of view, the parameters of the quasi Markov simplex can tell us something about the test or particular measuring instrument that we are using. In this context we gain information about the *reliability* of the instrument. Third, a hypothesis of a *stable* process over time gives us the possibility of examining change more closely. The concept of a stationary Markov process is somewhat confusing in this context. As Frederiksen & Rotondo (1979) point out, it does not mean that no change takes place, but that the process of change remains invariant.

In general, in order to test hypotheses about stabilities (such as stationarity) and reliabilities (such as equality) it is necessary to specify assumptions about the variances of the latent variables and about the error terms. In the context of four longitudinal assessments we presented a model which actually allows for imposing restrictions on the variances of latent variables. This model is suitable for disentangling *reliability* of the measurement of the developmental phenomena, such as intelligence, from features of the developmental process itself, such as *stability*. The separation of these commonly confounded, but in their essence different, concepts was demonstrated for a longitudinal study with four testings on a single variable (intelligence subtest). This approach can be generalized to more than four occasions as well as to multiple indicators for the latent construct. The model we develop for this purpose in the following section is of the autoregressive type again, in contrast to the models applied by Hertzog & Schaie (1986) and Schaie & Hertzog (1985).

However, this is not the end of the story for the situation of one variable. Having developed this model, one is also in the position to specify in a very general way inequalities among the parameters, and particularly inequalities between the variances (true score and/or error variances). Even proportional changes over time which do not affect the ratio of these variances can be modeled.

A reasonable hypothesis in psychometric intelligence research in old age might be the following one. The true score variances (of the construct) no longer change, i.e. the interindividual variability in old age remains constant over time. The reliabilities of the measurements, however, decrease, and additionally, as an independent process, stability *de*creases with increasing age. It is very important to re-emphasize that variance of the construct $[V(\eta_i)]$, stability (indicating the relative position of the subjects), and reliability are conceptually independent features of the system under study.

Another substantive hypothesis in intellectual development might aim for an increment of *interindividual* variability over time; the measurement instrument, however, should not change its reliability. Stability is expected to be invariant, i.e. in spite of increasing variances $V(\eta_i)$ the *correlation* between η_i and η_{i+1} is hypothesized to be unchanged. Of course, the key role is played again by the variances $V(\eta_i)$ and $V(\varepsilon_i)$. The basic assumption which has to be tested is that of equally proportional growth of both variances.

Even from these simple examples it becomes clear that different theories and models about development explicitly lead to different partitions of the total variance due to different sources, measurement errors included. Although these are well-known theoretical facts, they are nevertheless usually neglected in empirical research.

STRUCTURAL CHANGES OF INTELLIGENCE

Theory and data

In recent years some researchers have come up with the idea of transferring the theory of crystallized/fluid intelligence, which was developed following the Thurstonian-PMA tradition, to other concepts and test systems of intelligence, including Wechsler tests (Birren, Cunningham & Yamamoto, 1983; Botwinick, 1977; Horn & McArdle, 1980). The theory of crystallized and fluid intelligence has a strong developmental appeal, if one remembers Cattell's investment theory (Cattell, 1963, 1986; Horn, 1960, 1982; Horn & Cattell, 1966) and the trajectories of crystallized (Gc), fluid (Gf) intelligence, visuo-motor flexibility, and so forth, reported by Schaie (1979) and Schaie & Hertzog (1983).

One topic frequently addressed by developmental psychologists involves assessment of invariance of constructs over time or the invariance of developmental dimensions. From the traditional perspective the invariance definition of constructs over time is synonymous with definitions of factorial invariance. This involves the same relative magnitude of factor loadings of variables on factors as well as the same degree of relation between the factors (measurement equivalence). Emergence of 'qualitatively' new structures could emphasize the differential relative salience of a variable to a factor at a given time, or could postulate a change in the degree to which the postulated latent structures correlate (Cunningham, 1978, 1980*a*, *b*, 1981; Cunningham & Birren, 1980; Hertzog & Schaie, 1986; Schaie & Hertzog, 1986).

Table 13.3. *Covariance matrix of four intelligence subtests of WAIS/HAWIE measured at two occasions (1965, 1976). Data from BOLSA*

		t_1				t_6			
		AW1	GF1	ZS1	MT1	AW6	GF6	ZS6	MT6
t_1	AW1	5.371							
	GF1	3.547	5.040						
	ZS1	2.598	2.069	5.162					
	MT1	2.127	1.663	3.141	6.347				
t_6	AW6	4.606	3.484	2.732	1.868	6.943			
	GF6	3.838	3.470	2.161	1.716	4.074	6.037		
	ZS6	2.462	2.021	3.313	3.023	2.912	2.449	4.585	
	MT6	2.937	1.808	3.506	4.802	3.393	2.920	3.892	6.694

Notes: $t_1 = 1965$, $t_2 = 1976$. AW, Allegemeines Wissen/Information (IN); GF, Gemeinsamkeiten Finden/Similarities (SI); ZS, Zahlensymboltest/Digit Symbol (DS); MT, Mosaik Test/Block Design (BD); $N = 81$.

In line with these modelling ideas it is an essential precondition to separate clearly and distinctively the different sources of developmental change and the various facets of invariance and stability according to the theoretical viewpoints adopted. For example, if we stay within trait-oriented theories, we have to focus on 'stability' and structural 'invariance', particularly on the level of constructs. The only niche left in this invariant system is for change of the means (of the latent variables). Thus, in order to determine the means as hypothetical locus of quantitiative change, one has to make a 'nondevelopmental' point for invariance, equivalence, and stability of the other elements of the system under study, i.e. of the variances and covariances (see also Nesselroade, 1977; Labouvie, 1980).

Concerning the 'development' of intelligence in old age our main theoretical assumptions are the following: invariance of the measurement model over time, and structural stability of the Gf and Gc constructs. These assumptions will be elaborated, formalized and tested within the framework of two waves. In Table 13.3 the covariance matrix of the four subtests over time is presented. The model deals with just four observed HAWIE-subtests and two latent variables for the first assessment (1965), and symmetrically for the sixth assessment (1976) in BOLSA. 'Crystallized intelligence' (Gc) is measured by 'Information' and 'Similarities'; 'fluid intelligence' (Gf) by 'Digit Symbol' and 'Block Design'.

Hypotheses

The *prima facie* 'nondevelopmental' features are:

1. *Invariance of the measurement model over time.* By making

certain assumptions, constraints, and restrictions on the factor loadings and residual variances and covariances of the observed variables (see Bentler, 1973; Nesselroade, 1977), a variety of facets for the definition of invariance of the *measurement model* is available:

A. a certain invariant pattern of zero loadings,
B. the numerical values of the corresponding nonzero loading parameters over time,
C. the residual co/variances of the observed variables over time.

2. *Stability of constructs over time.* Stability refers to the structural part of the intelligence model, i.e., to the relations between the theoretical constructs. Given the assumption of high *temporal* stability, we expect high values for the paths from crystallized intelligence at time t_1 (Gc_1) to crystallized intelligence at time t_6 (Gc_6), and analogously from Gf at time t_1 to Gf at time t_6. A numerically high value β_{61} would indicate a reasonable predictability from latent variable at t_1 to latent variable at t_6. Furthermore, we expect the residual variances of η_3 and η_4 (i.e., Ψ_{33} and Ψ_{44}) to show low values (see Figure 13.3).

3. Another feature of stability refers to the variances of the latent variables and to their covariances within time i compared with these measures within time j. Given the assumption of this kind of structural invariances, we expect stable values of these parameters over time.

The classic longitudinal model

In order to test hypothese of this kind, two-wave models of the 'classic' type described below have been applied quite frequently to longitudinal data, for example by Bentler (1984), Cornelius (1984), Jöreskog (1979), Jöreskog & Sörbom (1976, 1977), Olsson & Bergman (1977), Rudinger (1985*c*), Sörbom (1976), and Weeks (1980).

For the sake of simplicity we begin with the smallest possible autoregressive longitudinal model with multiple indicators in which changes of structure can also be conceptualized: two occasions with two latent variables at each occasion. The two latent variables are indicated by two observed variables each. All current research questions, however, can be mapped onto this model and can be investigated in a prototypical way. Figure 13.3 reiterates the information about the relations between the observed subtests and the assumed latent variables (Gc, Gf) on the one hand (*measurement model*), and about the relations between the constructs (*structural model*) on the other hand. Relations among the constructs are defined by structural regression coefficients across time (β) and covariances within time.

Invariance of the measurement model is usually specified by pairwise equality constraints among the factor loadings (λ) and by pairwise equality constraints of the corresponding residual variances of the

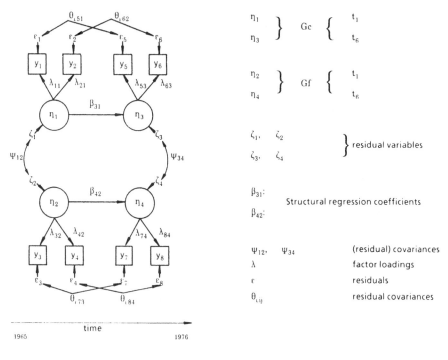

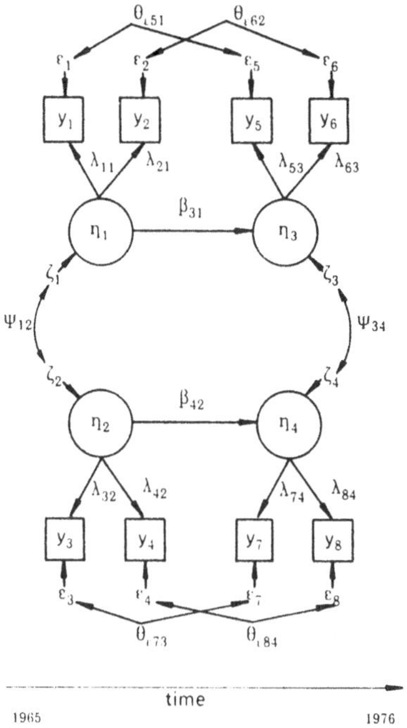

η_1, η_3 } Gc { t_1, t_6

η_2, η_4 } Gf { t_1, t_6

ζ_1, ζ_2, ζ_3, ζ_4 } residual variables

β_{31}: β_{42}: Structural regression coefficients

ψ_{12}, ψ_{34} (residual) covariances

λ factor loadings

ε residuals

$\theta_{\varepsilon ij}$ residual covariances

Note:
Variance/covariance matrix of the latent variables

	η_1	η_2	η_3	η_4
η_1	ψ_{11}	ψ_{12}	$\beta_{31}\cdot\psi_{11}$	$\beta_{42}\cdot\psi_{21}$
η_2	$\frac{\psi_{12}}{\sqrt{\psi_{11}\cdot\psi_{22}}}$	ψ_{22}	$\beta_{31}\cdot\psi_{12}$	$\beta_{42}\cdot\psi_{22}$
η_3	$\frac{\beta_{31}\cdot\psi_{11}}{\sqrt{\psi_{11}(\beta^2_{31}\psi_{11}+\psi_{33})}}$	$\frac{\beta_{31}\cdot\psi_{11}}{\sqrt{\psi_{22}(\beta^2_{31}\psi_{11}+\psi_{33})}}$	$\beta^2_{31}\psi_{11}+\psi_{33}$	$\beta_{31}\beta_{42}\psi_{12}+\psi_{34}$
η_4	$\frac{\beta_{42}\cdot\psi_{21}}{\sqrt{\psi_{11}(\beta^2_{42}\psi_{22}+\psi_{44})}}$	$\frac{\beta_{42}\cdot\psi_{22}}{\sqrt{\psi_{22}(\beta^2_{42}\psi_{22}+\psi_{44})}}$	$\frac{\beta_{31}\beta_{42}\Psi_{12}+\Psi_{34}}{\sqrt{(\beta^2_{31}\Psi_{11}+\Psi_{33})(\beta^2_{42}\Psi_{22}+\Psi_{44})}}$	$\beta^2_{42}\psi_{22}+\psi_{44}$

Diagonal: Variances
Upper Part: Covariances
Lower Part: Correlations

Figure 13.3. Minimized longitudinal model. Two measurement points, four subtests per occasion, and two latent variables (Gc, Gf) per occasion.

Table 13.4. *Selected LISREL results for the minimized longitudinal model: standardized solution*

$\lambda_{11} = 2.054 \neq \lambda_{53} = 2.247$
$\lambda_{21} = 1.674 \neq \lambda_{63} = 1.832$
$\lambda_{32} = 1.798 \neq \lambda_{74} = 1.917$
$\lambda_{42} = 1.867 \neq \lambda_{84} = 1.980$

$\theta_1 = \theta_5 = 1.129$
$\theta_2 = \theta_6 = 2.533$
$\theta_3 = \theta_7 = 1.364$
$\theta_4 = \theta_8 = 3.160$

$\left.\begin{array}{l}\beta_{31} = 0.956\\ \beta_{42} = 0.953\end{array}\right\}$ *Stability*

$\Psi_{12} = 0.648$ $\qquad 0.648 = \rho_{12}$

$\left.\begin{array}{l}\Psi_{33} = 0.087\\ \Psi_{34} = 0.142\\ \Psi_{44} = 0.092\end{array}\right\}$ $\qquad 0.732 = \rho_{34}$

Structural correlations

$V(\eta_1) = 4.218$
$V(\eta_2) = 3.233$
$V(\eta_3) = 5.050$
$V(\eta_4) = 3.674$

Notes:
$\left.\begin{array}{l}\rho_{12}\\ \rho_{34}\end{array}\right\}$ correlation between Gc and Gf at $\left\{\begin{array}{l}\text{time 1}\\ \text{time 6}\end{array}\right.$
$V(\eta_i)$ are variances of latent constructs: they are different! The pairwise equality constraints of the λ disappear in the standardized solution because of $V(\eta_i) \neq V(\eta_j)$, for all i, $j = 1, \ldots, 4$, $i \neq j$.

observed variables $[V(\varepsilon)]$, i.e.:

$$\lambda_{11} = \lambda_{53},\ \theta_{\varepsilon 1} = \theta_{\varepsilon 5} \quad \lambda_{32} = \lambda_{74},\ \theta_{\varepsilon 3} = \theta_{\varepsilon 7}$$
$$\lambda_{21} = \lambda_{63},\ \theta_{\varepsilon 2} = \theta_{\varepsilon 6} \quad \lambda_{42} = \lambda_{84},\ \theta_{\varepsilon 4} = \theta_{\varepsilon 8}$$

These equality constraints are considered to be a presupposition of 'measurement equivalence'.No hypothesis can be specified about 'stability' in this basic model, nor about structural regression coefficients (β), nor about variances and covariances of the latent constructs. This is partly because of the same reasons as with the simplex model, and partly because of additional hindrances, which have to be removed before this model is suitable for testing this class of hypotheses. The results are presented in Table 13.4.

The results of the eleven-year longitudinal study give us some evidence for the appropriateness of the measurement model specified *a priori* (Information, Similarities for *crystallized intelligence*; and Digit Symbol, Block Design, for *fluid intelligence*), and for the assumption of invariance of the measurement model over time. The model shows high structural regression coefficients (0.956 and 0.953). These results seem consentaneous with assumptions of high stability of crystallized and fluid intelligence.

We return now to the substantive hypothesis in developmental intelligence research. There is a rather distinct interest in testing whether the *structural* correlations remain invariant across time, i.e. to investigate whether correlation (Gc_1, Gf_1) is equal to correlation (Gc_6, Gf_6). In terms of our model this is the hypothesis $\rho_{12} = \rho_{34}$. When we apply the model shown in Figure 13.3, these correlations ρ_{12} and ρ_{34} are numerically different (0.65, and 0.73, see Table 13.4), but we have not yet tested any hypothesis, so, we do not know for sure whether these correlations are also statistically different. However, it is precisely invariance or change of these correlations which is the subject of the *differentiation/integration hypothesis* (Baltes *et al.*, 1980; Reinert, 1970). Therefore, it is supposed to be very crucial to test hypotheses about covariances and correlations between traits over time. These measures are the statistical counterparts of the theoretical conjectures.

Autoregressive vs non-autoregressive models

There are therefore some questions, such as: Why did the equality contraints of the factor loadings fade away? How can we really *test* hypotheses about structural features, such as structural invariance, i.e. ρ_{ij}, at t vs ρ_{ij}, at $t+1$?. Fortunately, answers can be given again, when we have a closer look at the equations of this model.

This problem is closely related to the problem with the Markov simplex model for covariances. With reference to the co/variance matrix in Figure 13.3, our hypothesis, $\rho_{12} = \rho_{34}$ can be displayed in the following equation:

$$\rho_{34} = \frac{\beta_{31}\beta_{42}\Psi_{12} + \Psi_{34}}{\sqrt{(\beta_{31}^2\Psi_{11} + \Psi_{33})(\beta_{42}^2\Psi_{22} + \Psi_{44})}} \stackrel{!}{=} \frac{\Psi_{12}}{\sqrt{\Psi_{11}\Psi_{22}}} = \rho_{12}$$

The variances, covariances, and correlations of the latent variables following the first assessment are functions of the variances of the latent variables at the first measurement, and of the structural regression coefficients connecting the first assessment with subsequent assessments. As long as there are no restrictions on these Ψ and β, the variances, covariances and correlations of the η are also free to a certain degree. So, in the autoregressive type of models, there is no direct way to test any assumptions about correlations or covariances between the latent variables. This holds for structural stability coefficients as well as for temporal stability coefficients.

However, as soon as one finds suitable restrictions on the Ψ and β, one also gets perfect control over the variances and covariances of the dependent latent variables (η_2, η_4). The problem can be narrowed to finding these suitable restrictions. With reference to the last equation, the hypothesis $\rho_{12} = \rho_{34}$ is specified by the following constraints:

$$V(\eta_1) = V(\eta_3); \qquad V(\eta_3) = \beta_{31}^2 V(\eta_1) + \Psi_{33} = \beta_{31}^2 \Psi_{11} + \Psi_{33}$$

i.e.

$$\Psi_{11} = \beta_{31}^2 \Psi_{11} + \Psi_{33},$$

and

$$V(\eta_2) = V(\eta_4),$$

i.e.

$$\Psi_{22} = \beta_{42}^2 \Psi_{22} + \Psi_{44},$$

and

$$\text{Cov}(\eta_1 \eta_2) = \text{Cov}(\eta_3 \eta_4),$$

i.e.

$$\Psi_{12} = \beta_{31} \beta_{42} \Psi_{12} + \Psi_{34}.$$

The problem which is inherent to these equations is well known to the reader: these equations are *nonlinear*. Following the same rationale as we applied for the simplex model we developed a new (superordinate) model to overcome this nonlinearity problem (Rudinger, 1986; Rudinger, Andres & Rietz, 1986). Before we demonstrate the possibilities of this new model, we turn to an alternate conceptualization of testing assumptions about co/variances and correlations of latent variables.

Nesselroade (1977), Schaie & Hertzog (1985), Hertzog & Nesselroade (1987) as well as McArdle (1988) and McArdle & Epstein (1987) make a plea for another type of model. They prefer models that just contain covariances among latent variables across time. In other words: their model implies no independent/dependent variable distinction, i.e. it is *not* the case that $\eta_{t+1} = f(\eta_t, \zeta_{t+1})$. It is just some kind of confirmatory factor analysis model (CFA) with correlated factors.

Rudinger, Andres & Rietz (1986) developed a more general model of this CFA type. It enables the researcher additionally to disentangle hypotheses about correlations from hypotheses about variances. The basic idea of the model is described in Figure 13.4. In our opinion it is a drawback of every CFA model that the essential feature of a *longitudinal* design is getting lost. The sequential *time order* of the assessments is no longer part of the model; it is now just part of the knowledge of the researcher. Of course, the researcher refers to this knowledge in interpreting the results, but no time-related assumptions are specified explicitly. Nevertheless, this model has some advantages and merits: it enables the researcher to *test* straightforward hypotheses about equality of variances, covariances and correlations of latent variables, although independent of their placing and spacing in time. This can be done quite easily because in the CFA model the design status of the latent variables is the status of independent variables; constraints refer just to variances and covariances of *in*dependent latent variables. Thus, the very complex and unsolved general problem in structural equation modeling, of how to specify *a priori* assumptions about variances and covariances of *dependent* variables, can be avoided this way. But one has to pay the price for this convenience; the time dimension is lost. The non-autoregressive model allows for testing measurement equivalence and *structural* invariance; the autoregressive model, however, yields information about *temporal* stability, conceptualized as predictability. From a substantive point of view as well as for mathematical reasons, we have a certain problem now. Both models are obviously qualitatively different. Both models, both sets of hypotheses cannot be rejected with our data: measurement equivalence, temporal stability, structural invariance including stable variances of the constructs, seem to be compatible with our data. However, they have been tested separately with two different models (these analyses are not presented here). Consequently, this allows no definite conclusion at all about whether the *conjunction* of the two sets of hypotheses can be accepted. The conjunction of these hypotheses can only be tested by a model which is a conjunction of the autoregressive and the non-autoregressive model. This hybrid model is expected to reparameterize both models. The attempt to integrate the features of both models leads to a complex model employing numerous phantom variables to deal with the nonlinearity problem effectively (for details, see Rudinger, Andres & Rietz, 1986; Rudinger *et al.*, 1989).

By applying this new model, a large variety of longitudinal hypotheses can be tested, concerning variances, covariances, and correlations of latent intelligence variables. Because of its generality this model allows for testing a hierarchy of partially nested hypotheses (see Figure 13.5). This will be demonstrated with the longitudinal intelligence data of BOLSA.

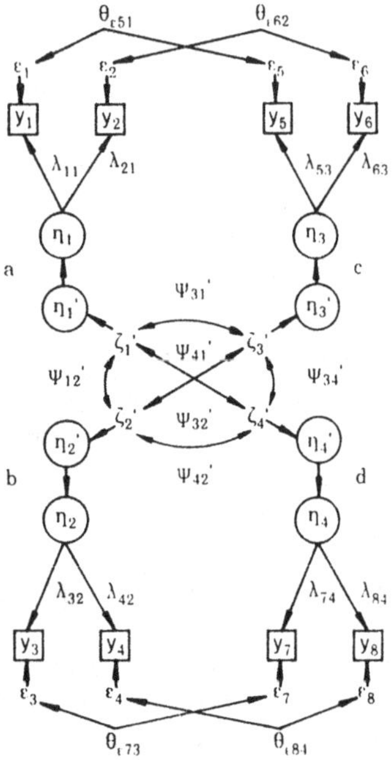

Note:
Variance/covariance matrix of the latent variables
for the minimized non-autoregressive model

	η_1	η_2	η_3	η_4
η_1	a^2	$a \cdot b\psi_{12}'$	$a \cdot c\psi_{13}'$	$a \cdot d\psi_{14}'$
η_2	$\frac{a\ b\psi_{12}}{\sqrt{a^2 \cdot b^2}} = \psi_{12}'$	b^2	$b \cdot c\psi_{23}'$	$b \cdot d\psi_{24}'$
η_3	ψ_{13}'	ψ_{23}'	c^2	$c \cdot d\psi_{34}'$
η_4	ψ_{14}'	ψ_{24}'	ψ_{34}'	d^2

Diagonal: Variances
Upper Part: Covariances
Lower Part: Correlations

$V(\eta_1') = V(\eta_2') = V(\eta_3') = V(\eta_4') = 1.0$

In this model the hypothesis

$$\rho_{12} = \rho_{34}$$

can be specified by the equality const

$$\psi_{12}' = \psi_{34}'.$$

In any case, i. e. with equal variances

$$a^2 = c^2, \text{ and}$$
$$b^2 = d^2,$$

or with unequal variances

$$a^2 \neq c^2$$
$$b^2 \neq d^2,$$

it holds $\psi_{12}' = \psi_{34}' \equiv \rho_{12} = \rho_{34}$

The coefficients a, b, d, c have to be greater than zero (0).

Equality of covariances is the sufficient condition, equality of values of variances are irrelevant conditions for the specification of the hypothesis of equal structural correlations.

Figure 13.4. Non-autoregressive longitudinal model.

Structural changes of intelligence in old age?

Our 'non-developmental' hypotheses concern the measurement part as well as the structural part of the intelligence model:

- measurement equivalence: invariant factor loadings of corresponding subtests across time,
- invariant reliabilities of corresponding subtests: invariant factor loadings, invariant residuals of the observed variables, and invariant variances of the latent variables Gc and Gf across time,
- structural invariance: invariant correlation between Gc and Gf across the time span of eleven years.

This specification leads to the most restrictive model placed at the top of the hierarchy of all possible models. The results of the analyses are presented in Table 13.5.

The model with invariant variances, invariant covariances, and pairwise constraints of the factor loadings, holds (column 1 in Table 13.5). The chi-square differences between this strong model and the weaker ones in columns 2, 3, and 4 are non-significant (see the bottom of the table). Thus, the most parsimonious model is preferred. The interpretation refers to this model, which is stable in all longitudinal aspects, probably except the means, but this is another story (Jöreskog & Sorbom, 1988; Sorbom, 1982). An invariant meaning of the intelligence constructs (Gc, Gf) can be assumed – even the relation between the intelligence constructs remains stable in time – and an almost unchanged relative position of the older persons in our sample over a time span of eleven years can be inferred (temporal stability). These results turn out to be very striking arguments for the justification of a trait-oriented perspective in evaluating developmental change in the field of psychometric intelligence.

CONCLUSION AND EVALUATION

The main attempt of this chapter was to illustrate our understanding of an appropriate mapping of substantive hypotheses in psychometric intelligence research onto features of structural equation models. This is primarily not at all a mater of computer software and data analysis. It is first of all subject matter of conceptual analysis and brain software. Thus, in order to *test* appropriately hypotheses about reliability, stability and interindividual differences in intelligence across time as well as about structural invariance and temporal stability of fluid and crystallized intelligence and measurement equivalence across time we have been forced to develop new models transcending the classic models of the autoregressive type.

Table 13.5. *Selected LISREL results (standardized solutions). Following Figure 13.5 a hierarchy of hypotheses has been tested, from stable variances and covariances across time to changing co/variances*

	Invariant variances		Changing variances	
	Invariant covariances	Changing covariances	Invariant covariances	Changing covariances (model shown in Figure 13.4 and Table 13.4)
$V(\eta_1)$	4.756	4.538	4.385	4.218
$V(\eta_2)$	3.610	3.461	3.357	3.232
$V(\eta_3)$	4.756	4.538	5.244	5.050
$V(\eta_4)$	3.610	3.461	3.753	3.674
Structural correlations				
ρ_{12}	0.685	0.644	0.684	0.648
ρ_{34}	0.685 $=$	0.727 \neq	0.684 $=$	0.732 \neq
Stability				
ρ_{13}	0.929	0.951	0.934	0.956
ρ_{24}	0.926	0.948	0.930	0.953
Measurement equivalence				
$\lambda_{11}, \lambda_{53}$	=	=	\neq	\neq
$\lambda_{21}, \lambda_{69}$	=	=	\neq	\neq
$\lambda_{32}, \lambda_{74}$	=	=	\neq	\neq
$\lambda_{42}, \lambda_{84}$	=	=	\neq	\neq
	Same reliabilities across time		Different reliabilities	
χ^2/d.f./p	19.10/21/0.579	16.38/20/0.693	17.59/19/0.550	14.81/18/0.675

χ^2 differences/d.f.:

2.72/1

1.51/2

2.78/1

1.57/2

4.29/3

By means of the new model type, a hierarchically ordered variety of hypotheses about stability of theoretical constructs and about differential or invariant reliability across time can be tested separately. More details about comparison of autoregressive models for one variable are given by Rudinger & Rietz (1988*a, b*). These authors present a partially ordered hierarchy of nested models.

At the top of this hierarchy, can be placed the model which employs only *three* parameters (β, $V(\varepsilon)$, $V(\eta)$) for the 'reconstruction' of the empirical co/variances. By means of specifying equal change processes (β) over time (stationarity) in connection with equal variances of true scores ($V(\eta)$) and equality of the error varlances ($V(\varepsilon)$), the strongest hypothesis possible has been set up: this implies the hypothesis of *invariant* stability and *equal* reliability over time. All other sets of hypotheses and all alternate models are less restrictive, since assumptions about β and/or $V(\varepsilon)$ and/or $V(\eta)$, and consequently about stability and/or reliability are *relaxed*. However, in doing so, there is a need for considerable interplay between theoretical notions of development and change, and the features of measurement devices. In the exemplified models a trait-oriented point for stability and invariance, particularly on the level of theoretical constructs, was made. This turns the focus to stability of *interindividual differences*. The classical simplex model (analyzing correlations) only yields information about relative interindividual differences. Our autoregressive model analyzing co/variances transcends the 'classic' correlational simplex modeling idea by modeling variances, too. What we can learn from *high* stability results is that subjects' time paths belong to the same family of developmental functions, i.e. the longitudinal trajectories exhibit a rather non-crossing pattern. The variances of the latent variables, which are 'under control' in the new model bear manifold information: in connection with stable variances high stability indicates a non-crossing parallel time paths pattern, i.e. there are no individual differences in change. In connection with, for example, increasing variances, high stability indicates a non-crossing fan spread pattern, i.e. increasing, individual differences that preserve subjects' ordering. These are well-known facts (see, e.g., Rogosa, Brandt & Zimowski, 1982; Rogosa & Willett, 1985). However, the models presented here are the first to allow for *testing* these assumptions. Until now it was not possible to test stability and reliability hypotheses separately in an *autoregressive* model. This was restricted to models employing only correlations or covariances in the structural part.

It is very important to remember that these models are designed to investigate either stability or change of interindividual differences across time. However, even in cases of 'high' stability (e.g., 0.90) and stable variances $V(\eta)$, clearly no information is provided about the function of the means across time. A stability model just indicates whether a large diversity of intraindividual time paths (low stability) exists or whether it makes sense to compare and to describe all subjects in terms of a common mean trajectory or function (high stability), for example non-decreasing crystallized, decreasing fluid intelligence in old age; or positively accelerated development of intelligence in childhood; or slow, but linear increasing, mental capacity in children with Down-Syndrome (Rudinger, 1988).

If one takes another perspective, for example that of a 'state' theory alternate assumptions about the relational system under study have to be considered, for example β close to zero (Hertzog & Nesselroade, 1987; Nesselroade & Bartsch, 1977). However, with the models presented here, no difficulties in also testing those assumptions will arise.

Stationarity, stability, stable variances, and invariant reliability over time do not mean that there is necessarily *no* change. The message is: if there are changes, these changes happen in a lawful, regular, predictable way; change can still occur in the domain of means. Nothing is said within the correlation/covariance models about the amount and form of changes of means. Consequetly, what is needed additionally is a model for the means.

The basic model for analyzing mean structures in a longitudinal context was introduced by Roskam (1976) and McArdle & Epstein (1987). The latter used structural equation modeling to combine traditional ideas from repeated-measures ANOVA (analysis of variance) with some traditional ideas from longitudinal factor analysis. McArdle & Epstein (1987) described a longitudinal model that includes correlations, variances, and means as a latent growth curve (LGC) model.

The most prominent feature of the McArdle & Epstein longitudinal model is the inclusion of (at least) one common factor. These latent growth factors are estimated from the repeated observations of a single variable, and are used to characterize longitudinal correlations and variances as well as the means. McArdle & Epstein consider it an advantage of their model that it is possible to study these longitudinal dynamic patterns without any need to reference time-to-time stability or autoregression coefficients. They prefer the (M)ANOVA type latent growth curves because they are interested in 'studying individual change as a function of time'.

According to McArdle & Epstein latent variables play a special role in growth curve models. In classical factor analysis the common factors represent systematic individual differences among sets of variables measured within a given longitudinal occasion. But here the many occasions are used to isolate systematic individual differences that connect the same individual between given longitudinal occasions. A single common factor score can be used to describe the broad similarity between an individual curve and the group curve. These interpretations led McArdle & Epstein to label these latent variables as *chronometric* factors.

By the introduction to the simplex model we referred to the problem of factor analyzing longitudinal correlations with T-technique. Of course, McArdle & Epstein comment upon this problem and try to refute Cronbach's (1967) position by two arguments: 'First, Cronbach's (1967) critique applies to the factor analysis of longitudinal correlations; but our latent growth models utilize information from longitudinal correlations, variances, and means. Second, Cronbach's (1967) critique applies to factor solutions that can be rotated; but our factor latent growth models are not rotatable and do not reflect an arbitrary pattern of change' (McArdle & Epstein, 1987: 112). They admit, however, that autoregressive models may also be fitted to the same longitudinal data, and comparison may be informative. From a mathematical point of view, it seems to be not without problems to compare the results of LGC and autoregressive models solely in a descriptive manner. In line with our philosophy, one has to construe another superordinate model which implies as subsets the models one wants to compare. The general LGC model consists of a mean part separated from a covariance part (Rudinger, 1988). For modeling the covariance part one can refer to page 282 and utilize the methods offered there. For modeling the mean part McArdle & Epstein (1987), Rietz (1988) and Rudinger (1988) offer a variety of designs, i.e. how to specify no growth, linearity, exponential growth, polynomial growth functions, etc. ready for LISREL or EQS-analysis (Rudinger & Rietz, 1987). Thus, the means can be modeled by a single chronometric factor, while the covariances can be modeled, for example, by an autoregressive structure with increasing variances, etc. The whole modeling idea is now turned to the analysis of moment matrices. There is actually *no genuine* difference in technical procedures.

In the second section of the chapter we turned to models with many dependent variables (y), with many individuals assessed over many times. The design enables the examination of many types of changes. Changes in variability and level, as in previous models, can also be examined here, but the *new* feature is that research can now focus on changes in *relationships* between variables and examine how these relationships change over time. This family of changes over time has been referred to as the 'structuring of change' as opposed to just 'measuring change' (Nesselroade, 1972). Figure 13.5 presents our hierarchy of models suitable for 'structuring change'.

The psychometric approach in its most advanced form of structural equation models makes it possible to distinugish different levels and types of change and invariance. There can be change or invariance in: (1) the number of latent constructs; (2) the values of 'factor' loadings; (3) the amount of error of measurement in the observed variables; (4) the variances of the latent constructs; (5) the relations (covariances)

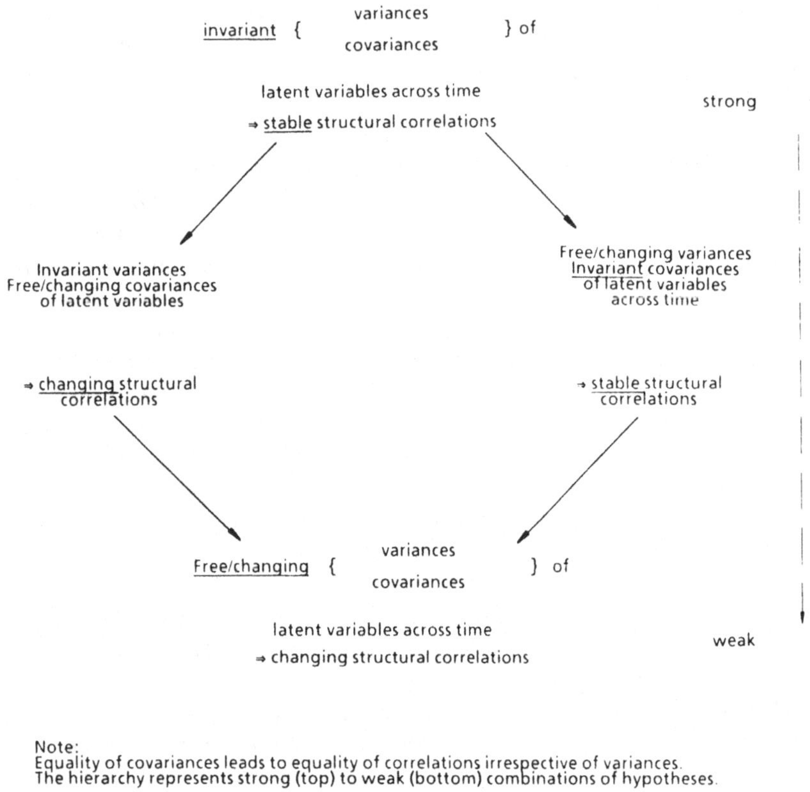

Figure 13.5. Structural changes, i.e. changes related to latent variables embedded into generalized autoregressive models.

between the latent constructs; and, last but not least, (6) the means of the constructs (see Nesselroade & Baltes, 1979; Hertzog & Schaie, 1986; Labouvie, 1980; Rudinger & Wood, 1989). The simultaneous consideration of (2), (3), and (4) is suitable to specify hypotheses about reliabilities of the observed variables as indices of latent processes under study. The consideration of (4) and (5) allows for hypotheses about correlations between the latent constructs. No matter which developmental model is chosen, what remains crucial is finding an appropriate mapping of theoretical *a priori* assumptions onto the model to be tested.

TECHNICAL APPENDIX 1

A simplex model with nonlinear constraints (adapted from Rudinger & Rietz, 1988)

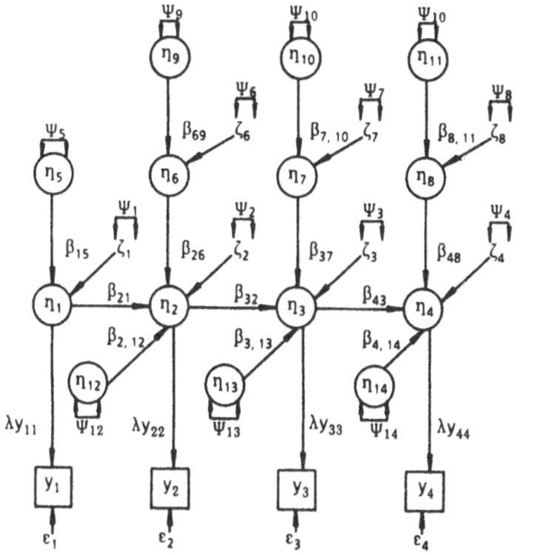

The "New Model" implies (in LISREL terms) the following restrictions:

1. $\lambda y_{11} = \lambda y_{22} = \lambda y_{33} = \lambda y_{44} = 1.0$
2. $\beta_{21} = \beta_{26}$
3. $\beta_{32} = \beta_{37}$
4. $\beta_{43} = \beta_{48}$
5. $\beta_{15} = \beta_{69} = \beta_{7,10} = \beta_{8,11} = \beta_{2,12} = \beta_{3,13} = \beta_{4,14}$
6. $\psi_1 = \psi_2 = \psi_3 = \psi_4 = \psi_6 = \psi_7 = \psi_8 = 0.0$
7. $\psi_5 = \psi_{12} = \psi_{13} = \psi_{14} = 1.0$
8. $\psi_9 = \psi_{10} = \psi_{11} = \underline{-1.0}$

These restrictions lead to the following variances:

$$
\begin{aligned}
V(\eta_1) &= \underline{\beta^2{}_{15}}(*1.0)\\
V(\eta_2) &= \beta^2{}_{21}(\beta^2{}_{15}*1.0) + \beta^2{}_{2,12}(*1.0) + \beta^2{}_{26}(\beta^2{}_{69}*(-1.0))\\
&= \beta^2{}_{21}(\beta^2{}_{15}) + \beta^2{}_{15} - (\beta^2{}_{21}(\beta^2{}_{15})) = \underline{\beta^2{}_{15}}\\
V(\eta_3) &= \beta^2{}_{32}(\beta^2{}_{15}*1.0) + \beta^2{}_{3,13}(*1.0) + \beta^2{}_{37}(\beta^2{}_{7,10}*(-1.0))\\
&= \beta^2{}_{32}(\beta^2{}_{15}) + \beta^2{}_{15} - (\beta^2{}_{32}(\beta^2{}_{15})) = \underline{\beta^2{}_{15}}\\
V(\eta_4) &= \beta^2{}_{43}(\beta^2{}_{15}*1.0) + \beta^2{}_{4,14}(*1.0) + \beta^2{}_{48}(\beta^2{}_{8,11}*(-1.0))\\
&= \beta^2{}_{43}(\beta^2{}_{15}) + \beta^2{}_{15} - (\beta^2{}_{43}(\beta^2{}_{15})) = \underline{\beta^2{}_{15}}
\end{aligned}
$$

The equality constraints

$$
\begin{aligned}
&\beta_{15} = \beta_{2,12} = \beta_{3,13} = \beta_{4,14} = a\\
&\beta_{21} = \beta_{32} = \beta_{43} = b\\
V(\varepsilon_1) = &V(\varepsilon_2) = V(\varepsilon_3) = V(\varepsilon_4) = c^2
\end{aligned}
$$

imply

$$
\begin{aligned}
V(\eta_1) &= V(\eta_2) = V(\eta_3) = V(\eta_4) = a^2\\
\mathrm{cov}(\eta_1\eta_2) &= \mathrm{cov}(\eta_2\eta_3) = \mathrm{cov}(\eta_3\eta_4) = a^2b
\end{aligned}
$$

This leads to <u>equal</u> reliabilities and to equal stabilities

$\mathrm{rel}_i = a^2/(a^2 + c^2)$, for all $i = 1, \ldots, 4$

$\rho_{ij} = a^2 b/(a^2a^2)^{1/2} = b$, for all $i = 1, \ldots, 3,\ j = i + 1$

ACKNOWLEDGEMENTS

Preparation of this chapter was facilitated by a German Research Foundation Grant RU 339/2-1. The first author is grateful to Peter M. Bentler, John R. Nesselroade, Wolfgang Schneider, and Phil K. Wood for providing insightful comments on earlier drafts of parts of this chapter. We wish to express our deep appreciation to Jane Janser for her invaluable assistance and helpful support in preparing this chapter.

REFERENCES

Anderson, T. W. (1960). Some stochastic process models for intelligence test scores. In K. J. Arrow, S. Karlin & P. Suppes (eds.), *Mathematical methods in the social sciences* (pp. 205–220). Stanford, CA: Stanford University Press.

Andres, J. (1986). *Analyse von Kovarianzmatrizen mit LISREL* (Bonner Methoden-Berichte, 5 (1)) University of Bonn, Dept of Psychology.

Andres, J. (1990). *Grundlagen linearer Strukturgleichungsmodelle.* Frankfurt: Lang.

Baltes, P. B., Cornelius, S. W., Spiro, A. H., Nesselroade, J. R. & Willis, S. L. (1980). Integration vs. differentiation of fluid-crystallized intelligence in old age. *Developmental Psychology, 16,* 625–635.

Bentler, P. M. (1973). Assessment of the development factor change at the individual level. In J. R. Nesselroade & H. W. Reese (eds)., *Life-span developmental psychology: Methodological issues* (pp. 145–174). New York/London: Academic Press.

Bentler, P. M. (1980). Multivariate analysis with latent variables: Causal models. *Annual Review of Psychologly, 31,* 419–456.

Bentler, P. M. (1984). Structural equation models in longitudinal research. In S. A. Mednick, M. Harway & K. W. Finello (eds.), *Handbook of longitudinal research,* (vol. 1, pp. 88–105). New York: Praeger.

Bentler, P. M. (1968*a*). Structural modeling and Psychometrika: A historical perspective on growth and achievements. *Psychometrika, 51,* 35–51.

Bentler, P. M. (1986*b*). *Theory and Implementation of EQS: A structural equations program.* Los Angeles: BMDP Statistical Software.

Bentler, P. M. (1988). Causal modeling via structural equation system. In J. Nesselroade & R. B. Cattell (eds.), *Handbook of multivariate experimental psychology.* New York: Plenum.

Birren, J. E., Cunningham, W. R. & Yamamoto, K. (1983). Psychology of adult development and aging. *Annual Review of Psychology, 34,* 543–575.

Botwinick, J. (1977). Intellectual abilities. In J. E. Birren & K. W. Schaie (eds.), *Handbook of the psychology of aging.* New York: Van Nostrand-Reinhold.

Buss, A. R. (1979). Toward a unified framework for psychometric concepts in the multivariate developmental situation: Intraindividual change and inter- and intraindividual differences. In J. R. Nesselroade & P. B. Baltes (eds.), *Longitudinal research and the study of behavior and development* (pp. 41–59). New York: Academic Press.

Cattell, R. B. (1963). Theory of fluid and crystallized intelligence: a critical experiment. *Journal of Educational Psychology, 54,* 1–22.

Cattell, R. B. (1986). Fluid and crystallized intelligence. *Psychology Today, 3,* 56–62.

Cliff, N. (1983). Some cautions concerning the application of causal modelling. *Multivariate Behavioral Research, 18,* 115–126.

Cornelius, S. W. (1984). Classic pattern of intellectual aging: Test familiarity, difficulty, and performance. *Journal of Gerontology, 39,* 201–206.

Cronbach, L. J. (1967). Year to year correlations of mental tests: A review of the Hofstätter analysis. *Child Development, 38,* 283–289.

Cunningham, W. R. (1978). Principles for identifying structural differences: Some methodological issues related to comparative factor analysis. *Journal of Gerontology, 33,* 82–86.

Cunningham, W. R. (1980*a*). Age comparative factor analysis of ability variables in adulthood and old age. *Intelligence, 4,* 133–149.

Cunningham, W. R. (1980*b*). Speed, age, and qualitative differences in cognitive functioning. In L. W. Poon (ed.), *Aging in the 1980's: Selected contemporary issues in the psychology of aging.* Washington, DC: American Psychological Association.

Cunningham, W. R. (1981). Ability factor structure differences in adulthood and old age. *Multivariate Behaviour Research, 16,* 3–22.

Cunningham, W. R. & Birren, J. E. (1980). Age changes in the factor structure of intellectual abilities in adulthood and old age. *Educational and Psychological Measurement, 40,* 271–290.

Dommel, N. & Rudinger, G. (1986). *Simplex analyses of longitudinal intelligence data.* Bonner Methoden-Berichte, 3(1), Universität Bonn.

Ecob, R. (1987*a*). Applications of structural equation modelling to longitudinal educational data. In P. Cuttance & R. Ecob (eds.), *Structural modelling by example: Applications in educational, behavioral, and social research.* Cambridge University Press.

Ecob, R. (1987*b*). Issues and problems in the application of structural modelling. In P. Cuttance & R. Ecob (eds.), *Structural modelling by example: Applications in educational, behavioral, and social research.* Cambridge University Press.

Frederiksen, C. H. & Rotondo, J. A. (1979). Time-series models and the study of longitudinal change. In J. R. Nesselroade & P. B. Baltes (eds.), *Longitudinal research and the study of behavior and development* (pp. 61–87). New York: Academic Press.

Guire, K. E. & Kowalski, C. J. (1979). Mathematical description and representation of developmental change functions on the intra- and interindividual levels. In J. R. Nesselroade & P. B. Baltes (eds.), *Longitudinal research in the study of behavior and development* (pp. 89–110). New York/London: Academic Press.

Guttman, L. A. (1954). A new approach to factor analysis: The radex. In P. F. Lazarsfeld (ed.), *Mathematical thinking in the social sciences* (pp. 258–348). Glencoe, Ill: The Free Press.

Guttman, L. A. (1955). A generalized simplex for factor analysis. *Psychometrika, 20,* 173–191.

Hayduk, L. A. (1988). *Structural equation modelling with LISREL: Essentials and advances.* Baltimore: The Johns Hopkins University Press.

Heise, D. R. (1969). Separating reliability and stability in test–retest correlation. *American Sociological Review, 34,* 93–101.

Hertzog, C. (1987). On the utility of structural regression models for developmental research. In P. B. Baltes, D. Featherman & R. M. Lerner (eds.), *Life-span development and behavior.* Hillsdale, NJ: Erlbaum.

Hertzog, C. & Nesselroade, J. R. (1987). Beyond autoregressive models: Some implications of the trait-state distinction for the structural modeling of developmental change. *Child Development, 58*(1), 93–109.

Hertzog, C. & Schaie, K. W. (1986). Stability and change in adult intelligence: I. Analysis of longitudinal covariance structures. *Psychology and Aging 1*(2), 159–171.

Hofstätter, P. R. (1954). The changing composition of intelligence: A study in T-technique. *Journal of Genetic Psychology, 85,* 159–164.

Horn, J. L. (1960). Integration of structural and developmental concepts in the theory of fluid and crystallized intelligence. In R. B. Cattell (ed.), *Handbook of multivariate experimental psychology.* Chicago: Rand McNally.

Horn, J. L. (1982). The aging of human abilities. In B. B. Wolman (ed.), *Handbook of developmental psychology.* Englewood Cliffs, NJ: Prentice Hall.

Horn, J. L. & Cattell, R. B. (1966). Refinement and test of the theory of fluid and crystallized general intelligences. *Journal of Educational Psychology, 57,* 253–270.

Horn, J. L. & McArdle, J. J. (1980). Perspectives on mathematical/statistical model building (MASMOB) in aging research. In L. W. Poon (ed.), *Aging in the 1980's* (pp. 503–541). Washington, DC: American Psychological Association.

Humphreys, L. G. & Parsons, C. K. (1979). A simplex process model for describing differences between cross-lagged correlations. *Psychological Bulletin, 86,* 325–334.

Jagodzinski, W. & Kühnel, S. M. (1987). Estimation of reliability and stability in single-indicator multiple-wave models. *Sociological Methods and Research, 15,* 219–258.

Jöreskog, K. G. (1970). Estimation and testing of simplex models. *British Journal of Mathematical and Statistical Psychology, 23,* 121–145.

Jöreskog, K. G. (1974). Analyzing psychological data by structural analysis of covariance matrices. In D. H. Krantz, R. C. Atkinson, R. D. Luce & P. Suppes (eds.), *Contemporary developments in mathematical psychology: Measurement, psychophysics, and neural information processing* (Vol. 2, pp. 1–55). San Francisco: W. H. Freeman.

Jöreskog, K. G. (1979). Statistical estimation of structural models in longitudinal developmental investigations. In J. R. Nesselroade & P. B. Baltes (eds.), *Longitudinal research in the study of behavior and development* (pp. 303–351). New York: Academic Press.

Jöreskog, K. G & Sörbom, D. (1976). Statistical models and methods for test-retest situations. In D. N. M. de Gruijter & L. J. Th. van der Kamp (eds.), *Advances in psychological and educational measurement* (pp. 135–157). New York: Wiley.

Jöreskog, K. G. & Sörbom, D. (1977). Statistical models and methods for analysis of longitudinal data. In D. J. Aigner & A. S. Goldberger (eds.), *Latent variables in socio-economic models* (pp. 285–325). Amsterdam: North-Holland Publishing Co.

Jöreskog, K. G. & Sörbom, D. (1985). Simultaneous analysis of longitudinal data from several cohorts. In W. M. Mason & S. E. Fienberg (eds.), *Cohort analysis in social research: Beyond the identification problem* (pp. 323–341). New York: Springer-Verlag.

Jöreskog, K. G. & Sörbom, D. (1988). *LISREL VII – A guide to the program and applications.* Chicago, Ill: SPSS Inc.

Labouvie, E. W. (1980). Identity versus equivalence of psychological measures and constructs. In L. W. Poon (ed.), *Aging in the 1980's: Selected contemporary issues in the psychology of aging.* Washington, DC: American Psychological Association.

Long, J. S. (1983*a*). *Confirmatory factor analysis: A preface to LISREL.* Beverly Hills: Sage.

Long, J. S. (1983*b*). *Covariance structure models: An introduction to LISREL.* Beverly Hills: Sage.

McArdle, J. J. (1988). Dynamic but structural equation modeling of repeated measures data. In J. R. Nesselroade & R. B. Cattell (eds.), *The handbook of multivariate experimental psychology.* New York: Plenum Press.

McArdle, J. J. & Epstein, D. (1987). Latent growth curves within developmental structural equation models. *Child Development, 58,* 110–133.

Molenaar, P C. M. (1985). A dynamic factor model for the analysis of multivariate time series. *Psychometrika, 50,* 181–202.

Nesselroade, J. R. (1977). Issues in studying developmental change in adults from a multivariate perspective. In J. E. Birren & K. W. Schaie (eds.), *Handbook of the psychology of aging* (pp. 59–69). New York: Van Nostrand-Reinhold.

Nesselroade, J. R. & Baltes, P. B. (eds.). (1979). *Longitudinal research in the study of behavior and development.* New York: Academic Press.

Nesselroade, J. R. & Bartsch, T. W. (1977). Multivariate perspectives on the construct validity of the trait-state distinction. In R. B. Cattell & R. M. Dreger (eds.), *Handbook of modern personality theory.* New York: Wiley.

Olsson, U. & Bergman, L. R. (1977). A longitudinal factor model for studying change in ability structure. *Multivariate Behavioral Research, 12,* 221–242.

Rindskopf, D. M. (1983). Parameterizing inequality constraints on unique variances in linear structural equation models. *Psychometrika, 48,* 73–83.

Rindskopf, D. M. (1984). Using phantom and imaginary latent variables to parameterize constraints in linear structural models. *Psychometrika, 49,* 37–47.

Rogosa, D. (1979). Causal models in longitudinal research: rationale, formulation, and interpretation. In J. R. Nesselroade & P. B. Baltes (eds.), *Longitudinal research in the study of behavior and development* (pp. 263–302). New York: Academic Press.

Rogosa, D. & Willett, J. D. (1985). Understanding correlates of change by modeling individual differences in growth. *Psychometrika, 50,* 203–228.

Rogosa, D., Brandt, D. & Zimowski, M. (1982). A growth curve approach to the measurement of change. *Psychological Bulletin, 90,* 726–748.

Roskam, E. E. (1976). Multivariate analysis of change and growth: A critical review. In D. N. M. de Gruijter & L. J. Th. van der Kamp (eds.), *Advances in psychological and educational measurement* (pp. 111–134). London: Wiley.

Rietz, C. (1988). Latente Wachstumskurven: Theorie und empirische Studien am Beispiel der Intelligenzentwicklung im Alter. Diploma Thesis, University of Bonn.

Rudinger, G. (1985*a*). Struktur-Analysen. In T. Hermann & E.-D. Lantermann (eds.), *Persönlichkeitspsychologie – Ein Handbuch in Schlüsselbegriffen.* München: Urban & Schwarzenberg.

Rudinger, G. (1985*b*). Prozeß-Analysen. In T. Herrmann & E.-D. Lantermann (eds.), *Persönlichkeitspsychologie – Ein Handbuch in Schlüsselbegriffen.* München: Urban & Schwarzenberg.

Rudinger, G. (1985*c*). intelligence in a longitudinal perspective. In J. M. A. Munnichs, P. Mussen & P. G. Coleman (eds.), *Life-span and change in a gerontological perspective* (pp. 63–74). New York: Academic Press.

Rudinger, G. (1988). *Methodological issues in analyzing special populations.* Paper presented at the 22nd International Congress of Psychology, Sydney, August 28–September 3, 1988.

Rudinger, G. & Rietz, C. (1987). Intelligenzentwicklung über einen Zeitraum von 35 Jahren. Paper presented at 8. Deutsche Tagung fuer Entwicklungspsychologie, September 13–16, 1987, Bern.

Rudinger, G. & Rietz, C. (1988*a*). Stability and reliability of developmental phenomena. Poster presented at the 5th Australian Developmental Conference, Sydney, August 25–27, 1988.

Rudinger, G. & Rietz, C. (1988*b*). *Testing hypotheses about stability and reliability in autoregressive models by linear structure equation techniques.* Bonner Methodenberichte, 5(2). Universität Bonn.

Rudinger, G. & Wood, P. K. (1989). *N's times, and number of variables in longitudinal research.* In D. Magnusson & L. Bergman (eds.), *Longitudinal research: Quality of data.* New York: Cambridge University Press.

Rudinger, G., Andres, J. & Rietz, C. (1986). Structures of change and changes of structure in longitudinal designs. Paper presented at the International Conference on Longitudinal Methodology: Budapest.

Rudinger, G., Andres, J., Rietz, C. & Schneider, W. (1989). Structural equation models for studying intellectual development. Paper presented at the European Science Foundation's 2nd workshop on methodological issues in longitudinal research 'Stability and change: Methods and models for data treatment.. Soria Moria, Norway, April 1989.

Saris, W. E. & Stronkhorst, L. H. (1984). *Causal modelling in non-experimental reserach.* Amsterdam: Sociometric Research Foundation.

Schaie, K. W. (1979). The primary mental abilities in adulthood: An exploration in the development of psychometric intelligence. In P. B. Baltes & O. G. Brim, jr (eds.), *Life-span development and behavior* (vol. 2). New York: Academic Press.

Schaie, K. W. & Hertzog, C. (1982). Longitudinal methods. In B. B. Wolman (ed.), *Handbook of developmental psychology* (pp. 91–115). Englewood Cliffs, NJ: Prentice Hall.

Schaie, K. W. & Hertzog, C. (1983). Fourteen-year cohort-sequential analyses of adult intellecutal development. *Developmental Psychology, 19*, 531–543.

Schaie, K. W. & Hertzog, C. (1985). Measurement in the psychology of adulthood and aging. In J. E. Birren & K. W. Schaie (eds.), *Handbook of the psychology of aging* (2nd edn, pp. 61–92). New York: Van Nostrand Reinhold.

Schaie, K. W. & Hertzog, C. (1986). Toward a comprehensive model of adult intellectual development: Contributions of the Seattle Longitudinal Study. In R. J. Sternberg (ed.), *Advances in human intelligence*, (Vol. 3, pp. 79–118). Hillsdale, NJ: Erlbaum.

Sörbom, D. (1976). A statistical model for the measurement of change in true scores. In D. N. M. de Gruijter & J. L. Th. van der Kamp (eds.), *Advances in psychological and educational measurement* (pp. 159–169). New York: Wiley.

Sörbom, D. (1982). Structural equation models with structured means. In K. G. Jöreskog & H. Wold (eds.), *Systems under indirect observation: Causality, structure and observation* (pp. 183–195). Amsterdam: North-Holland Publ. Co.

Weeks, D. G. A. (1980). A second order longitudinal model of ability structure. *Multivariate Behavioral Research, 15*, 353–365.

Werts, C. E. & Linn, R. L. (1970). A general linear model for studying growth. *Psychological Bulletin, 73*, 17–22.

Werts, C. E., Jöreskog, K. G. & Linn, R. L. (1971). Comment on 'The estimation of measurement error in panel data'. *American Sociological Review, 36*, 110–115.

Werts, C. E., Linn, R. L. & Jöreskog, K. G. (1977). A simplex model for analyzing academic growth. *Educational and Psychological Measurement, 37*, 745–756.

Werts, C. E., Linn, R. L. & Jöreskog, K. G. (1978). Reliability of college grades from longitudinal data. *Educational Psychological Measurement, 38*, 89–95.

Wheaton, B., Muthén, B., Alwin, D. & Summers, G. (1978). Assessing reliability and stability in panel models. In D. R. Heise (ed.), *Sociological methodology* (pp. 84–136). San Francisco: Jossey-Bass.

Wiley, D. E. & Wiley, J. A. (1970). The estimation of measurement error in panel data. *American Sociological Review, 35*, 112–117.

Wohlwill, J. F. (1973). The study of behavioral developmental. New York: Academic Press.

14 Longitudinal studies for discrete data based on latent structure models

ERLING B. ANDERSEN

INTRODUCTION

This chapter is intended to be partly an exposition of some selected discrete data models for longitudinal data, and partly an illustration of their applicability. It is not the intention to give a complete survey of existing models, and the list of references is not complete in any sense. The interested reader will, however, by consulting one or more of the listed references, quickly be guided into the literature on the subject.

Firstly, two data examples are presented. Secondly, a number of latent structure models are presented with emphasis on model structures and very little on the more technical aspects such as estimation methods, test statistics and numerical procedures. Thirdly, the given models are applied to the two examples.

TWO DATA SETS

Longitudinal data are data where individual characteristics or individual responses are observed for the same individuals at various points in time. In this chapter, we shall, for ease of presentation, limit ourselves to two and three time points.

Data set 1 is presented in Table 14.1. The table shows the observed score on a psychiatric questionnaire with 12 items. The score was observed for 1460 individuals in 1974 and again in 1978. The table shows the observed frequencies of the joint observed score (i, j) where i is the score in 1974 and j the score in 1978.

The problem under study in Table 14.1 is the change in the individual psychiatric vulnerability between 1974 and 1978.

Data set 2 is presented in Table 14.2. A Danish Survey Company carried out three consecutive polls, two before the time in 1972 when Denmark joined the EEC, and one after. The polls were taken in August 1971, October 1971 and December 1973. On each occasion the interviewed persons were asked whether they would vote for or against Danish membership of the EEC, or if they were still undecided. Table

Table 14.1. *Joint score distribution for a psychiatric questionnaire with 12 items, observed for 1460 individuals in 1974 and again in 1978*

Score 1976	1978 score (j)													
(i)	0	1	2	3	4	5	6	7	8	9	10	11	12	*Total*
0	137	60	32	27	8	0	0	0	3	3	2	0	0	272
1	58	78	38	16	19	6	3	3	0	0	0	0	0	221
2	39	29	43	29	13	19	10	10	0	0	0	0	0	192
3	17	24	27	19	35	20	13	1	5	1	0	0	0	162
4	13	14	22	23	30	30	14	9	4	6	2	0	0	167
5	6	9	17	20	29	22	22	13	3	5	2	0	0	148
6	2	4	6	14	18	21	19	11	7	3	3	2	0	110
7	1	2	3	6	7	19	16	10	6	5	2	2	0	79
8	1	1	1	3	5	6	6	5	5	3	1	1	0	38
9	0	0	1	1	2	2	4	10	1	8	5	1	0	35
10	0	1	1	1	0	2	2	3	2	1	6	3	1	23
11	0	0	0	2	0	0	2	4	0	0	0	2	1	11
12	0	0	0	2	0	0	0	0	0	0	0	0	0	2
Total	274	222	191	163	166	147	111	79	36	35	23	11	2	1460

Note: For technical reasons the 1978 data are adjusted to have about the same marginals as the 1976 data. See Andersen (1985) for more details.

Table 14.2. *The observed responses for a sample of 493 persons, who were asked on three occasions whether they would vote for Danish membership of the EEC*

		December 1973		
August 1971	October 1971	Yes	No	Undecided
Yes	Yes	148	15	13
	No	2	30	1
	Undecided	20	15	5
No	Yes	11	9	1
	No	14	73	7
	Undecided	9	21	2
Undecided	Yes	8	12	1
	No	3	28	2
	Undecided	16	14	13

14.2 shows the number of persons observed for each of the 27 possible response patterns. The problem is here to describe the way the sample (and, if representative, accordingly the population) has changed its view on Danish membership of the EEC between August 1971 and December 1973.

A LATENT STRUCTURE MODEL

Many longitudinal data sets in psychology, education and psychiatry look like Table 14.1. The observed data for an individual at a given point in time is the score on an attitude or attainment test or on a rating scale. Such score data are often described by a suitable latent trait model, where the observed score is the empirical measurement of an unobservable latent variable. If we limit ourselves to two points in time, such a latent trait model is visualized in Figure 14.1. As the same people are observed at both time points, we must allow for a correlation between the results at the two time points. This correlation is very much in evidence in Table 14.1. We shall assume, however, that the correlation between the scores can be adequately described by a correlation between the values of the latent variables at the two time points. This assumption is indicated in Figure 14.1 by a correlation ρ between the values θ_1 and θ_2 of the latent variables, while the observed scores r_1 and r_2 are only correlated through their dependencies on θ_1 and θ_2. In order to formulate a statistical model for the data, we then only need to specify statistical models for the three links in Figure 14.1, i.e. for the joint distribution of θ_1 and θ_2, for the distribution of r_1 given θ_1 and for the distribution of r_2 given θ_2.

In Figure 14.1, the assumed models are indicated by the symbols $N_2(\theta_1, \theta_2)$ for a two-dimensional normal distribution and $R(r \mid \theta)$ for a Rasch model. The parameters of the complete model are accordingly

$$
\begin{aligned}
N_2(\theta_1, \theta_2):\quad & E[\theta_1] = \mu_1 \\
& E[\theta_2] = \mu_2 \\
& \mathrm{var}[\theta_1] = \sigma_1^2 \\
& \mathrm{var}[\theta_2] = \sigma_2^2 \\
& \mathrm{corr}(\theta_1, \theta_2) = \rho. \\
R(r_1 \mid \theta_1):\quad & \text{Item difficulties } \alpha_{11}, \ldots, \alpha_{1k}. \\
R(r_2 \mid \theta_2):\quad & \text{Item difficulties } \alpha_{21}, \ldots, \alpha_{2k}.
\end{aligned}
$$

Here k is the number of items in the test.

It is obvious that the parameter of primary interest is the correlation coefficient ρ between θ_1 and θ_2, since ρ measures the extent to which there is a connection between the responses at time 1 and time 2. If

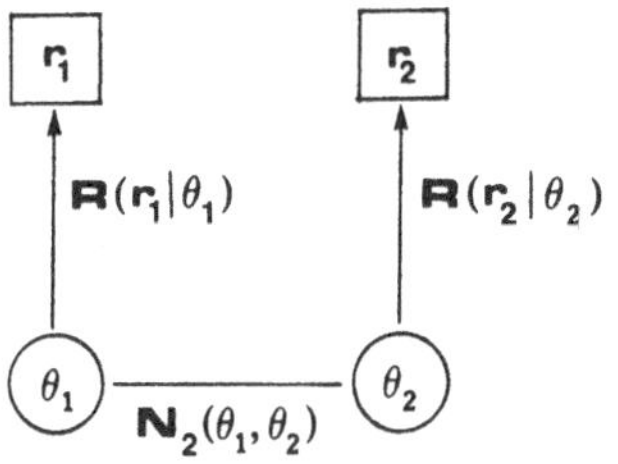

Figure 14.1. Diagram of a latent structure model with correlated latent variables.

$\rho = 0$ the responses are independent, while if $\rho = 1$ the values of the individual latent variables have not changed and differences between the responses at time 1 and time 2 are due to the random variation inherent in the Rasch model, not to a change in latent attitude.

We shall not go into technical details with the statistical methods necessary for estimating the parameters and evaluating the fit of the model. The analysis can be summarized in points 1–3 below.

1. The item parameters of the two Rasch models are estimated in the usual way (see Andersen, 1980: Ch. 6 or Andersen, 1990: Ch. 12).
2. The parameters of the normal latent distribution $N(\theta_1, \theta_2)$ are estimated as described in Andersen (1985). In principle the method is to formulate a parametric multinomial model for the joint score distribution $f(r_1, r_2)$; $r_1 = 1, \ldots, k$, $r_2 = 1, \ldots, k$, of which μ_1, μ_2, σ_1^2, σ_1^2 and ρ are parameters and then apply the maximum likelihood method to this distribution.
3. The fit of the model is evaluated based on the parametric multinomial model described point 2. Thus if

$$\pi(r_1, r_2) = \text{probability of observed joint scores } r_1 \text{ and } r_2$$

and

$$x(r_1, r_2) = \text{observed number of joint scores } r_1 \text{ and } r_2,$$

the goodness-of-fit test statistic is

$$Q = 2 \sum_{r_1} \sum_{r_2} (x(r_1, r_2) - n\hat{\pi}(r_1, r_2))^2 / (n\hat{\pi}(r_1, r_2))$$

where $\hat{\pi}$ is the value of π with the maximum likelihood estimates of the parameters inserted.

Table 14.3. *Parameter estimates for data set 1*

Item (j)		Difficulty α_j
1		1.19
2		0.92
3		−1.26
4		−0.85
5		−1.64
6		0.67
7		0.50
8		0.28
9		−0.34
10		−0.48
11		0.00
12		−1.00
Time point	Mean	Variance
1	−1.5	2.2
2	−1.5	2.2
Correlation	0.856	

ANALYSIS OF DATA SET 1

For data set 1, the parameter estimates are summarized in Table 14.3. It is no coincidence that $\hat{\mu}_1 = \hat{\mu}_2$ and $\sigma_1^2 = \sigma_2^2$. In fact a special selection of the sample at time point 2 was used, which was based on the score r_1 at time point 1. Hence the data shown in Table 14.1 are those obtained after adjustment has been made for the special selection procedure. It is a side effect of this procedure that $\hat{\mu}_1 = \hat{\mu}_2$ and $\sigma_1^2 = \hat{\sigma}_2^2$. More details are given in Andersen (1985). The analysis of Table 14.1 thus reveals that there is correlation of about 85% between the values of the latent variables at time points 1 and 2. It is important to stress that it is a population correlation, such that a correct interpretation of the number $\hat{\rho} = 0.856$ is that the values of θ_1 and θ_2 vary in the given population according to a two-dimensional normal distribution with correlation coefficient 0.856. Figure 14.2 shows the 95% contour ellipse of such a distribution. Thus with probability 0.95 the values of θ_1 and θ_2 for a randomly chosen person from the given population will fall within the shown ellipse.

It is also important to stress that a latent correlation is generally larger than the correlation between the observed scores, since the latter also accounts for the random variability in the Rasch model. For the numbers in Table 14.1, the empirical correlation between r_1 and r_2 is 0.645, i.e. more than 20% lower than the latent correlation.

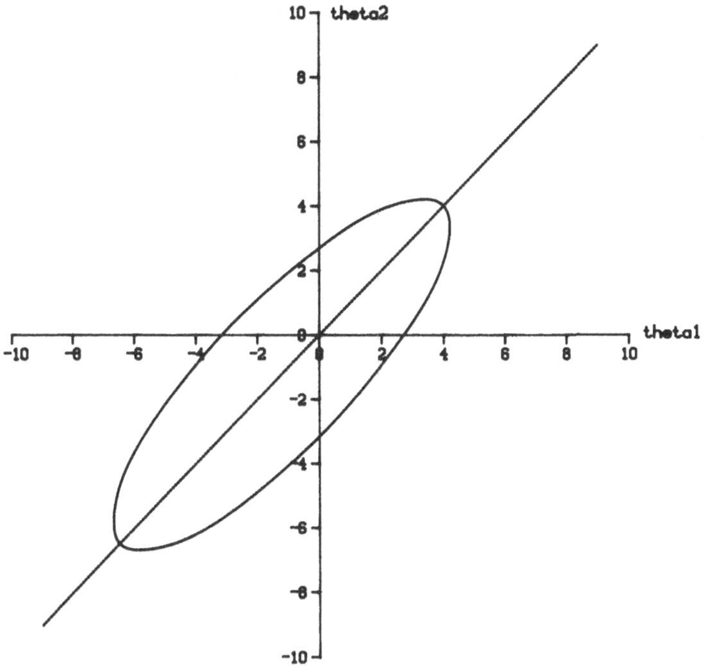

Figure 14.2. The 95% contour elipse for a two-dimensional normal distribution with $\mu_1 = \mu_2 = -1.1$, $\sigma_1^2 = \sigma_2^2 = 2.2$ and $\rho = 0.856$.

LATENT CLASS MODELS

In the model described on page 310 and applied on page 312, the latent variable had a variation in the population that was described by a continuous probability distribution. In order to estimate the parameters of such continuous latent distributions it is necessary to make rather detailed assumptions about the distribution of the observed variable. Thus in the analysis on page 312, the probability distribution of the score r given latent variable θ was assumed to be a Rasch model. Parameterwise the Rasch model is a model with a very simple structure. For latent class models such restrictive model assumptions are not imposed on the probability distribution of the observed response. It is then necessary, however, to make rather strong and in fact unrealistic assumptions about the distribution of the latent variable in the population. The basic assumption of latent class analysis is that any individual in the population belongs to one of a few **latent classes.** Within a latent class all individuals have the same value of the latent variable. The parameters of a latent class model are thus the latent class frequencies, and the conditional probabilities of the response, given the latent class.

In order to describe specific latent class models for longitudinal data, we consider a very simple situation, where a categorical variable is observed at three points in time for a sample of n individuals. To make the notation as simple as possible we denote the variable observed at time point 1 variable A, while B and C are the variables observed at time points 2 and 3. The observed responses at time points 1, 2 and 3 are denoted i, j and k, where each variable has I categories. In Table 14.2, variable A is thus the response in August 1971, variable B is the response in October 1971 and variable C the response in December 1973. The number of categories in Table 14.2 is $I = 3$ and $i = 1$, $j = 1$, $k = 1$ if an individual has answered yes on all three occasions.

The observed data are thus x_{ijk}, $i = 1, \ldots, I$, $j = 1, \ldots, I$, $k = 1, \ldots, I$, where

$$x_{ijk} = \text{number of individuals with response } (ijk).$$

We must then formulate a model for

$$\pi_{ijk} = \text{probability of response } (ijk) \text{ for a random individual.}$$

Suppose now that there are M latent classes. We can then formulate the basic latent class model as

$$\pi_{ijk}^{ABC} = \sum_{m=1}^{M} \pi_{im}^{A} \pi_{ijm}^{AB} \pi_{jkm}^{BC} \varphi_m, \tag{1}$$

where the parameters have the following interpretations

(a) φ_m = frequency of individuals in latent class m.

(b) π_{im}^{A} = probability of response i at time 1 for an individual in latent class m.

(c) π_{ijm}^{AB} = probability of response j at time 2 given response i at time 1 for an individual in latent class m.

(d) π_{jkm}^{BC} = probability of response k at time 3 given response j at time 2 for an individual in latent class m.

Formula (1) expresses that, if attention is restricted to individuals within a latent class, then the probability π_{ijk} of response (ijk) follows the probability law

$$\begin{aligned}\pi_{ijk} &= P(A = i, B = j, C = k)\\ &= P(A = i)P(B = j \mid A = i)P(C = k \mid B = j)\end{aligned}$$

provided an individual response only depends on his or her response at the previous time point. The basic assumption of a latent class model is thus that response probabilities only vary within a population, when we cross a line between latent classes. The latent class model is illustrated in Figure 14.3.

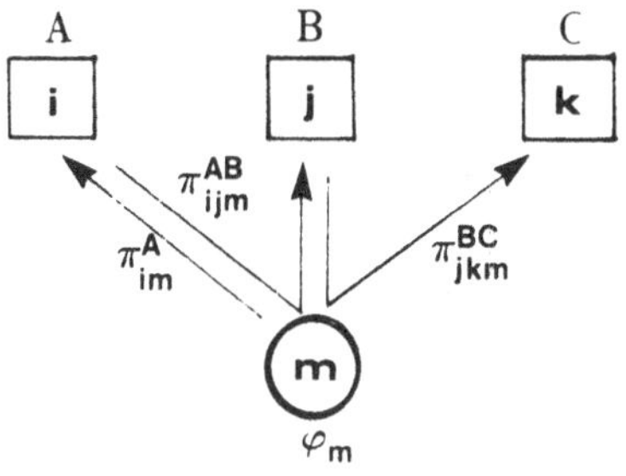

Figure 14.3. Diagram of latent class model.

In Markov chain language, one would denote the π^A_{im}s as initial probabilities and the π^{AB}_{ijm}s and π^{BC}_{jkm} as transition probabilities. It is not possible to estimate the parameters of model (1) without making further assumptions. We shall consider three special cases denoted models I, II and III. For the three models the parameters of (1) are restricted in the following way:

Model I: (i) $m = (m_1, m_2)$

(ii) $\pi^A_{im} = \pi^A_i$

(iii) $\pi^{AB}_{ijm} = \pi^B_{jm_1}$

(iv) $\pi^{BC}_{jkm} = \pi^C_{km_2}$

(v) $\varphi_m = \varphi_{m_1m_2}$

Model II: (i) $\pi^{AB}_{ijm} = \pi^B_{jm}$

(ii) $\pi^{BC}_{jkm} = \pi^C_{km}$

Model III: (i) $m = (m_1, m_2, m_3)$

(ii) $\pi^A_{im} = \pi^A_{im_1}$

(iii) $\pi^{AB}_{ijm} = \pi^B_{jm_2}$

(iv) $\pi^{BC}_{jkm} = \pi^C_{km_3}$

(v) $\varphi_m = \varphi^A_{m_1}\varphi^{AB}_{m_1m_2}\varphi^{BC}_{m_2m_3}$

The three models are illustrated in Figure 14.4.

Much of the literature on application of latent class models to longitudinal data is relatively recent. According to Clogg (1979), who applied latent class models to mobility tables, the idea was advocated by Boudon (1972, 1973). The famous reanalysis of the Coleman data by Goodman (1974) is an early example of a latent class model applied to longitudinal data. But also in the fundamental book by Lazarsfeld & Henry (1968) there is an application of a latent class model to longitudinal data. Important recent contributions are a series of papers by Clogg & Goodman (1984, 1985, 1986) and by Langeheine (1988). Within marketing research there seems to be a special interest in the

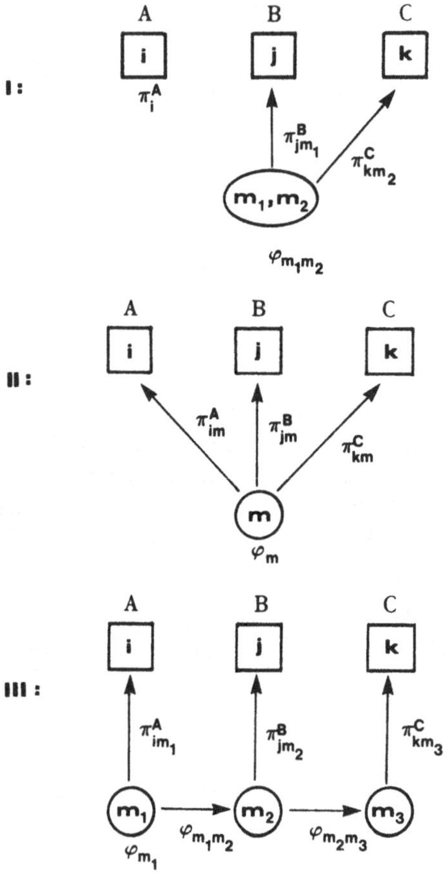

Figure 14.4.

application of latent class models to brand choice theory. Selected references are Green, Carmone & Wachspress (1977), Madden & Dillon (1982) and Poulsen (1982, in press).

As for the model on page 314, we shall not go into details with the statistical methods for latent class analysis. The estimation of the parameters is carried out by means of the so-called EM-algorithm, developed by Dempster, Laird & Rubin (1977), but first proposed for latent class analysis by Goodman (1974).

The goodness-of-fit of a latent class model is evaluated by means of the Q-test statistic

$$Q = \sum_{ijk} (x_{ijk} - n\hat{\pi}_{ijk})^2 / (n\hat{\pi}_{ijk}),$$

where $\hat{\pi}_{ijk}$ is given by (1) with the maximum likelihood estimates of the model parameters inserted. Q is approximately chi-square distributed with I^3-1-q degrees of freedom, where q is the number of unrestricted parameters under the model. For models I, II and III, the values of q and the degrees of freedom are:

Model I: $q=(I-1)(1+M_1+M_2)+M_1M_2-1$
$\text{d.f.}=I^3-I(M_1+M_2+1)-(M_1-1)(M_2-1)+2$

Model II: $q=3(I-1)M+M-1$
$\text{d.f.}=I^3-3IM+2M$

Model III: $q=(I-1)M+(M_1-1)+M_1(M_2-1)+M_2(M_3-1)$
$\text{d.f.}=I^3-(I-1)M-M_1M_2-M_2M_3+M_2,$

where $m_1=1,\ldots,M_1, m_2=1,\ldots,M_2,\ m_3=1,\ldots,M_3$ and $M=M_1+M_2+M_3$.

ANALYSIS OF DATA SET 2

We shall now apply models I, II and III to the data in Table 14.2.

It makes sense to try to apply a model with a latent variable to the data in Table 14.2, since the change in attitude towards the EEC may vary with the individuals. An analysis by a latent class model is thus an attempt to identify groups of persons, or *segments* (as is the commonly used phrase in marketing), which have similar change behavior. In order to ensure identifiability of the model in terms of the parameters, only a few classes can be identified for the numbers in Table 14.2. From the expressions for the degrees of freedom given above, it follows that, since $I=3$, the numbers M_1 and M_2 in model I must both be less than or equal to 3, yielding 9 latent classes. If, however, $M_1=M_2=3$, the number of parameters is 22 and there remains only 4 degrees of freedom to check the model. For $M_1=M_2=2$ where the model can be checked on 13 degrees of freedom, the number of latent classes is 4.

For model II, the number of latent classes M must be less than or equal to 3.

For model III, M_1 as well as M_2 and M_3 must be less than or equal to 2, yielding 8 latent classes, but at each time point a person's latent variable can only be at two levels. Without going into details we present in Tables 14.4 and 14.5 the results of the analysis of the data in Table 14.2, based on models I, III and II with m equal to 2 and 3. The two versions of model II are denoted II_2 and II_3.

Table 14.4 shows the estimates of the model parameters for all four models, while Table 14.5 shows the expected numbers and goodness-of-fit test statistics for the models. Clearly model I fits the data very badly.

Table 14.4. *Parameter estimates for models I, $II_2 II_3$ and III*

		Latent class			
		$m = 1$	2	3	4
Model I:		$(m_1, m_2) = (1, 1)$	(1, 2)	(2, 1)	(2, 2)
$\hat{\pi}^A_{im}$:	$i = 1$	0.438	0.438	0.438	0.438
	2	0.327	0.327	0.327	0.327
	3	0.235	0.235	0.235	0.235
$\hat{\pi}^B_{jm}$:	$j = 1$	0.057	0.057	0.575	0.575
	2	0.481	0.481	0.251	0.251
	3	0.462	0.462	0.174	0.174
$\hat{\pi}^C_{km}$:	$k = 1$	0.327	0.417	0.327	0.417
	2	0.347	0.536	0.347	0.536
	3	0.326	0.047	0.326	0.047
$\hat{\varphi}_m$:		0.091	0.157	0.073	0.679

Model II_2:		$m = 1$	2
$\hat{\pi}^A_{im}$:	$i = 1$	0.207	0.889
	2	0.492	0.049
	3	0.301	0.062
$\hat{\pi}^B_{jm}$:	$j = 1$	0.109	0.871
	2	0.577	0.000
	3	0.314	0.129
$\hat{\pi}^C_{km}$:	$k = 1$	0.165	0.859
	2	0.732	0.065
	3	0.103	0.076
$\hat{\varphi}_m$:		0.563	0.437

Model II_3:		$m = 1$	2	3
$\hat{\pi}^A_{im}$:	$i = 1$	0.303	0.210	0.937
	2	0.129	0.582	0.052
	3	0.568	0.208	0.011
$\hat{\pi}^B_{jm}$:	$j = 1$	0.262	0.088	0.931
	2	0.000	0.741	0.000
	3	0.738	0.171	0.069
$\hat{\pi}^C_{km}$:	$k = 1$	0.436	0.124	0.878
	2	0.332	0.819	0.058
	3	0.232	0.058	0.064
$\hat{\varphi}_m$:		0.179	0.438	0.383

Table 14.4. (*cont.*)

Model III:		$m_1 = 1$	2
$\hat{\pi}^A_{im_1}$:	$i = 1$	0.100	0.950
	2	0.562	0.009
	3	0.338	0.041
$\hat{\varphi}^A_{m_1}$:		0.523	0.477
		$m_2 = 1$	2
$\hat{\pi}^B_{jm_2}$:	$j = 1$	0.109	0.871
	2	0.577	0.000
	3	0.314	0.129
$\hat{\varphi}^{AB}_{m_1m_2}$:	$m_1 = 1$	0.939	0.061
	2	0.149	0.851
		$m_3 = 1$	2
$\hat{\pi}^C_{km_3}$:	$k = 1$	0.124	0.921
	2	0.771	0.005
	3	0.105	0.074
$\hat{\varphi}^{BC}_{m_2m_3}$:	$m_2 = 1$	0.948	0.052
	2	0.078	0.922

A possible major explanation is that the assumption of constant initial response probabilities in August 1971 is too restrictive. Of models II_2 and II_3, II_3 fits best. The fit is even satisfactory. A latent structure model thus seems to explain the variation in the data in a satisfactory way, although the number of parameters necessary (20) is close to the available degrees of freedom in the model (26). The parameters of model II_3 are easy to interpret. The next largest latent class, $m = 3$, which covers 38.3% of the population, is a segment which has predominantly has been in favour of the EEC on all three occasions. The largest latent class, $m = 2$, is a segment of the population where the attitude has changed from about 60% against, 20% in favour and 20% undecided in August 1971 to about 80% against, 10% in favour and 5% undecided in December 1973. This segment covers 43.8% of the population. The smallest segment covering 17.9% of the population shows a somewhat confusing behaviour, first moving heavily towards undecided, then moving towards yes and no in about the same magnitude. The behaviour of this last segment can partly be explained by the fact that Denmark actually joined the EEC between time points 2 and 3. But the main picture that emerges from the parameter estimates for model II_3 is

Table 14.5. *Observed numbers, expected number and test statistics for models I, II_2, II_3 and III*

Response pattern	Observed numbers	Expected numbers: Model I	II_2	II_3	III
111	148	39.30	144.35	148.28	144.43
112	15	49.70	15.42	15.08	15.39
113	13	7.33	13.27	12.43	13.41
121	2	26.58	5.47	4.15	5.49
122	30	33.14	24.26	27.50	24.26
123	1	6.85	3.43	1.93	3.43
131	20	21.07	24.25	20.23	24.22
132	15	26.18	14.82	13.59	14.80
133	5	5.77	3.74	5.80	3.76
211	11	29.37	10.35	10.74	10.42
212	9	37.14	11.51	10.62	11.47
213	1	5.48	2.24	1.92	2.25
221	14	19.87	12.98	11.51	13.02
222	73	24.77	57.56	76.30	57.54
223	7	5.12	8.13	5.36	8.14
231	9	15.75	8.24	6.91	8.26
232	21	19.57	31.44	20.42	31.40
233	2	4.31	4.53	3.23	4.53
311	8	21.06	11.58	7.86	11.62
312	12	26.63	7.44	7.69	7.40
313	1	3.93	1.83	3.38	1.84
321	3	14.24	7.95	4.11	7.95
322	28	17.76	35.24	27.23	35.13
323	2	3.67	4.98	1.91	4.97
331	16	11.29	5.82	17.21	5.82
332	14	14.03	19.31	18.57	19.23
333	13	3.09	2.84	9.04	2.84
q		566.87	83.41	12.43	83.42
d.f.		13	13	6	9
Level of significance		0.000	0.000	0.053	0.000

a large group of loyal supporters of the EEC, but an even larger group, who are increasingly against membership in the EEC. The parameters of model II_2 are consistent with this picture. With only two classes in model II_2 it seems that classes $m = 1$ and 2 for model II_3 are merged into class $m = 1$ for model II_2. The fact that model II_2 fits the data so much worse than model II_3 is a clear indication of the importance of the small segment in model II_3 with attitudes that are markedly different from those in segments $m = 2$ and 3.

The parameter estimates of model III are consistent with the estimates of model II_2. Nor has the fit of model III improved in comparison with model II_2. Thus nothing is gained by assuming the existence of transition probabilities in latent space. The estimated transition matrices between latent levels at time points 1 and 2 and between time points 2 and 3 actually shows that people with very low probabilities change the level of their latent variable. Note that people with the latent variable at level 1 corresponds to segment $m = 1$ in II_2, i.e. those individuals who move towards being opponents. On the other hand, a person with the latent variable at level 2 is a loyal supporter of membership.

CONCLUSIONS

Both latent class models and latent structure model with a continuous latent variable (often termed latent trait models) are useful tools for the statistical analysis of longitudinal data from a wide range of the social sciences. Latent class models have the advantage of being a very flexible framework for model modifications and model reformulations. Latent trait models do not rely on the often unrealistic assumption of constant value of the latent variable within a few latent classes. These models are, however, more complicated as regards numerical calculations and statistical procedures. Hence tempting model reformulations can not in many cases be tested because of numerical difficulties.

The main advantage of both types of models, which they share with the LISREL models, is that time-related dependencies can be formulated in terms of the latent variables, where realistic models would locate such dependencies. Thus changes over time in a latent variable can be studied in isolation from randomness due to the observation technique.

REFERENCES

Andersen, E. B. (1980). *Discrete statistical models with social science applications.* Amsterdam: North Holland Publishing Co.

Andersen, E. B. (1985). Estimating latent correlations between repeated testings. *Psychometrika, 50,* 3–16.

Andersen, E. B. (1990). *Statistical models for categorical data.* Heidelberg: Springer Verlag.

Boudon, R. (1972). Note on a model for the analysis of mobility tables. *Social Science Information, 11,* 179–188.

Boudon, R. (1973). *Mathematical structures of social mobility.* San Francisco: Jossey-Bass.

Clogg, C. C. (1979). Latent structure models of mobility. *American Journal of Sociology, 86,* 836–868.

Clogg, C. C. & Goodman, L. A. (1984). Latent structure analysis of a set of multidimensional contingency tables. *Journal of the American Statistical Association, 79,* 762–771.

Clogg, C. C. & Goodman, L. A. (1985). Simultaneous latent structure analysis in several groups. In N. B. Tuma (ed.), *Sociological methodology.* San Francisco: Jossey-Bass.

Clogg, C. C. & Goodman, L. A. (1986). On scaling models applied to data from several groups. *Psychometrika, 51,* 123–135.

Dempster, A. P., Laird, N. M. & Rubin, D. B. (1977). Maximum likelihood estimation from incomplete data via the EM-algorithm. *Journal of the Royal Statistical Society B, 39,* 1–22.

Goodman, L. A. (1974). Exploratory latent structure analysis using both identifiable and unidentifiable models. *Biometrika, 61,* 215–231.

Green, P. E., Carmone, F. J. & Wachspress, D. P. (1977). Consumer segmentation via latent class analysis. *Journal of Consumer Research, 3.*

Langeheine, R. (1988). Manifest and latent Markov chain models for categorical panel data. *Journal of Educational Statistics, 13,* 299–312.

Lazarsfeld, P. F. & Henry, N. W. (1968). *Latent structure analysis.* Boston: Houghton Mufflin.

Madden, T. J. & Dillon, W. R. (1982). Causal analysis and latent class models. *Journal of Marketing Research, 19,* 472–490.

Poulsen, C. S. (1982). *Latent structure analysis with choice modelling applications.* Aarhus: The School of Business Administration and Economics.

Poulsen, C. S. (in press). A latent structure approach to brand choice modelling. *International Journal of Research in Marketing.*

15 Stability and change in patterns of extrinsic adjustment problems

LARS R. BERGMAN AND DAVID MAGNUSSON

INTRODUCTION

Research on individual development has been strongly dominated by an interest in variables; in the characteristics of and interrelationships among person variables, and in the relationships between person variables and environmental variables (Thomae, 1988; Wohlwill, 1973). However, if the focus is on an analysis of the character of the structures and processes involved in the total functioning of an individual – in a current and in a developmental perspective – it is easy to see that this approach to the study of individual development has clear limitations (Magnusson, 1985, 1988).

Individual functioning can be described as a multidetermined stochastic process partly unique to the individual; a characteristic that is reflected in strong interactions and nonlinearity in data across individuals. This view leads to the conclusion that we have to complement the variable-oriented approach with one in which the person as a *gestalt* is the central object of interest. Operationally, such a person orientation implies that individuals are studied on the basis of their patterns of individual characteristics relevant for the study of the problem under consideration.

Several methodological approaches are possible for the study of individual development in terms of patterns. The aim of the present chapter is to illustrate the applicability of a cluster analysis oriented methodology to research on individual development, by presenting an empirical study concerned with the issue of early maladjustment behaviors as precursors of later adjustment problems.

Our choice of a proper methodology for the elucidation of the problem is clearly theory-based. Thus the study presents a link between substantive theory and a relevant method for treatment of data. As an illustration of the methodology the study presented here is descriptive. However, it is also applicable using a confirmatory or theory-testing approach.

A person-oriented view of the adjustment process

Basic to the present approach is an interactional view of the adaptation process which lies behind the emergence of adjustment reactions, with different individuals being characterized by different process characteristics. For expositions of the interactional view the reader is referred to, for instance, Magnusson (1988) and Magnusson & Allen (1983*a*,*b*). The following basic properties are assumed to hold for the kind of adaptation processes being considered here.

1. The process is partly specific to individuals.
2. The process is complex and is conceptualized as containing many factors on different levels which may have complicated relations to each other; the adjustment reactions are considered to be one central aspect of the process.
3. There is a meaningful coherence and structure (a) in individual growth in terms of the process, and (b) in differences in individuals' process characteristics. Assumptions (a) and (b) are similar to those made by Magnusson (1988) when characterizing an interactional approach to psychology.
4. It is reasonable to believe that, although there is an infinite variety of individual differences with regard to process characteristics, if viewed at a detailed level; there will also be a number of rather common types, if viewed at a more global level. The reason for this belief lies in analogies with other kinds of systems, for example, with biological systems where a number of distinct types are often found (e.g. of plant systems, ecotypes; see Colinvaux, 1980). With regard to classification, a similar point has also been made by Gangestad and Snyder (1985). They argue for the existence of distinct types, each sharing a common source of influence.

Although the adaptation process should mainly be viewed as a whole, in each specific case of empirical research a basic and meaningful delineation of subspaces of the individual's total functioning can and must be made. It was decided here to concentrate on the external manifestation in behavior of the adaptation process. The interest is focused on out-directed adjustment problems and the degree of presence of such problems. Then adjustment problems can be treated as a configuration of elements where each element achieves its importance only in relation to all the other ones. Of course, this delineation is only one possible approach within the general framework presented above.

The above person-oriented view of the adjustment process forms the broad theoretical background of the present empirical study, which specifically concerns the structure and development of extrinsic adjustment problems. For the sake of brevity, the literature about the substantive fields involved is not reviewed here, and is only commented upon rather briefly in the results and discussion sections.

METHOD

Measuring adjustment problems

When studying adjustment problems one often uses strictly relative scales, on which each person's value for a certain aspect of individual functioning derives its meaning only in relation to the other persons' values in the groups studied. For many purposes, this may be an adequate scaling, but for studying the development of patterns of adjustment problems within the present context it is not adequate (Magnusson & Bergman, 1984; Bergman & Magnusson, in preparation).

Consider the following example. Within the longitudinal research program Individual Development and Adjustment (IDA; Magnusson, 1988) a pupil's questionnaire was given at ages 10, 13 and 16. At age 10, 88% of the girls were positive about school as judged from their answers to several items in the questionnaire. We believe that this mainly reflected a genuinely positive attitude towards school at this age (at a higher age more negative attitudes were found). It then does not appear reasonable to rank all girls according to the score obtained and to say that, for instance, the lowest 20% of the girls had an adjustment problem in this respect. Apart from the fact that irrelevant response sets may well be the most important source of variation in the scores of the 88% with a clearly positive attitude, which makes it highly questionable to separate the pupils into two groups, it should be realized that knowing that 88% reported positive attitudes towards school is an important piece of information. It can be compared with the frequency of girls who reported the absence of psychosomatic reactions, which was 51%, indicating that, at this age, psychosomatic problems were more frequent than negative school attitudes. Such information is lost if relative scaling is used. In the study of several adjustment problems at several points in time this loss would include the inability to see whether one adjustment problem is more common than another at a given age and to see whether an adjustment problem becomes more or less common with age.

For our purposes, this loss of comparability is of decisive importance and cannot be accepted regardless of technical and other advantages of a purely relative scaling. What is needed is some kind of extrinsic tally that allows us to produce measurements on, at least, the level of a quasi-absolute scale. With this we mean a scale whereby meaningful comparisons are possible with respect to the prevalence of the different adjustment problems under study at a given age and with respect to the manifestation of the same adjustment problem at different points in time. In one sense this situation is shared by most epidemiological studies in the behavioral sciences, although the nature of the quasi-absolute tally varies. For instance, a measurement procedure developed for a certain segment of the population (e.g., a psychiatric classification system) is sometimes used to measure the general population.

However, there are also important differences between the purpose of quasi-absolute scaling suggested in the present connection and the epidemiological endeavor to measure prevalence of symptoms. There the aim is an absolute prevalence statement for a given behavior problem whereas in the present context the aim is to produce a scaling that is comparable across problems and over time but it is not necessary that any adjustment problem considered singly can be given an absolute interpretation. Thus, it is the *multivariate* scaling of all the problems that is the focal point together with achieving the above-mentioned comparability; there is no interest here in interpreting an adjustment problem in isolation from other problems.

Obviously, there are difficult problems in constructing quasi-absolute scales, and we know of no generally 'best' procedure; the procedure that will be used here (page 330) is only one alternative believed to be appropriate for our specific purpose.

Cross-sectional classification analysis based on pattern data

Classification is more basic to people than measurement (see Zubin, 1968 for a historical overview). It can also be considered as a less advanced endeavor, open to various kinds of error (Whitehead, 1956). However, to qualify this last statement, there is a crucial distinction between classification as a method for providing the basic data, for instance, a typologist's directly assigning the subjects to different types, as in Jung's (1921) topology, and classification as a method for finding dense points or natural clusters based on analysis of dimensional data (which, of course, presupposes that measurement has taken place).

The first kind of classification has been criticized. For instance, given the assumption that reality is adequately represented by a multi-dimensional vector of numbers it has been shown that only under special circumstances can such a multidimensional system be adequately represented by a small number of types (Ekman, 1951, 1952). Thus, under certain circumstances using classification to produce the basic data has drawbacks in that no comprehensive dimensional data are ever produced and the analysis of typological data is hostage to the appropriateness of restrictive assumptions that are difficult to check after the data have been collected.

Against the second kind of classification, these objections are no longer valid. Since it is based on dimensional data, this kind of classification is naturally viewed as only one kind of analysis of these data; the results can also be checked and complemented by ordinary dimensional kinds of analyses.

The classifications performed here used descriptive cluster-analytic methodology. The straightforward classification of subjects on the basis of observed characteristics has been criticized by some authors. For instance, Gangestad & Snyder (1985) have argued against this kind of classification, which they call phenetic, and in favor of a genetic classification which defines clusters that share a genotypic source of influence (latent classes, cf. the latent structure analysis of Lazarsfeld). Although their suggested approach opens up interesting possibilities, we disagree with their two main arguments against phenetic classification, namely (a) the fact that different cluster-analytic methods and options can give different results and (b) the frequently occurring situations in which clusters are not tight.

With regard to (a) above, the counterargument is that a complex reality can be described in different ways without there necessarily being anything wrong with any description (this argument is further elaborated in the discussion). With regard to (b) above, it is true that in many situations the clusters are not tight, with some subjects falling 'in between' and with a lack of clear structure. However, this often reflects the complicated patterns and multivariate outcomes that exist in reality, and the fact that the method fails to give an orderly picture of a multivariate reality which is not orderly is not a valid argument against the method *per se*. In fact, Monte Carlo studies have shown that when samples are generated from populations with a clear structure, without adding large errors, most major clustering algorithms are reasonably good at finding this structure (see, e.g., Milligan, 1980). An additional consideration here is that the use of a residue, that is, not demanding all subjects to be classified (less than 100% coverage) can enhance the possibilities of finding the structure in the data. In this way the clustering solution is less affected by outliers which can be caused by errors of measurement or can represent true but unique response patterns. (Bergman, 1988; Bergman & Magnusson, 1984; Edelbrock, 1979; Milligan, 1981, to be further discussed below). As discussed by Bergman (1988) there are also theoretical reasons for using a residue. The main argument is that often it is not reasonable to expect *all* subjects to fit into a small number of syndromes or typical patterns. There may be individuals who because of special circumstances exhibit very unique patterns and they should not be forced into the classification system.

To sum up, for our present purposes, we find it useful to use a phenetic approach to classification, one in which subjects are grouped according to their patterns of observed values. It is then important to pay close attention to the choice of clustering algorithm, similarity measure, and to the existence of outliers. Perhaps the choice of which variables to include in the analyses is the most important one. We have there been guided by theoretical considerations and have also tried to use as few and reliable indicators as possible to diminish the influence of errors of measurement on the profiles (regarding the last point, see also Bergman & Magnusson, 1983).

A survey of the literature on cluster analysis led to the conclusion that useful solutions often are obtained by *k*-means relocation cluster analysis, using squared euclidean distance and with a start classification obtained by Ward's method (see Milligan, 1981; Morey, Blashfield & Skinner, 1983). This method has been combined here with the concept of using a residue to produce a RESIDAN analysis (Bergman, 1988), which is briefly described in the next section.

Finally, we make a comment on the use of an appropriate dissimilarity measure. In the present application it is necessary to take both form and level of the profile into account (cf. Cronbach & Gleser, 1953), since otherwise essential information is lost that is contained in the quasi-absolute scaling. Therefore, the well-known squared euclidean distance measure was used.

Cross-sectional classification using RESIDAN. The RESIDAN rationale is briefly characterized as follows:

1. The starting point is the matrix of (dis)similarity measures to be used in the main analysis.
2. Based on this matrix, all subjects who are similar to at most *k* other subjects are identified. These subjects constitute the *residue*. For small samples, the value of *k* may often be set to zero, whereas, for larger samples, a value of 1–5 might be appropriate. The threshold value for considering two subjects as similar naturally depends upon the type of (dis)similarity measure used (in this case squared euclidean distance) and on the researcher's subjective decision about the level in the similarity value needed to consider two cases as similar. For instance, two cases can be considered as similar by the researcher if they are as similar as two average cases belonging to the same cluster tend to be.
3. The residue is removed from the data set, and the cluster analysis is performed on the reduced data set. Different cluster-analytic methods are, of course, possible; Ward's hierarchical method (Ward, 1963), using squared euclidean distance, was used here to provide the start classification. It is widely

used and is perhaps the method that most often has been judged to have the highest validity and recovery of known structure in methodological studies (Morey, Blashfield & Skinner, 1983; see also Milligan, 1981, for a slightly different view). The solution obtained from Ward's method is then subjected to a *k*-means analysis (using procedure RELOCATE in CLUSTAN, Wishart, 1982) to relocate subjects that ended up in the wrong cluster (an additional small residue is also formed, in which subjects who are far from all cluster centroids are placed).

4. The residue is then analyzed both descriptively and by testing theories about rare patterns (antitypes). For a further discussion of the RESIDAN rationale the reader is referred to Bergman (1988). Owing to lack of space, the aspects of RESIDAN that concern analyzing and interpreting the residue are omitted in this presentation.

Longisectional classification analysis

Longisectional classification analysis is a rather fancy name for the simple strategy of cross-tabulating categorizations pertaining to two different points in time (Lienert & Bergman, 1985). (Of course, there are other, more sophisticated methods for longitudinal analysis in this context but for the present illustration this method is sufficient.) For example, in longisectional cluster analysis, cluster solutions for the same longitudinal sample but from two different points in time are cross-tabulated. In this way, frequent cluster value combinations (frequent longitudinal streams) as well as infrequent streams can be studied by examining the cells. Usually one also wants to obtain information about which streams are more frequent than expected by chance and which streams are less frequent than expected by chance. A natural first step is then to construct a table of expected frequencies for each cell, with which the observed frequencies are compared. This could be done within the framework of ordinary contingency table analysis and the significance of a deviance between the observed and the expected value of a cell could be tested using, for instance, adjusted residuals (Haberman, 1973).

A problem with using the adjusted residual approach is that it is based on normal approximations. It has been shown that such approximations are not good when extreme tail probabilities are being considered (Bergman & El-Khouri, 1986; Bergman & von Eye, 1987). Since one normally performs tests of several cells and thus is interested in evaluating very small probabilities, it may be preferable to use exact hypergeometric probabilities (see Bergman & El-Khouri, 1986). For this purpose, a program EXACON was used here, in which each cell frequency is tested using exact hypergeometric probabilities (Bergman & El-Khouri, 1987).

DATA

Sample

The sample used here comes from the longitudinal research program Individual Development and Adjustment (IDA; Magnusson, 1988). It includes a school grade cohort of children who were followed from age 10 to adult age. This cohort is the sample studied here. Two different kinds of data were used; namely, behavioral data from age 10 and age 13, and data from official records from the age of 18 to the age of 24. At age 10, the sample size was $n = 517$ and at age 13 the sample size was $n = 540$. For $n = 435$ boys, data were available at both age 10 and 13. The data from each age included almost the whole school grade cohort at that age with a negligible drop-out (below 1%; further discussed below). Since the data from adult age were based on official records they were almost without drop-out (less than 1%).

Variables

The adjustment problems at age 10 and age 13, respectively, were studied using data for the adjustment problems described in Table 15.1. As can be seen from Table 15.1, the same problems were studied at the two ages. The reliability of each of the raw score indicators is estimated to be above 0.80 for all indicators (see Magnusson, Dunér & Zetterblom, 1975).

In line with the reasoning indicated above, a quasi-absolute four-point scale was constructed for each adjustment problem in the following manner:

Value code	*Description*
0	no adjustment problem of this kind
1	the adjustment is not good but no clear problem
2	an adjustment problem of this kind
3	a pronounced adjustment problem of this kind

For each adjustment problem, quantitative information from one or more raw score indicators was used. A fixed mechanical procedure was then used to arrive at the scaling which involved no subjective decisions (see Bergman & Magnusson, in preparation).

Table 15.1. *Adjustment problems studied at age 10 and age 13*

Adjustment problem	Information used to measure the adjustment problem
Aggression	Teachers' ratings
Motor restlessness	Teachers' ratings
Lack of concentration	Teachers' ratings
Low school motivation	Teachers' ratings
Poor peer relations	Sociometric ratings by peers
Low school achievement	School marks in Swedish and mathematics

Naturally, it was difficult to decide the cut-off point in the raw score distributions for some of the indicators in order to define the values in the four-point scale. The decisions were made by the authors after careful consideration and consultation with other experts and also included interrater comparisons with a satisfactory outcome. The guidelines for the decisions regarding cut-off points were: (a) a psychological analysis; (b) indications from other empirical studies regarding critical cut-off points; and (c) properties of the raw score variables (both statistical/technical and in reference to the measurement process). As mentioned earlier, the aim of this quasi-absolute scaling was to achieve code values approximately matching the above absolute descriptions rather than to obtain fixed percentages having different values. In addition to the childhood data, data from official records for criminal offences and alcohol abuse covering the age period 18–24 years were used in one specific analysis (reported in Table 15.6). A simple dichotomous variable was then formed which indicated inclusion in at least one of the registers of criminality and alcohol abuse, or absence from both these registers. Analyses made by Bergman & Magnusson (in preparation) indicated the usefulness of this simple dichotomy for the present purposes.

As in most other studies involving multivariate non-experimental data, the present data set contains a partial drop-out in the form of a number of cases having missing values in one or a few variables. It was possible to keep this drop-out very low by careful data collection and by using only indicators with a low drop-out rate. Also when using the quasi-absolute scaling procedure it was possible to use other pertinent information for scaling an indicator in some cases when the first-hand information was missing.

For a few persons, cases with almost complete data were imputed using a 'twin' procedure within MPREP (multivariate preparatory analysis: see Bergman & El-Khouri, in preparation). In this way, temporary data files for cluster analyses were constructed, separately at age 10 and age 13. At age 10, 40 cases were imputed following the procedure described above (37 missed information about poor peer relations and three missed information about low achievement). For three cases no twin was found. At age 13, 12 cases were imputed and in one case no twin was found. We believe that the gain in retaining these almost complete cases for the analyses far out-weighed the problem of having some cases that were, to a small extent, artificial. Thanks to this procedure (as well as to the high coverage of the data originally collected and the scaling procedure), the analyses at each point in time could be performed on almost the whole school grade cohort with negligible drop-out. For a further discussion of the problems of imputation in the present context, the reader is referred to Bergman & Magnusson (1984) and to Bergman & El-Khouri (1986).

RESULTS

The cross-sectional patterning of adjustment problems

Patterning at age 10. At age 10, the boys were grouped on the basis of their patterns of adjustment problems, using the cluster analytic procedure described earlier. The six extrinsic adjustment problems presented in Table 15.1 were then included.

The earlier described RESIDAN method was used in the analyses. First a residue of deviant subjects that were not to be classified was formed to be analyzed separately ($k = 1$ and threshold 0.50: the residue analysis is not included in this presentation). The residue consisted of nine subjects. Then the cluster-analytic procedure described earlier was applied (in the relocation step a threshold of 1.50 was used to eliminate subjects that did not fit any cluster centroid; in this way the residue was increased by three subjects to a total of 12 subjects). Following the quasi-absolute scaling rationale described earlier, the variables were not standardized. A nine-cluster solution was found which 'explained' 72% of the total error sum of squares (described in Table 15.2).

Table 15.2 demonstrates that cluster 1 ($n = 161$) was characterized by no problems in any of the indicators. For all indicators the cluster mean is below 1 on the four-point scale. Cluster 2 ($n = 88$) was characterized by almost no problems (only a weak indication of poor peer relations). There was also a cluster characterized by pronounced poor peer relations and no other problems (cluster 4, $n = 40$). Two clusters characterized by a severe pattern of adjustment problems emerged, namely cluster 8 ($n = 37$), which was labeled 'hyperactivity syndrome' and cluster 9 ($n = 25$), which was labeled 'multi-problem syndrome'.

Table 15.2. *Final clustering solution for extrinsic adjustment problems at age 10*

				Cluster mean of					
Cluster	Size	Average coefficient	Description	Aggr.	Motor restl.	Lack conc.	Low school motiv.	Poor peer rel.	Low school achiev.
1	161	0.04	No problems	—	—	—	—	—	—
2	88	0.08	Almost no problems	—	—	—	—	1.0	—
3	64	0.23	Weak motor restl.	—	1.4	—	—	—	—
4	40	0.29	Poor peer rel.	—	—	—	—	2.5	—
5	31	0.20	Low achiev.	—	—	—	—	—	2.4
6	23	0.50	Low school motiv. syndrome	—	—	2.4	1.5	—	1.2
7	33	0.51	Aggr. and motor restl.	2.2	1.8	—	—	—	—
8	37	0.46	Hyperactivity syndrome	1.0	2.3	2.2	1.3	—	—
9	25	0.65	Multi-problem syndrome	2.0	2.5	2.8	2.4	1.0	2.0
Residue	12								
All	517								

Note: — means that the cluster mean of a variable is less than 1 in the four-point scale coded 0, 1, 2, 3. As was described in the method section, cluster analysis of the type RELOCATE was used which was based on a start classification from a hierarchican analysis of type Ward. Average coefficient means average error sum of squares within the cluster. Three cases were removed to the residue in the final analysis making a total of 12 residue cases.

The results will be discussed further at a later stage, in terms of a longitudinal perspective. However, we will make two additional comments here. First, the pattern description given by the cluster analysis indicates that the behaviors that here fall under the general heading of conduct problems or hyperactive behavior did not emerge as single-problem clusters in their strong manifestations; they occurred only in multi-problem patterns. Secondly, three groups of children emerged who were characterized by a syndrome including low school achievement: one group manifested low achievement as a single problem, while for two of the groups it was only one aspect of a multi-problem panorama. It may well be that the prognoses for these groups are very different, as we shall see later. A similar point can be made for poor peer relations.

These observations point to the potential danger in interpreting the relationship between a single aspect of early conduct problems and, for instance, an adult outcome in terms of antisocial behavior (see Magnusson & Bergman, 1988).

Patterning at age 13. At age 13, a second cluster analysis was performed using the RESIDAN rationale described earlier. The same procedure as at age 10 was used. An eight-cluster solution was found which 'explained' 71% of the total error sum of squares. The number of residue subjects after the final grouping was eight. The cluster solution is described in Table 15.3.

Table 15.3 shows that a large cluster characterized by no problems emerged (cluster 1, $n = 245$). Two clear single-problem clusters also emerged, one of which was characterized by poor peer relations as a single problem (cluster 4, $n = 32$) and the other which reflected low achievement as a single problem (cluster 5, $n = 39$). Three multi-problem clusters were found, namely cluster 6 ($n = 47$), which was labeled 'low school motivation syndrome', cluster 7 ($n = 44$), which was labeled 'aggression and hyperactivity', and cluster 8 ($n = 24$), which was labeled 'multi-problem syndrome'.

Generalizability of the cluster solutions. Obviously, a different variable content and a sample with different properties can be expected to lead to a different clustering solution. Nevertheless, it is an important question to what extent the results are robust to moderate changes in different respects. With regard to this, two sets of findings are notable:

1. When the results of this cluster analysis at age 13 were compared with the results from another analysis of the same sample, using a different method (RESCLUS) and a slightly different variable content (low achievement was replaced by

Table 15.3. *Final clustering solution for extrinsic adjustment problems at age 13*

				Cluster mean of					
Cluster	Size	Average coefficient	Description	Aggr.	Motor restl.	Lack conc.	Low school motiv.	Poor peer rel.	Low school achiev.
1	245	0.06	No problems	—	—	—	—	—	—
2	60	0.25	Weak motor restl.	—	1.4	—	—	—	—
3	41	0.30	Weak aggr.	1.6	—	—	—	—	—
4	32	0.35	Poor peer rel.	—	—	—	—	1.9	—
5	39	0.24	Low achiev.	—	—	—	—	—	2.5
6	47	0.52	Low school motiv. syndrome	—	1.3	2.3	1.9	—	1.0
7	44	0.42	Aggr. and hyperact.	2.2	2.3	1.9	1.3	—	—
8	24	0.55	Multi-problem syndrome	1.9	2.8	2.7	2.4	2.0	—
Residue	8								
All	540								

Note:—means that the cluster mean of a variable is less than 1 in the four-point scale coded 0, 1, 2, 3. As was described in the method section, cluster analysis of the type RELOCATE was used which was based on a start classification from a hierarchical analysis of type Ward. Average coefficient means average error sum of squares within the cluster. One case was removed to the residue in the final analysis making a total of 8 residue cases.

Table 15.4. *Comparison between the clustering solutions for the main group at age 13 and for the pilot group at age 13*

Main group clusters			Pilot group clusters			Squared distance between cluster centroids
No.	Size	Description	No.	Size	Description	
1	245	No problems	1	144	No problems	0.00
2	60	Weak motor restlessness	2	68	Weak motor restlessness	0.02
3	41	Weak aggression	3	26	Weak aggression	0.03
4	32	Poor peer relations	4	49	Weak poor peer relations	0.14
5	39	Low school achievement	5	24	Weak low school achievement	0.24
6	47	Low school motivation syndrome	6	47	Weak low school motivation syndrome	0.28
7	44	Aggression and hyperactivity	7	39	(Aggression) and hyperactivity	0.28
8	24	Multi-problem syndrome	8	26	Multi-problem syndrome	0.37

underachievement), similar results were obtained (Bergman & Magnusson, 1987).

2. Within IDA there also exists a pilot group, aged 13 in 1965, for which approximately the same information was collected. The pilot group is of almost the same size ($n = 442$) and is also a school grade cohort of the same kind as the main group, although 42 children attending special classes (mostly because of learning problems) were not included in the pilot group sample. This sample was used for a replication study. For the pilot group the same six indicators as used for the main group could be studied, although poor peer relations and low achievement were measured slightly differently. Exactly the same kind of RESIDAN analysis that was performed on the main group was performed on the pilot group. In the main group analysis an eight-cluster solution was chosen; for the pilot group this number of clusters also met reasonably well the criteria for deciding the number of clusters, although the nine-cluster solution, in this case, was somewhat better. Nevertheless, the eight-cluster solution, with an 'explained' error sum of squares of 67.0%, was chosen. In Table 15.4 the solution for the pilot group is compared with that for the main group. The squared euclidean distances between the cluster centroids are also given.

Table 15.4 demonstrates that the clustering solutions of the main group and the pilot group were very similar. For each cluster in the main group solution there existed an identical or very similar cluster in the pilot group solution. The squared distances between a cluster centroid in the main group and the corresponding cluster centroid in the pilot group was in every case less than the average distance in the main group between a subject in a cluster and that cluster's centroid (= average coefficient, see Table 15.3).

Longitudinal analyses

Does the patterning of adjustment problems change with age? In this section the focus is on stability and change in the typical patterning of adjustment problems. What are the similarities and differences between the subgroups or clusters that are obtained at the different ages? To clarify this issue, a comparison is made in Table 15.5 between the patterning of adjustment problems at age 10 (the cluster solution given in Table 15.2) and the patterning of adjustment problems at age 13 (the cluster solution given in Table 15.3).

As can be seen in Table 15.5 the typical patterns at the different ages were similar, as was expected. For instance, the single-problem clusters characterized by pronounced poor peer relations and pronounced low

Table 15.5. *A comparison between the cluster solutions at age 10 and age 13*

Cluster at age 10		Most similar cluster at age 13	
Description	Size	Description	Size
1. No problems	161	1. No problems	245
2. Weak poor peer relations	88		
3. Weak motor restlessness	64	2. Weak motor restlessness	60
4. Poor peer relations	40	4. Poor peer relations	32
5. Low school achievement	31	5. Low school achievement	39
6. Low school motivation syndrome	23	6. Low school motivation syndrome	47
7. Aggression and motor restlessness	33	7. Aggression and hyper-activity	44
8. Hyperactivity syndrome	37		
9. Multi-problem syndrome	25	8. Multi-problem syndrome	24

achievement, respectively, emerged at both ages as did the multi-problem clusters low school motivation syndrome and multi-problem syndrome. The multi-problem syndrome was slightly different at the two ages: at age 10 low achievement was more characteristic of the members of the cluster than was poor peer relations, but at age 13 the pattern was reversed. Clusters 7 and 8 at age 10 corresponded to some extent to cluster 7 at age 13, which was characterized by aggression and motor restlessness as the core symptoms but which also included other conduct problems. One cluster at age 13 was not found at age 10 (3. weak aggression).

That the low school motivation syndrome became twice as common at age 13 as it was at age 10 points to the possibility of an early onset of a mechanism by which more and more children become alienated from school as they grow older. One can also speculate concerning the result that the multi-problem syndrome was slightly different between ages. It may be that poor peer relations became more of a core problem leading to other problems at age 13 than at age 10, perhaps because teenagers are more peer-oriented.

How do patterns of adjustment problems evolve? How do the typical patterns of adjustment problems evolve; what kind of patterns at age 10 are connected to what kind of patterns at age 13? This was studied by cross-tabulating cluster membership at the two ages. Since such a table is rather cumbersome because of its size, only the significant streams are depicted in Figure 15.1. For each (cluster at age 10) × (cluster at age 13) combination it was tested whether the observed frequency was significantly in excess of what could be expected

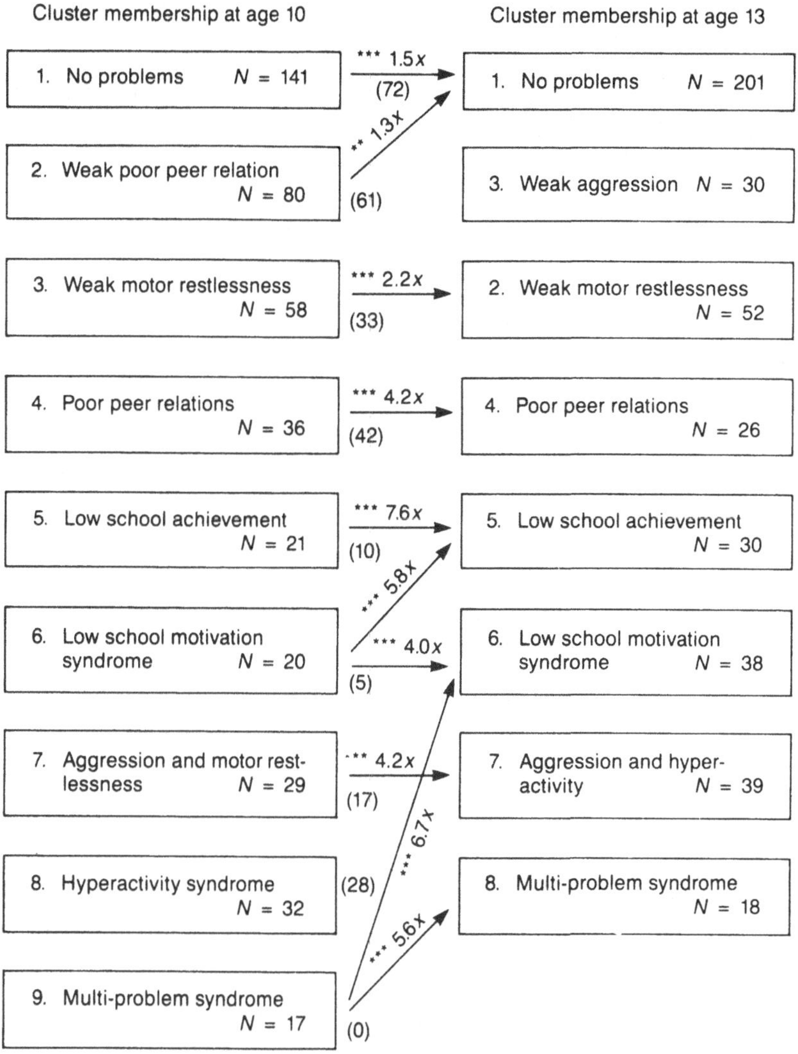

Figure 15.1. Significant longitudinal streams between age 10 and age 13. Figures on arrow indicate how many times larger the probability of having that cluster combination is from what is expected by chance. (Percentage of members in a specific cluster at age 10 who are in cluster 1 at age 13 within the parenthesis.) $N = 434$. Note. *, **, and *** mean that $p < 0.05$, $p < 0.01$, $p < 0.001$ respectively using a one-tailed hypergeometric test.

according to an independence model (significant types). It should be noted that, since a large number of dependent test were performed ($9 \times 8 = 72$ tests), the significance levels must be interpreted with caution. In Figure 15.1 an arrow is drawn for each cluster combination that was a significant type ($p < 0.05$).

The results demonstrated that being in the 'no problems' cluster at age 10 was significantly related to being in the same cluster at age 13 ($p < 0.001$). Other clusters for which there was a significant stability were: weak motor restlessness, poor peer relations and low school achievement, low school motivation syndrome, and multi-problem syndrome. The 'aggression and motor restlessness' cluster was significantly related to a similar cluster at age 13 (aggression and hyperactivity). Thus, not only were similar clusters found at the different ages indicating *structural stability* over time, as was shown in a previous section; there was also a reasonable *individual stability*.

In some cases there was also a significant relationship between different kinds of clusters at the two ages, for instance the multi-problem syndrome at age 10 was related to the low school motivation syndrome at age 13, and the low school motivation syndrome at age 10 was related to the 'low achievement' cluster at age 13. These developmental paths seem logical. For instance, it is natural that even if a child characterized by a low school motivation syndrome at age 10 leaves these problems behind, he may well continue to have problems with school achievement in Swedish and mathematics since knowledge in these subjects is cumulative; if one starts off badly it is difficult to compensate for the loss of knowledge later on. Thus, it is reasonable that he will end up in the low school achievement cluster at age 13.

It is also noteworthy that for the most severe syndrome at age 10 (cluster 9), *no one* was found in the well-adjusted cluster at age 13 and also for clusters 5, 6 and 7 this figure was very low (10, 5, and 17%, respectively). These results support, and even amplify, Rutter and his co-workers' findings of a high degree of stability in conduct disorders during this phase of development (Rutter, 1981). In addition, it should be noted that the prognosis for those characterized by the low school motivation syndrome is worse than for those characterized by the hyperactivity syndrome. Perhaps the loss of knowledge in the basic school subjects that often goes with the first syndrome has more serious long-term consequences than does (moderately) hyperactive behavior, which may be more age-specific.

Adjustment problems in childhood and adult maladjustment. The question was raised as to what extent adult maladjustment is mainly related to belonging or not belonging to a severe maladjustment cluster at age 13, without the presence or absence of maladjustment at age 10 making much of a difference. To elucidate these issues, Table 15.6 was constructed. For three main types of adjustment patterns at age 10 and age 13, the percentage characterized by some kind of adult maladjustment is given (interpreted in 1–3 below; the adult maladjustment variable is described on page 331).

Table 15.6. *Percentage characterized by some kind of adult maladjustment according to official records after type of adjustment problem pattern at age 10 and at age 13*

	Adjustment problem configuration at age 13			
	No problem (cluster 1)	Some problems (clusters 2–6)	Severe conduct pr. (clusters 7, 8)	All
Type of adjustment problem pattern at age 10				
No problems (cluster 1)	8	16	33	11
Some problems (clusters 2–6)	16	21	67	24
Severe conduct pr. (clusters 7–9)	36	30	58	40
All	14	22	57	23

Table 15.6 can be used as a basis for the following conclusions:

1. There was a strong relation between belonging to the severe adjustment problem configurations at age 10 or at age 13, on the one hand, and adult maladjustment, on the other hand.
2. The relation between the adjustment problem configurations at age 10 and adult maladjustment was moderated by the adjustment configuration at age 13.
3. The relation between the adjustment problem configuration at age 13 and adult maladjustment was moderated by the adjustment configuration at age 10.

The results reported above indicate that the maladjustment pattern at age 10 makes a difference for adult maladjustment even after the maladjustment pattern at age 13 has been taken into account. A logit model with the age 10 grouping and the age 13 grouping as the independent variables and the log odds ratio of adult maladjustment as the dependent variable provided an acceptable fit to the data, indicating that the irregularities that could be seen in the table might be attributed to random fluctuations.

DISCUSSION

It is interesting to note how theoretical concepts like 'structure', 'change', and 'stability' get intermingled with the corresponding methodological translations. This is seen clearly here where these vague concepts have been given methodological translations within a person-oriented framework, focusing on patterns or configurations and using clustering procedures as the statistical method instead of being given a more common methodological translation within a variable–oriented framework. For example, 'structure' is translated here as 'the typical adjustment reaction profiles', compared with a factor-analytic variable-oriented application in which 'structure' often implies 'the factor structure resulting from a factor analysis of the adjustment reactions'. Similarly, in the present investigation the term 'individual change' denotes that 'a person is characterized by one type of pattern at age 10 and by another type of pattern at age 13'. In a factor analysis oriented setting, 'individual change' might mean 'a difference between the factor scores at two different ages for the same factor'.

This underscores the intimate relation between the theoretical level and the methodological/empirical level from which our models/analogies/experiences originate. The theoretical reasoning often derives its meaning from analogies and models taken from the methodological/empirical level. (Note that this is something different from the often legitimate operalization of concepts by the measurement procedure used.) For instance, when talking about 'structure' and 'change' on a theoretical level one often, implicitly, makes the theoretical concepts meaningful by associating them with some statistical method for studying them. One might, however, question the extent to which our theoretical thinking is overly influenced by existing method and models for data treatment, in part because of the mechanism discussed above and in part because the existing methods provide the only window to the empirical world.

In this chapter a descriptive approach was used in the empirical illustration. The following comments are pertinent to this choice. The importance of careful observation and description should be emphasized as a precursor and complement to theory construction and testing in the study of individual development (Magnusson, in press). Of course, theory construction and building statistical models for testing theories are of primary importance. However, theories and models must not be generated at the expense of skipping the preliminary (and recurrent) step of carefully observing and describing the complex reality reflected in the data (cf. Cronbach, 1975). If this step is skipped, research runs the risk of producing and maintaining sterile theories without sufficient contact with reality: the theory-testing procedure itself might create blinkers which prevent the researcher from seeing important aspects of reality (cf. the so-called 'confirmation bias'; Greenwald, Pratkanis, Lieppe, & Baumgardner, 1986). Careful observation and description, using reliable methods, yield results of importance not only for further theoretical formulations but also for research methodology and strategy. It is hoped that the present study gives an example of this.

The study of individual development is a complex undertaking. Perhaps the most difficult issue then is how to introduce time or age in a study: at a theoretical, a methodological, and a measurement level. This issue has many aspects; one of which concerns the manner in which biological maturation is taken into account, since individual differences in maturational tempo can influence the results of a developmental study (Magnusson, 1985). Another issue concerns how to handle age as an independent variable. Should measurements be performed at fixed chronological ages (which ages?) with the measurements at the different ages providing the variables, or should age be the main independent variable in the statistical model with the necessary information provided by, for instance, noting the exact age at which certain events occur? From certain points of view, a process-oriented theoretical and methodological approach is preferable, but in practice one often first studies each age separately and then tries to link the results or structures from the different ages, as was done here. In the present context, it is a natural next step to describe individual development directly by forming longitudinal types based on longitudinal patterns. This can be done by longitudinal cluster analysis, which is under development by us, among others. However, this area contains many technical problems (for instance how to separate individuals with similar trajectories but with a different outcome).

It has sometimes been argued that a drawback of cluster-analytic methodology is that different methods can render different results. Differences have sometimes been observed depending on the choice of clustering algorithm, of similarity measure, of sample, and, above all, of the variables included in the analyses (Milligan, 1980). However, these differences in results should not be over-interpreted. *First*, it should be noted that a judicious choice of variables (including the avoidance of unreliable indicators) and of clustering method would reduce the method and sample variation. Here we would like to emphasize the usefulness of a residue approach in which not everyone is classified. Our faith in the generalizability of the results presented here receives certain support from results of the previously mentioned methodological studies. *Second*, it should be noted that different methods leading to different descriptions does not necessarily mean that there is something wrong with any of the methods; the same complex multivariate reality can be described in different ways. To make a univariate analogy: the arithmetic mean and the median are sometimes different when computed for the same data set, but this difference does not invalidate either of the 'methods'.

Measurement is inextricably related to theory and to methods for data treatment. Measurement models should be made explicit, relating the data produced to the theoretical concepts that are introduced (Rudinger & Wood, 1990; Rutter & Pickles, 1990). Often measurement and scaling issues entail difficult problems that too often are neglected (Harris, 1963). We do not pretend to have solved these problems in our application but we believe that we have pointed to one possible way of handling them; a way which is consistent with our person-oriented view.

It is obvious that the cluster analysis oriented methodology used here normally means that important aspects of the input information are lost in the resulting description of individuals according to cluster membership. To a certain extent this problem is alleviated through the use of a residue which is analyzed separately, but the basic fact remains that k-dimensional information cannot generally be assumed to be perfectly represented by one categorical variable (see page 327 for a further discussion of this). However, any meaningful and understandable description of a complex reality must build on simplification; non-essential aspects of the information must be ignored in order to highlight the essential aspects. In the present application, the most important aspect was the pattern-as-a-whole, and the chosen method focused on this pattern. It may often be a sound procedure to complement this kind of analysis with some variable-oriented method of analysis to obtain a binocular view. However, the results of the different approaches provide fundamentally different pictures, each providing important information (Magnusson & Bergman, 1988).

REFERENCES

Bergman, L. R. (1988). You can't classify all of the people all of the time. *Multivariate Behavioral Research, 23,* 425–441.

Bergman, L. R. & El-Khouri, B. (1986). On the preparatory analysis of multivariate data before (longitudinal) cluster analysis. Some theoretical considerations and a data program. Department of Psychology, University of Stockholm, Report no. 651.

Bergman, L. R. & El-Khouri, B. (1987). EXACON – a Fortran 77 program for the exact analysis of single cells in a contingency table. *Educational and Psychological Measurement, 47,* 155–161.

Bergman, L. R. & El-Khouri, B. (in preparation). MPREP: A Fortran 77 computer program for the preparatory analysis of data before multivariate analysis.

Bergman, L. R. & von Eye, A. (1987). Normal approximations of exact tests in configural frequency analysis. *Biometric Journal, 29,* 849–855.

Bergman, L. R. & Magnusson, D. (1983). The development of patterns of maladjustment. The IDA project, Department of Psychology, University of Stockholm, Report no. 50.

Bergman, L. R. & Magnusson, D. (1984). Patterns of adjustment problems at age 10: An empirical and methodological study. Department of Psychology, University of Stockholm. Report no. 615.

Bergman, L. R. & Magnusson, D. (in preparation). Longitudinal patterns of adjustment problems: a methodological and empirical study.

Bergman, L. R. & Magnusson, D. (1987). A person approach to the study of the development and adjustment problems: An empirical example and some research strategy considerations. In D. Magnusson & A. Öhman (eds.), *Psychopathology: An interactional perspective.* New York: Academic Press.

Colinvaux, P. (1980). *Why big fierce animals are rare.* Pelican Books.

Cronbach, L. J. (1975). Beyond the two disciplines of scientific psychology. *American Psychologist, 30,* 116–127.

Cronbach, L. J. & Gleser, G. C. (1953). Assessing similarity between profiles. *Psychological Bulletin, 50,* 456–473.

Edelbrock, C. (1979). Mixture model tests of hierarchical clustering algorithms. The problems of classifying everybody. *Multivariate Behavioral Research, 14,* 367–384.

Ekman, G. (1951). On typological and dimensional systems of reference in describing personality. *Acta Psychologica, 8,* 1–24.

Ekman, G. (1952). *Differentiell psykologi.* Stockholm: Almqvist & Wiksell.

Gangestad, S. & Snyder, M. (1985). To carve nature at its joints: On the existence of discrete classes in personality. *Psychological Review, 92*(3), 317–349.

Greenwald, A. G., Pratkanis, A. R., Lieppe, M. R. & Baumgardner, M. H. (1986). Under what conditions does theory obstruct research progress. *Psychological Review, 93*(2), 216–229.

Haberman, S. J. (1973). The analysis of residuals in cross-classified tables. *Biometrics, 29*(1), 205–220.

Harris, C. W. (1963). *Problems in measuring change.* Madison, Wisconsin: University of Wisconsin Press.

Jung, C. G. (1921). *Psychologische Typen.* Zürich: Rascher & Cie.

Lienert, G. A. & Bergman, L. R. (1985). Longisectional interaction structure analysis (LISA) in psychopharmacology and developmental psychopathology. *Neuropsychobiology, 14,* 27–34.

Magnusson, D. (1985). Implications of an interactional paradigm for research on human development. *International Journal of Behavioral Development, 8*(2), 115–137.

Magnusson, D. (1988). Individual development from an interactional perspective. A longitudinal study. Vol. 1 in D. Magnusson, (ed.), *Paths through life.* Hillsdale, NJ: Lawrence Erlbaum.

Magnusson, D. (in press). Back to the phenomena. *Zeitschrift für Psychologie.*

Magnusson, D. & Allen, V. (1983*a*). Implications and applications of an interactional perspective for human development. In D. Magnusson & V. Allen (eds.), *Human development: An interactional perspective.* New York: Academic Press.

Magnusson, D. & Allen, V. (1983*b*). An interactional paradigm for human development. In D. Magnusson & V. Allen (eds.), *Human development: An interactional perspective.* New York: Academic Press.

Magnusson, D. & Bergman, L. R. (1984). On the study of the development of adjustment problems. In L. Pulkkinen & P. Lyytinen (eds.), *Human action and personality*. Jyväskylä: University of Jyväskylä.

Magnusson, D. & Bergman, L. R. (1988). Longitudinal studies: Individual and variable based approaches to research on early risk factors. In M. Rutter (ed.), *Risk and protective factors in psychosocial development*. New York: Cambridge University Press.

Magnusson, D., Dunér, A. & Zetterblom, G. (1975). *Adjustment: A longitudinal study*. New York: Wiley. Stockholm: Almqvist & Wiksell.

Milligan, G. W. (1980). An examination of the effect of six types of error perturbation on fifteen clustering algorithms. *Psychometrika, 45* (3).

Milligan, G. W. (1981). A review of Monte Carlo tests of cluster analysis. *Multivariate Behavioral Research, 16*, 379–407.

Morey, L. C., Blashfield, R. K. & Skinner, H. A. (1983). A comparison of cluster analysis techniques within a sequential validation framework. *Multivariate Behavioral Research, 18*, 309–329.

Rudinger, G. & Wood, P. K. (1990). *N*'s, times and number of variables in longitudinal research. In D. Magnusson & L. R. Bergman (eds.), *Data quality in longitudinal research*. New York: Cambridge University Press.

Rutter, M. (1981). Longitudinal studies: A psychiatric perspective. In S. A. Mednick & A. E. Buert (eds.), *Prospective longitudinal research: an empirical basis for the primary prevention of psychiatric and social disorders*. Oxford University Press.

Rutter, M. & Pickles, A. (1990). Improving the quality of psychiatric data: Classification, cause and course. In D. Magnusson & L. R. Bergman (eds.), *Data quality in longitudinal research*. New York: Cambridge University Press.

Thomae, H. (1988). *Das Individuum und seine Welt: Eine Persönlichkeitstheorie*. Göttingen, West Germany: Hogrefe.

Ward, J. H. (1963). Hierarchical grouping to optimize an objective function. *Journal of American Statistical Association, 58*, 236–244.

Whitehead, A. N. (1956). Mathematics as an element in the history of thought. In J. R. Newman (ed.), *The world of mathematics*. New York: Simon & Schuster.

Wishart, D. (1982). *CLUSTAN: User manual*. Edinburgh: Program Library Unit, Edinburgh University.

Wohlwill, J. F. (1973). *The study of behavioral development*. London: Academic Press.

Zubin, J. (1968). Classification of human behavior. Read before Canadian Psychological Association Institute on Measurement, Classification and Prediction. University of Calgary, Alberta, Canada.

Index

adjustment problems, extrinsic 323–44
  childhood, adult maladjustment associated 340–1
  cross-sectional classification analysis 326–9: RESIDAN 328–9, 332
  data 330–2: sample 330; variables 330–2
  longitudinal classification analysis 329–30
  measurement 325–6
  person-oriented view 324–5
  results 332–41: cross-sectional patterning 332–7; longitudinal analyses 337–41
adult social functioning, parameter estimates from recursive models 145–7
aging 47
alcohol drinking, mortality associated 103
anxiety state 72

Beck Depression Inventory 75
behavioral genetic concepts 236–48
  future directions 247–8
  genetic/environmental contributions to stability/change 241–2
  genetic/environmental stability/change 239–41
  models 242–7: common factor model 244–5; genetic simplex model *see* genetic simplex behavioral model; latent growth curve model 245–7; longitudinal model 236–8; transmission-factor model 245, 247; two-occasion model 241 (fig.), 242
  parameters of interest 236–42
  partition of variation at each time point 238–9
  Swedish Adoption/Twin Study of Aging 238
bereavement 134
body mass index (BMI) 103
body weight, and mortality 103
Bonn Longitudinal Study of Aging 274, 276 (table)
bully/victim problems (Scandinavia) 106–31
  alternative interpretations 123
  cohort effects 111–13
  dosage-response relationship 125–6
  hierarchical nature of data 127–9
  methodology 108–11
  outcome variables 113–15
  program package 131 note
  quality of data 123
  residual change scores or simple difference scores? 126–7
  results 115–23
  statistical analyses 115
  time by cohort analysis 123–5

caseness threshold 72
categorical data, direct/indirect effects for 160
causal inferences making 8–9
central tendency, individual's 62
change 49
childhood disorder/adult disorder, continuity comparison 151 (table)
childhood 'life-span' cohort study 98–9
children
  behavioral disturbance 140
  birth of younger sibling 137
  reaction to step-parent 137
  responsibility taking 137
classification 326
  cross-sectional, based on pattern data 326–9
  phenetic 327
cluster analysis 19, 328
  k-means relocation 328
  longitudinal 343: applications 19–22
  methodology 343, 344
coding point in time 6–7
cognitive operations emergence, sequentiality in 167–8

cohort
  definition 108
  effects 111: non-genuine 112–13
collection point in time 6
Colorado Adoption project 247
concepts-measurement models, matching 8
configural frequency analysis 22–3
confirmation bias 342
confirmation *vs* exploration 9–10
confirmatory approach 9
  limitations 9
constraints inherent in specific problem 190–4
  nature of data 191–2: subjects 191; variables 191–2
  requirements for data analysis 192–4: constraints arising from qualitative nature of data 193; constraints created by establishing correspondence between item grouping and subject grouping 193; constraints imposed by longitudinal nature of study 193–4
  theoretical issues 190–1
constraints on development, external/internal 187
continuous initial symptom score 77 (table), 87
correspondence analysis 193–4, 194–209
  comparison of different kinds of individuals/tasks 201
  identification of contrasts (factors) revealing individual-task hierarchies 201
  incorporation of supplementary individuals into completed analysis 201
  results 202–8: analysis of first occasion (cross-sectional approach) 203–5; longitudinal analysis 205–8
  'supplementary individuals' technique 206–8
  treatment of categorized data in descriptive manner 201
  use with individual data 202
covariance matrices, structural equation models 278–9
covariance structural model, general 252
Cox model 224
  hazard rate 223
'critical questioning' technique (Piaget) 191–2
cross-sectional studies 3–4

décalages
  in development/developmental sequences 166, 176
  individual 192, 193, 204
  intraindividual 191, 206
  universal 192, 193
depression 47
  aetiological model 69
  aetiology 68
  basic result in continuous terms 75–83
  basic vulnerability result 78 (table), 79 (table), 80 (table), 84 (tables), 85 (tables)
  borderline 71, 72
  continuous measures 75–86, 88
  diagnosis 72
  interactive effects 73–5
  intraindividual variability in older adults' depression scores 47–63
  multiple regression analysis *see* multiple regression analysis neurotic 69
  Present State Examination (PSE) 71, 75: Index of Definition (ID) 85–6, 87
  provoking agents 70, 74
  psychological factors 89
  psychotic 69
  relative size beta weights of initial symptom score/vulerability factor 82 (table)
  social variables 74
  treated interval variable (CES-D)/dichotomy 91
  vulnerability factors 70–1, 74
developmental behavior genetics 250–71
developmental functions 275
developmental process
  character 2–4
  coherence 5
  lawful continuity 5
  multidetermined, stochastic process 2–3
  stability 4–5: absolute 4; relative 4
developmental sequences
  analysis, conceptual/methodological implications 167–71
  conceptual arguments 167
  precursor 167
  prerequisite structures 167
diachronous profiles 168
difference-testing procedures 168–9
differentiation/integration hypothesis 291
discontinuity tests between childhood/adulthood 150 (table)
discrete data, longitudinal studies 308–21
  latent class models 313–17
  latent structure models 310–11, 312 (table)
  two data sets 308–11

event-history data 213–14
  cost 232
event-oriented collection design 214
EXACON 329–30
exploration 9

fat indicators 18

generation 'life-span' study 103
genetic profiles, individual, simulation studies 255–7
genetic simplex behavioral model 242–4, 247, 250–71
  application to real data 263–9
  general covariance structure model 252
  latent genetic/environmental trends 251
  latent time-dependent profiles of genetic/environmental influences 250–1
  monozygotic/dizygotic twin data 252–5 *passim*
  simulation study of individual genetic profiles 255–7
  specifications as LISREV VI model 259–61
  structural means 257–63
German Life History Study 215–17, 225–31
growth, human 28–44
  biological parameters 31
  curve fitting 32–3: average growth 39–43; residual variance 32
  individual growth pattern 29–32
  JPPS model 36–8
  peak height velocity ages 42–3
  polynomials 32–3
  Preece–Baines model 33 (fig.), 34–6
  skeletal dimensions in pathological situations 44
  spurts 31
  structural models 43–4
  triple logistic model 38, 39 (fig.)
growth curves 275

Hamilton Rating Scale 75
hazards for women 153–7
health, differential development, in life-span perspective 95–105
health screening (Värmland) 13–18
hierarchical cluster-analysis method (Ward) 328–9
higher-order cross-tabulations 22
hyperactivity syndrome 332, 333 (table), 339 (fig.)

intellectual development
  reliability of assessment 275–95
  simplex property 276–7
  stability 275
  structural equation models of study 274–301
Individual Development and Adjustment (IDA) 330, 337
intelligence
  crystallized 291
  differentiation/integration hypothesis 291
  fluid 291
  structural changes 286: autoregressive *vs* non-autoregressive models 291–3, 294 (fig.); classic longitudinal model 288–91; in old age 295; minimized longitudinal model 289 (fig.)
interdependency 135
interindividual differences 48, 49
'intra-analysis' (Escofier & Pages) 202
intraindividual change 168
intraindividual variability 47–55
  Cornwall Manor study 55–60: analysis/results 57–60; methods/procedures 55–7; purpose 55
  longitudinal research 62–3
  models of developmental change 61–2
  P-technique and 53–5
  research implications 52–3
  significance of change patterns 61

knowledge development (Piaget) 191

latent class 313–14
latent class model of continuity in disorder, measurement characteristics/ prevalence estimates 149 (table)
latent class transition (Markov model) 147–52
latent structure analysis 23
liability (proneness) 61
linear structural relations 1–2
logarithm of cell frequency 23
logit analysis 23
log linear analysis 2
log linear modeling 22, 23
longisectional classification analysis 329–30
Louisville Twin Study 247
low school achievement 334, 336 (table), 338 (table), 339 (table)
low school motivation syndrome 334, 335 (table), 336 (table), 338 (table), 339 (table), 340

marital support
  definition 140
  paths 153 (fig.)
Markov model (latent class transition) 147–52
Markov simplex 277
  quasi 277–81
marriage
  effect on male delinquent 135
  non-delinquent woman 135
maternal employment 136
mathematical problems, simple, test 7
measurement models 344
midlife crisis 133
military service 136
mobility tables 212
moving house 135–6
MREP (preparatory multivariate analysis) 331–2
multiple regression analysis 67–92
  forced-entry 81, 83, 87
  Index of Definition 90
  standardized regression coefficients 81
  use as dictomy 89
  used with dichotomous dependent variation 88
multiple-problem syndrome 332, 333 (table), 334, 335 (table), 336 (table), 338 (table), 339 (table)

nondeviant spouse 140, 142, 151 (table)
Norway
  bullying in schools *see* bully/victim problems
  childhood 'life-span' cohort study 98–9
  coronary heart deaths 96–7
  generation 'life-span' study 103–4
  longitudinal *vs* cross-sectional findings 102–3
  mortality 95–8: children 98–9
  record linkage studies 104
  reproductive 'life-span' cohort study 99–102
  student satisfaction with school life 115

old age, intelligence in 283, 285–6, 287
  structural changes 295
order-theoretical analysis 186, 187
order-theoretical statistical procedures 172–3

path analysis 3, 212
pattern analysis (Zubin) 22
planning 141–3, 143 (table)
  frequency 142
prediction analysis 172
  unconditional 172–3
Present State Examination (PSE) 71, 75
  Index of Definition (ID) 85–6, 87
probabilistic validation procedures (scalability model) 172
profile
  diachronous 168
  synchronous 168
profile-oriented methods 19–23
  descriptive 19
  longitudinal application of cluster analysis 19–22
  longitudinal application of studying all possible patterns 22–3
  model-based 23
proneness (liability) 61
prospective approaches to longitudinal research 5–7
psychiatric disorder 69
P-technique 53–5
puberty, early (girls) 136–7

qualitative analyses of individual developmental trajectories in cognition 166–87
  conservation of area 173–4, 175–81: developmental hypothesis 175–6; formulation of developmental model 176–7; synchronous model 176–7; statistical examination of model/results 177–81; task-analysis 175
  design 173–5
  developmental model: syllogistic reasoning 181–6: developmental hypothesis 181; formulation of model 181–2; statistical examination of model/results 182–6; task analysis 181
  instruments 173–5
  method 173–5
  subjects 173–5
  syllogistic deductions 174–5
quality change with time 7–8

record linkage studies 104
recruitment probabilities 172
reference point in time 6–7
regression analysis 68
relative importance index 81
reliability 281
RESCLUS 334
RESIDAN 328–9, 332, 334, 337
residuals decomposition 202
resilience 62
retrospective approaches to longitudinal research 5–7

scalability model (probabilistic validation procedure) 172
school leaving 133, 135
  early 137
sequence hypothesis 169–70
  difference-testing procedures 168–9
  unidimensional Guttman scaling 170
simplex model with nonlinear constraints 301
simplex property 276–7
simulation of individual genetic profiles 255–7
social mobility 212–33
  estimation 223–5
  event-history analysis, statistical concepts 217–23: covariates 222–3; cumulative hazard function 221; hazard rate 220; intensity (risk) functions 220; regression models 222–3; survivor function 220
  event-history data 213–14
  event-oriented collection design 214
  event-oriented observation plan 215–17
  feedback processes 215
  German Life History Study (GLHS) 215–17, 225–31
  labour market research 213
  path analysis 212
  results 225–31
  status attainment research 212–13
socioeconomic panel 232
sources of error, assumption-oriented 14–15 (table), 16–18
spurious duration dependency 135
stability 49, 281
standardized regression coefficients 81
state(s) 50
  intraindividual variability 51–2
  normal daily variability 51
statement calculus 170
state–trait distinction 49–52
statistics
  analysis of survery material 67–9
  complex multivariate 67
status attainment research 212–13
structural equation models
  for covariance matrices 278–9
  for studying intellectual development 274–301
'supplementary individuals' technique 206–7
Swedish Adoption/Twin Study of Aging 238
Swedish twins, adolescent 247
syllogistic proposition, basic forms 175 (table)
synchronous profiles 168
system of simultaneous equations/structural model 144

teenage mother 134, 136
temperament attributes 51
trait 50
  stability 51
trait-like attributes 51
trait–state distinction 49–52
transient distress responses 90
triangular system of simultaneous equations 144
triangulation of age, period, cohort effects 247–8
T-technique (Catell) 176–7
turning points in developmental processes 133–61
  children reared in institutions 138–9
  cross-tabulation analysis 138–44
  event-history model for gaining supportive relationship 152–7
  timing 136
  transition to early adult life for young people in care 138
  women's transition risks 153–7

unemployment 134
unidimensional Guttman scaling 170
usage point in time 6

variable-oriented methods 10–18
  applications 10–18
  assumptions 10–18: testing 18
  assumption oriented sources of error 11–18
  design aspects of specification 18

Weibull competing risk mode 161
Weibull distribution (exponential) 223
Weibull hazards 153, 154 (table)
Weibull regression model hazard rate 223

Printed in the United States
By Bookmasters